End the Yo-Yo

End the Yo-Yo

*The Eat As Much
As You Want System*

Jim Frith

A "Must Read if you seriously want to

- Feel better
- Be slender for the rest of your life
- Stop gaining weight back after losing it
- Reach your weight goal without a plateau
- Lose weight without ever feeling hungry
- Change your life for the better
- Sleep better
- Live longer
- Boost your metabolism
- Eliminate many triggers for depression
- Keep your mind sharp every day

Contents

Acknowledgements

Researching and writing this book was the culmination of a years-long quest for me, but I only got to my destination with the help of friends. I want to thank several who carefully read my various drafts and gave invaluable feedback: Elizabeth Law, Nancy Grojean, Claire Danielson, and Tina Thayll. There are many others who helped me, and I want to thank each of you as well. You know who you are. Special thanks also goes out to my weight-loss and fitness clients who trusted me enough over the years to follow my guidance.

Introduction and Overview

Lose Weight and Keep It Off

This claim has become such a cliché that many people no longer believe it's possible, but I will prove to you that you realistically can keep weight off with the Eat As Much As You Want system. Many diets out there can help you lose weight, but the "keep it off" part is truly what's missing in almost every plan.

These ubiquitous claims are based either on theoretical possibilities or on a minority of people keeping weight off or on a higher percentage keeping weight off for less than a year. The truth is that keeping weight off is typically reported by the general population as much more difficult than losing it in the first place. The fact that it is actually easy to do with the Eat As Much As You Want system sets this system apart.

This book challenges a lot of the diet myths and assumptions that permeate our culture. I invite you to have an open mind as you read. There is ample scientific evidence for what I am asserting which will be laid out fully in later chapters. You will notice throughout this book that I carefully dissect why different approaches to weight loss lead to the inevitable regaining of weight. I present real life stories as well as scientific studies. You will see that subtle changes in what you are doing make a massive difference in whether you end up bingeing your way back to obesity or easily maintaining your lost weight.

The differences are not willpower or absolute consistency, and I will show you that you can make mistakes and recover easily. The true difference is whether you use your body's own built-in mechanisms to satisfy hunger and speed your metabolic rate, or if you pick a fight with your body, trying to force yourself to endure repeated and chronic hunger. Cooperation with your own body is the key!

Avoid hunger!

Who among us has not made ourselves hungry while losing weight? I know I have. And it works! For a few weeks, simply by severely limiting your food intake and making yourself hungry, you can lose lots of weight. It all seems so easy… until it isn't.

Gradually, the hunger increases, but the weight loss slows down. Soon the growing feeling of chronic hunger morphs into food fantasies and a severely slowed metabolism. Depression may creep in. Interest in sex or social interaction may drop off. This is the onset of "starvation mode", an innate hormonal change that the body uses to prevent you from starving to death when food becomes scarce.

Next, you hit a wall. You have all of the bad and none of the good, because the weight stops coming off no matter how hungry you make yourself. This is called a "weight-loss plateau". It is extremely common and terribly frustrating.

After that, you are in a grind. No weight comes off, but the yearning for fatty, sweet, calorie-packed foods continues to grow. You desperately want to lose weight, but your body will not cooperate. Over a period of weeks, willpower begins to erode. You look at the people you know who have never had a weight problem, and you envy their unfair genetics.

Finally, you reach a breaking point. Suddenly, you are bingeing on all those delectable foods you have been dreaming about. You can't get enough of them, no matter how full your stomach gets. You feel guilty, and you try to hide it from other people. They may not see your binges, but the secret is out because you are gaining weight.

You try to fight it. Binge. Starve. Binge. Starve. But your slowed metabolism keeps you from being able to effectively lose weight anymore. There is no winning that battle.

Gradually, overeating becomes a continuum. All that weight you lost comes back. This is called "yo-yo weight loss." What an awful experience!

The war is lost, yet you tell yourself you will return to fight another day. You convince yourself you lack the willpower to lose the weight. Or you listen to others who promise a step-by-step path to develop that personal motivation that has gone missing. It's all in your head, they tell you. Find your motivation and believe in your ability to lose weight, and the weight will come off. That is what the popular culture tells you.

The Truth

The truth is that your inability to keep weight off is not in your head. If it were a lack of willpower or motivation, you would have lost the weight already and kept it off. You have proven your motivation time and again as you waded into the battle against your body.

Rather, it is physical. It is the very fact that you are fighting your body instead of working with it that is causing this great difficulty. The truth is that your body is genetically set up to make you slender, but you have to learn to work with your body instead of against it. This book will teach you how to end the yo-yo by enlisting your body's own hormonal system, so you can lose weight without hunger, without a plateau, and with no yo-yo.

Hunger and Your Metabolism

Your metabolism is too slow. In fact, you can probably tell me how old you were when you first recognized that you have a slow metabolism. To keep weight off, you need to work with your body's natural mechanism to speed up your metabolism. That is why hunger is so bad: When you allow yourself to become hungry, you are actively slowing down your metabolism.

Once you understand the innate survival mechanisms of the body, you can begin to use them to help you instead of fighting a losing war. When they are working for you, they will vanquish that excess weight for you, and you will coast to your weight-loss goal. Willpower and personal motivation are certainly great and admirable, but they are far more effective when they are fighting alongside your body's hormone system instead of against it.

So let's start with the basics. Any diet that makes you hungry sets you up to gain the weight back. The hormones that control hunger also control your metabolic rate. Hunger for even a few hours slows your metabolism. When you make yourself hungry for large parts of every day for an extended period of time, your metabolism slows way, way down, and it can stay slow for many years.

Hunger can come from multiple sources. It may be from chronic inflammation, lack of chewing, going too long between meals, not eating sufficient bulk and phytonutrients, and not eating the right balance of protein and slow-digesting carbohydrates spaced out throughout the day. Another hunger source is eating too many "calorically-dense" foods, which are foods containing a lot of calories in a small volume (such as oil or pasta or rice). Calorically-dense foods can put a large number of calories into your stomach without filling you up.

A hunger-driven, slowed-down metabolism is a double-edged sword: Hunger makes you crave too much of the wrong kinds of food. A slow metabolism causes you to stop losing weight even if you have dramatically cut calories. But when you learn how to vanquish hunger with fewer calories and more nutrients, you can speed up your metabolism and easily burn more calories than you consume.

Get to the point

I've been coaching weight-loss clients for a long time, and this is the first thing some people say to me:

"Just tell me how to eat!"

So I'll tell you: Eat a balanced diet of whole foods. Have lots of nutrient-dense low-calorie fruits and vegetables with every meal. Eat a little bit of high quality protein with each meal from natural sources such as lean meats, dairy, soy, eggs, fish or poultry. Eat a little bit of higher-caloric density, low Glycemic Index ("low-GI") carbohydrates with each meal such as beans, coarse whole-grained breads, dairy, pears and quinoa.

The Glycemic Index is a measure of how quickly the carbs you eat enter your bloodstream as blood sugar. Low-GI carbs send sugar to your bloodstream slowly. High-GI carbs send sugar quickly.

Is there science behind this concept of eating high-quality, balanced meals for weight loss, health and longevity? Yes, there is. A lot of science. This is what makes it possible for you to lose weight without hunger.

Can you eat as much as you want? Yes, you can. But there are rules you'll need to follow to balance all of these foods for the right proportions and amounts of proteins, higher-caloric density carbs, water or beverages, and the fruits and vegetables you will consume in unlimited quantities.

And there are other lifestyle choices to ensure the pounds you lose stay lost. These include sleep strategies, alcohol moderation, sugar elimination, probiotics, reduction in fats intake, establishment of your life's purpose, and social support. We'll talk more on all of these topics later in the book.

If you do not want a slender body, good health, longevity, and a high quality of life, then read no further. If you are unwilling to make habit changes, this book is not for you. But if you are ready to immediately improve your life, I am happy to share my knowledge.

My Story

When I was in high school, I was a wrestler, and I had to cut weight to get to my weight class. Periods of that were brutal, because I was trying to do what everyone else was doing: cutting back on my quantities of food, cutting down on carbohydrates, and eating lots of protein. I constantly felt terrible hunger, had food fantasies, and felt tired. My mother became very worried about me.

"You need to eat!" she insisted.

She started to push me to eat more, including carbs. "You can't keep up your strength without a balanced diet," she said.

I pushed back and said I couldn't eat more, or I wouldn't make weight. Being a wise mom, she didn't push too hard.

A few years earlier, she had announced that she was "retired" from motherhood when the youngest of my six older sisters was nearing the end of high school. She stopped cleaning the house and mostly stopped cooking, so I usually cooked my own food. My siblings and I were definitely not committed to housework, so our house became a progressively bigger mess.

So here I was trying to cut weight, and Mom began to cook again. Not only that, but she made some of my favorite dishes! How cunning she was! She knew I loved spaghetti and some other dishes no one in the world made except my mom. These were tomato-based meat sauces poured over rice or spaghetti.

She also knew I couldn't have these foods and still make weight. The fight she couldn't win with words she was trying to win with temptations.

What a quandary! But I was stubborn and determined not to let my team down. I sadly refused to eat my favorite dishes.

Mom's face fell when I turned away from spaghetti. I began to leave the kitchen resigned to another hungry night.

"Wait!" she said.

I turned around.

 "Why don't you have the sauce over something that won't make you gain weight?" she offered.

She spooned lima beans onto a plate and handed it to me. I greedily dished Mom's spaghetti sauce over the limas.

It was delicious! This kind of eating quickly became a pattern.

Amazingly, my weight stayed where I needed it, but I had much greater energy. It was clear to me that she was right that a balanced diet was the way to go. The added energy went with added strength. My senior year, I was a State Champion.

Fast-forward 33 years to 2008. I gained a lot of weight. I spent many years being very out of shape, but by 2008, I had been working out for several years. Still, I was 40 pounds too heavy. I had made good progress in increasing strength. My blood pressure was high, but I did not want to give up on any of the muscle and strength gains I had made.

Then I remembered those dishes Mom lured me into when I was a wrestler. I buried myself in research, and the Eat As Much As You Want system was born. I lost 40 pounds and gained even more strength. I have kept it off ever since, and I am stronger now than I was when I started.

The Role of Hormones

Life is short. Moving toward greater health should feel good. Being hungry or having constant cravings feels terrible.

This book teaches you to boost your metabolism. You will not only gain the tools to lose weight, but also to keep the weight off, have a high quality of life, live longer, sleep better, and be happier -- all without hunger.

Metabolic hormones

Many hormones influence your metabolism. They include insulin, leptin, ghrelin, testosterone, estrogen, and growth hormone, among others. Any diet program that does not work with these hormones to diminish hunger, increase metabolic function, and improve feelings of wellness fails to give you a sustainable solution.

Most diets help you to lose weight, but few of them optimally work with your natural hormones to make your experience pleasant, your weight loss steady, and your outcome sustainable. I will teach you how to do all of that without pills, supplements, or surgery.

A critical part of sustainable weight loss is learning how to be the master of your endocrine system, the body's metabolism control network made up of glands, your own hormones, and your brain. I will teach you how. It's not difficult once you know how.

Unhealthy diets

You may be surprised at how many extremely popular diets are bad for you. It is also surprising to a lot of people how weight regain (the "yo-yo") is spurred by those diets. The diet plans typically claim to be "safe and effective" because participants lose weight, and they do not get sick during the three, six, or 12-month period after they start. However, any diet you go on will fail you in the long term if you do not keep your hunger satisfied and your metabolism strong.

Eat As Much As You Want

If you eat the right way, your lack of hunger will keep you from eating more calories than you burn. This means eating the right foods in the right proportions and frequency to give your body all the nutrients it needs, to avoid or resolve inflammation, to avoid hunger, and to keep your metabolism strong.

"Ad libitum" eating is the scientific term for eating as much as you want. Studies on ad libitum eating have taught us how the human body navigates hunger. These studies have shown that animals and humans alike stop being hungry when they have gotten the nutrients their bodies need.

The balance of nutrients in your meal, mix of foods that you eat, and timing of meals are a huge part of determining whether your hunger will cease before you have eaten as many calories as you are burning. This book will teach you how to keep your hunger satisfied and your metabolism strong while still losing weight.

Unhealthy sleep patterns, excessive drugs or alcohol, unnatural foods, and inappropriate balances of nutrients can all interfere with our bodies' hunger satisfaction-signaling systems (Chapters 9,11,12, 13, 15, and 17). Also, when we don't get the nutrients we need even though we've already consumed enough calories, we eat to excess and gain weight.

When our endocrine systems are getting the right signals, we don't have to rely on willpower to stop eating because our hormones tell us when we have had enough to eat even if we have not consumed as many calories as we are burning. We simply don't want any more food. Learn how to use ad libitum eating to your advantage. We will extensively discuss the science behind this.

Set point theory

Each person's body has a genetic "set point" for weight. Your body, when healthy, will always defend your genetic set point. This process is governed by your endocrine system.

When our endocrine systems are healthy, our set points are at weights we would consider slender. Unfortunately, the American diet has short-circuited our set points. In this book, you'll learn how to repair the short circuits.

Poor Choices Have Led Us Here

Obesity is an epidemic. 42.4% of American adults are obese. The majority of the rest are overweight. People often ask me how we got here. The answer: Our short-circuited endocrine systems have collided with a society that has us sitting more. We are consuming more calories than we used to, and we are burning fewer.

We Americans eat more inflammatory foods than we did 60 years ago, subject ourselves to inflammatory fragrances and other toxins, sleep more poorly (Chapter 17), watch more TV (Chapter 14), spend more time on computers, and lead substantially more sedentary lives. We sit more and move less. As a result, we are heavier, more tired, more prone to diabetes, depression and other ailments.

We are eating about 800 more calories per day than our counterparts in 1961! (Chapter 22.) Inflammation and processed foods are luring us to be out of control in our caloric intakes.

We shouldn't even have the appetite to eat that many calories. Our bodies can and should tell us when to stop. This book is the path out of this nightmare. I will connect you with your innate ability to be happily satisfied with fewer calories and no hunger.

Vegetables in our culture

"We need more balance in what we're eating," I said to my family a few years ago.

We were on a family trip, and the consensus was to stop at yet another fast-food restaurant.

"We *are* eating balanced meals," one family member insisted.

"Really? Where are the veggies, then?"

"French fries are made of potatoes, and ketchup is made from tomatoes!"

This brought giggles all around.

No one would seriously argue that a burger and fries is nutritious or healthy eating. Yet, it has become an American staple.

I am reminded of how integral vegetable consumption was to my ancestors.

"I would never marry a man who likes onions," declared my grandmother.

It was 1918. Her dislike for onions was legendary in the family.

So when she announced she was bringing a man home to meet the family, everyone knew what the final test would be. They made two versions of squash casserole, one with onions and one without.

"Which would you like," my great grandmother asked, "the squash with onions or the squash without?"

"Oh, without please," answered my grandfather.

Giggles erupted all around the table. He was the one!

I have heard that story many times, and it always got a laugh as a silly way to decide on a spouse. My grandparents obviously had more in common than that. But it strikes me now that fruits and vegetables had a far more exalted place in the typical meal in those days. Good health now demands that we bring them back to their prominent place at our tables.

Not just a diet

This book is about a systematic approach to life and eating. It's a holistic approach to life for optimal weight and health. Whether you count calories, follow a Mediterranean, anti-inflammatory, or low-GI diet, this approach teaches you how to avoid yo-yo weight loss, how to stop and reverse weight-loss plateaus, and how to avoid hunger and cravings. It is also flexible enough to use with many dietary restrictions.

Bad advice

Our popular culture has convinced us that certain unhealthy choices are good and that willpower and self-imposed hunger provide the surest path to weight loss. Or we're told to unbalance our diets or starve ourselves for long portions of every day. These bad choices lead us over and over again into yo-yo weight loss. You'll learn the science of why these are bad choices.

Sleep

Inadequate sleep leads to obesity, high blood pressure, chronic fatigue, and cognitive dysfunction including dementia. Too much or too little sleep is associated with substantially diminished life expectancy. Any weight-loss program that does not address sleep habits is incomplete. The science of naturally attaining restful and adequate sleep has markedly advanced in recent years. Chapter 17 provides 18 science-based strategies to help you to get the rest you're dreaming of.

Refined sugar, processed foods, and fat

Certain foods that permeate our society and culture actually disrupt our ability to satisfy our hunger. When we eat refined sugars, certain processed foods, and fats, our bodies crave more (Chapters 5, 6, 11, and 20).

Whole foods contain natural sugars and carbohydrates in lower concentrations along with bulk that triggers natural hunger satisfaction. Contrast that with refined sugars, which hyper-stimulate appetites, are addictive, and can lead to numerous health problems in addition to chronic overconsumption of calories. (Chapter 11)

High amounts of fat in foods taste good, but they do not satisfy, so they lead to overeating in real-world ad libitum meals (Chapter 10). Processed foods often contain inflammatory chemical additives, are less nutritious, and do not efficiently satisfy your appetite (Chapter 20).

Lean proteins and low-caloric density, nutrient-rich, low-Glycemic Index carbohydrates give you the greatest satisfaction per calorie (Chapter 12). Your body needs certain amounts of both in each meal for you to feel satisfied.

Move away from excessive fat consumption, especially of unhealthy fats such as saturated and trans fats. Substantially cut back on refined sugars, foods that put lots of sugar into your blood in a short period of time (high-Glycemic Load), and processed foods. The Eat As Much As You Want system food lists categorize foods and favor the ones that improve health and satisfaction (Chapters 9, 12 and 20).

If you have a refined-sugar habit, kick it! Chapter 11 will explain why a high-sugar diet is so dangerous and bad for you. It will walk you through the process of ending that habit step-by-step and will provide you with the tools you need to be successful.

Speed is a bad mantra

New clients typically come to me only after they realize they are constantly yo-yoing. They have often concluded that they have no willpower when in fact they have used their tremendous willpower to battle self-imposed hunger. When I convince them to work with their bodies instead of against them, that is when they start to lose weight again (Chapters 5, 6, 9, 12, 20 and 21).

Speed is an all-American mantra. We worship the idea of getting to our goals quickly, and weight loss is no different in people's views. Unfortunately, fast weight loss does not lead to sustained weight loss. Instead, it leads to a metabolic crash. Studies have shown that losing one to two pounds a week is realistically sustainable.

Avoid directing your motivation and willpower into a losing strategy. This book teaches you what actually works. Do not fight your natural hormonal survival mechanisms. Work with your body to get to a healthier you.

Losing weight the right way requires patience and discipline. Super fast weight loss almost always backfires. One to two pounds per week still adds up to 50 to 100 pounds a year! Steadily lose the excess weight the right way so you never gain it back. As you do, your entire life will become better, healthier, and richer.

The Eat As Much As You Want System

This book will teach you what you need to know to lose weight and keep it off without any hunger. It will require you to take some actions and change some habits, but the rewards will far surpass the costs. You may eat more frequently than you are used to, and you may have to abandon many popular beliefs about how to lose weight and improve health. But it will work, and you'll feel great!

I am not asking you to take a leap of faith. Read the book. Look at the studies referenced in the footnotes if you wish. Reach an understanding of why what you have done in the past did not work, why this approach does work, and why it is so easy to do when you have struggled so hard in the past. Change your habits only when you fully grasp why you should.

Super-quick meals

Part of the system is to eat every three to four hours, which is generally five times a day. If you are concerned that you do not have time to eat five times a day, you can lay that concern to rest. Meals do not have to take longer than five minutes, and there are no specific times that your mealtimes need to be. You can fit them into your day wherever they fit best. Your meals can be as quick as you want them to be, and you use part of each meal as something you snack on while you work or play (Chapters 21, 22 and 24). Plan ahead, and eating right can be very time efficient.

What Mom Taught Me

After our showdown back in high school, Mom recognized how much "making weight" and doing well in wrestling meant to me. She became very supportive and helpful.

"Lima beans give you starch," she said. "The meat in the sauce gives you protein. You need both to stay strong and have energy."

"That makes sense," I said.

"But you should have some broccoli too," she continued.

"Why?"

"Because that gives you nutrients neither of the others do to keep you healthy, and at the same time it will fill you up, so you're not hungry."

She was right.

This lesson stuck with me, and it became the basic foundation of the Eat As Much As You Want system. In this system, the meat and lima beans are "Countables" because we limit the amount we eat of those, and the broccoli is an "Unlimited" because we can eat as much of it as we want.

Unlimiteds

There are many foods to choose from called "Unlimiteds" that you can eat in unlimited quantities (Chapter 9) because they provide valuable nutrients and fill you up long before you have eaten more calories than you should. These are divided into lists. Certain lists are called "Must Haves" because it is important to eat some foods from these lists in every meal. Broccoli, for example, is on one of the Must Haves lists.

The nutrients from Unlimiteds help to keep you healthy, reduce inflammation, and extend your life. And they are vitally important in making ad libitum eating work for you.

Countables

Some foods are called "Countables" in this system. In Countables, some or all of the grams of protein, carbohydrate and fat are countable (Chapter 12). These are higher-caloric density foods that we need for good health. Countables are foods that you eat in limited quantities because they are nutritionally important, but are too calorically dense to efficiently satisfy your appetite.

You might think it would be a good idea to skip the Countables so you can just eat everything in unlimited quantities, but this would be a mistake. Countables play a key role in making sure that your macronutrient balance is healthy and sustainable, and that your hunger is fully satisfied. Countables and Unlimiteds together give you the nutrition you need in quantities that keep hunger away.

Caloric minimums

With this system, there are no caloric maximums, but it is recommended that your meals and your daily consumption meet certain caloric minimums. When you eat correctly, your own lack of hunger will tell you when to stop eating. The minimums are there to help make sure you consume enough calories to keep your hormones healthy and your metabolism burning as strongly as it can.

Never finish a meal still hungry! (Chapters 1 through 3, 5 and 24)

Logging

Studies have shown that when you regularly keep a record of your weight, what you eat, and your activities, this habit makes it more likely that you will be successful. Logging this data enhances mindfulness. When you know there will be a record, you'll think twice about what you eat. This helps you to stick with your strategic plan.

The records you keep also enable you to see your behaviors and compare them to your results. That makes it easier to see what behaviors to change to strategically enhance the effectiveness of your efforts.

Adjustments for a changing metabolism and goals

When you reach your goal weight and it is time to stop losing weight, you will increase your Countables. You can also increase them if you are losing weight too fast. Unlimiteds are always unlimited (Chapter 9), and you will always eat enough to stay satisfied.

Limiting weight loss to only fat

The typical American dieter loses about three pounds of muscle for every 10 pounds of weight loss. This can lead to being weak and gaunt. Not so with the Eat As Much As You Want system.

Exercise and activity are a vital component of healthily making sure that your body is burning more calories than you are consuming (Chapter 7). When you are ready to take exercise to the next level, go to Chapter 18. There, you will learn exercise principles that help to maximize the preservation of muscle with the goal of losing only fat. This is the Holy Grail of weight loss: Get stronger and more solid and lose no muscle while you shed pounds of fat.

Clients have tended to lose inches faster than pounds when following the Eat As Much As You Want system and exercising in accordance with Chapter 18. They have also measurably gained strength.

Special dietary needs

Whether you are omnivorous, vegan, or insulin resistant, or if there are certain animal proteins that you want to avoid, this system can work for you.

However, the information in this book should not be taken as specific dietary advice, because I have no way of knowing what medical or other special needs you may have. Consult a Registered Dietician or Medical Doctor if you have any concerns about how various foods may affect you.

Chapter 1

Eat As Much As You Want

of the Right Kinds of Foods.

Free Yourself from Harmful Myths

Scientific research keeps revealing new truths and debunking old myths. Do you remember the movie "Groundhog Day" with Bill Murray? He kept reliving the same day over and over. In my work as a weight-loss coach, I have relived this conversation times. In fact, I just had it again yesterday.

"I know what I need to do. I just don't do it," my new client said.

"Why not?" I ask.

"I *have* done it -- plenty of times," she said.

"Done what?"

"Lost weight."

"So why are you heavier than you want to be now?"

"I lose weight for awhile, then I get tired of being good. Then I gain it all back."

"Why?"

"I get tired of the discipline, and I don't like being hungry."

"Okay," I said. "So what happens next?"

"I splurge. Then I start eating what I want to, and I gain it all back."

This is yo-yo weight loss. It always starts with the belief that you already know what you need to do. Then comes hunger. The breakdown always relates to an end to willpower.

Today, I had a conversation with another client.

"I can lose weight," she said. "That's not the hard part."

"Yeah?" I said. "What's the hard part?"

"Maintenance," she said. "Keeping it off."

As a society, we have been led to believe that if a weight loss plan causes us to lose weight, it is effective. The fact that we gain all of the weight back does not change many people's minds.

Let's judge weight-loss plans by a new standard. Weight loss is only one component. Whether you kept the weight off while enhancing your quality of life and life expectancy is more important. And the most important factor is whether you were comfortable maintaining the discipline necessary to keep the weight off.

The turning point

When my clients have come to the realization that they actually *don't* know what to do, that's when the turning point has always come. That is when they have opened their minds to changing their approaches to weight loss. That is when they have gone from struggling and battling their own bodies to working with the innate mechanisms that control their weight. When the turning point comes, they abandon self-imposed torment, and they transition from yo-yo to sustained weight loss.

That is when self-imposed hunger stops being acceptable.

Science has progressed

The science of weight loss has advanced dramatically in recent years, but popular beliefs have not. As you read in this book about peer-reviewed research studies published by the National Institutes of Health (NIH) on dieting and weight loss, you will see that making yourself hungry when losing weight is a very bad idea.

Our popular culture has duped us with some terribly false information about weight loss that millions now believe as fact. Our society says that to lose weight we must be hungry. Wrong! If you accept this false lesson, you will conclude that eating as much as you want and losing weight without hunger is nonsense or a scam. I invite you to think carefully about your own experiences, and about the research I will be sharing with you. The research will show you the truth, and rest assured: eating the way I will teach you in this book really works.

As you read this, I hope you will begin a journey toward better long-term health and a trimmer you. This journey should be a pleasure. Yes... a pleasure. We have been fooled into believing that losing weight must be an awful experience. The truth is that greater health should feel good. It feels awful to be hungry for big parts of each day and to suffer from frequent cravings. Worse still, as I will show you, hunger and metabolic slowdown go hand in hand, so when you allow yourself to feel hungry, your body is slowing itself down to save calories. You definitely don't want that to happen when you are trying to lose weight. Never deprive yourself of enough nutrients to keep you satisfied unless you are actively withdrawing from a food addiction.

Sustainability Must Be Comfortable

Every diet plan out there claims to be sustainable. On what do they base their claims? In some cases, the claims are completely baseless. In others, they are made based on studies showing people keeping weight off for less than a year. Truly sustained weight loss should stay gone for many years if not permanently.

In this book, I will share from a tremendous number of scientific studies. These studies teach us lessons. What I am sharing with you

4

is how to apply those lessons to make your weight-loss journey truly sustainable.

Hunger avoidance is vital to weight-loss sustainability. Making yourself hungry to lose weight works for a few weeks, and it may result in significant weight loss, but it is unnecessary and it is a terrible idea. Hunger is the main reason why more than 80% of dieters regain the weight they lose.

Look back at the conversations I had with my clients yesterday and today. I hear these same comments *all the time*. In America, we live in the land of plenty. If our bodies tell us we need to eat more, it is extremely difficult to resist this urge.

Hunger is part of how your body protects you from starving to death. The same hormones that make you hungry also slow down your metabolism to preserve energy. A slowing metabolism makes weight loss much more difficult, and it leads to a weight-loss plateau followed by a yo-yo weight re-gain. We'll discuss this in great detail in subsequent chapters.

When hunger continues over a period of weight loss, it doesn't go away with one big meal. "Discipline" breaks down because an innate desire for calorically-dense foods has accumulated over a period of weeks, and it remains until you have gained back all of the lost weight. This is a survival mechanism that we all have.

Anytime you are hungry, it takes more food to satisfy your appetite. Hunger that has been chronic during a long period of weight loss eventually becomes unbearable, and it ultimately causes people to break their diets. Hunger clouds judgment and causes poor food choices even when you have the best of intentions.

In short, any weight-loss plan that does not strategically avoid hunger is destined for failure. Hunger cannot simply be satisfied periodically, say once or more than once a day. It must be AVOIDED. I cannot say that strongly enough. And the avoidance must continue throughout the weight-loss period and into weight maintenance.

What discipline is intolerable?

Remember yesterday's conversation with my new client where she said she always gains weight back because she grows tired of being disciplined and hungry? I continued my intake interview with her:

"What is it about the discipline that becomes intolerable?" I asked.

"Have you every endured hunger day after day for months at a time? Hey, I like going out with my friends, and I want to eat what they eat and drink what they drink."

"You mean after you've lost the weight?" I asked.

"Yes, I can usually last until I reach my weight goal, or at least I get close to it, but all the while I am thinking about the celebration when I get there."

"Is one celebration enough?" I asked.

"No!!" she said emphatically. "After putting myself through all that hunger, it usually takes several weeks of bingeing for my appetite to return to normal. That's why I always put the weight right back on."

That in a nutshell is what is wrong with allowing yourself to become hungry during weight loss. Once the hunger monster is let loose, it can't be put back into a cage easily.

"Do you keep weighing yourself after you start bingeing?" I asked.

"No, what's the point of that? I already know I'm gaining weight by then. I really don't want to know how much."

"How would your experience have been different if you were never hungry while you lost weight?" I asked.

She looked at me like I was crazy for a moment, then she became thoughtful.

"Wow, that would be awesome," she answered. "I'd still go out and celebrate with my friends when I reached my goal weight, but I could go back to eating the right way immediately afterwards."

"So you wouldn't binge for several weeks?"

"I don't think so." She paused thoughtfully, then continued. "No, why would I? If I wasn't hungry to begin with, then I wouldn't have fantasized so much about food, and I wouldn't have endured that gnawing desire to go berserk with eating. I'd be able to enjoy actually staying at my goal."

"Would you keep weighing yourself daily then?"

"Yes, for sure. If I was able to avoid the intense urge to binge, then I would want to know if my weight increased by two or three pounds, so I could make sure it didn't get out of control."

There you have it. My new client could not have made the case for hunger avoidance better if she had tried. So now I'd like you to try to wrap your head around how to lose weight without ever getting hungry. I have a lot of clients who have proven that it works.

Caloric Intake vs. Satiety

First, it's important to understand that calories do not automatically satisfy your appetite. It is a huge mistake to equate caloric intake with hunger satisfaction. Some foods satiate dramatically more effectively than others.

Fats, for example, do not satiate. Instead, they enhance palatability, which makes you want to eat more. The same is true of salt, refined sugar, bleached flour products and most highly processed foods. Eating the wrong kinds of foods will enhance your appetite and lead you to still want more when you have already eaten too many calories for weight loss.

For example, have you ever eaten a bowl of nuts as you sat talking with friends or family? Or while watching television? I have. When I got to the end of the bowl, I reached for more, but it was empty. My hunger felt no more satisfied than when I started. Nuts are primarily fat. Salted nuts especially go down quickly and easily. Yet, at 800 calories per cup, that bowl may have had 1000 to 1500 calories.

Instead of filling your plate with foods that make you want more calories, get most of the volume of your meals from fruits and vegetables that are very bulky and nutrient rich compared to the number of calories. "Satiety"—that wonderful sense of peace that comes from having your hunger completely satisfied—is driven by a variety of mechanisms built into your body to make sure you are getting the nutrients you need. Satiety partly comes from chewing, partly from a full stomach, and partly from internal sensors that measure the nutrients themselves.

The two macronutrients that satiate are protein and low-Glycemic Index (low-GI) carbohydrates. Later, you'll see the science behind this statement. Most of your calories should come from these two sources. For healthy balance, consume small amounts of calorically-dense foods such as beans, whole grains, various protein sources, and healthy fats.

Foods that are low-GI (meaning the carbohydrates in the foods turn to blood sugar slowly) will keep your hunger satisfied longer and keep your energy higher. Non-caloric nutrients in fruits and vegetables are vital to health and help speed your metabolism. Thus, most of your carbohydrate intake should be from nutrient-rich, low-

GI fruits and vegetables. I am going to share lots of studies about these facts in later chapters.

High-Glycemic Index (hi-GI) carbohydrates are foods such as sugar, white bread and desserts. They can spike your blood sugar, which ultimately leads to low energy, drowsiness and renewed hunger 30 to 45 minutes later. It may seem strange that sugar would make you drowsy. Within a few minutes after a sugar rush, insulin in your bloodstream pushes the sugar to your fat.

This causes your blood sugar level to suddenly drop. A sudden drop in blood sugar is a hunger cue, so your brain tells you that you're hungry again even though you ate less than an hour earlier.

Sustainability requires satiety. By eating the right mix of foods, you satisfy hunger before you have eaten as many calories as you are burning. And you will have more energy throughout the day, which means you are likely to feel like moving more. That is the healthy and sustainable way to lose weight.

Weight loss should not only be sustainable, but it should enhance quality of life and support greater longevity. How you achieve these goals is a big part of what you will learn by reading this book.

How fast should I lose weight

If you weigh 200 pounds and you're trying to lose 40 pounds, then 20 weeks is about the fastest amount of time you should allow yourself to reach your goal. The CDC says *"evidence shows that people who lose weight gradually and steadily (about 1 to 2 pounds per week) are more successful at keeping weight off."*[1]

---

[1] "Losing Weight." Centers for Disease Control and Prevention, https://www.cdc.gov/healthyweight/losing_weight/index.html

A 1995 study[2] showed that the risk of formation of gallstones increases exponentially in obese people when they lose more than 3.3 pounds per week.

For many years, I have recommended to my clients that they target a weight loss in the range of between ½% and 2% of bodyweight per week. I have emphasized that 2% must be the absolute upper limit of weight loss, and I have generally been a lone voice telling them not to lose weight too fast. For most people, about 1% per week is more ideal.

The right mix of foods, combined with regular exercise and a variety of other healthy habits, can comfortably produce weight loss of ½% to 2% per week without hunger. The trick is to choose the correct balance of foods that will keep you satiated without a lot of calories, which is what you will learn to do here.

What happens if I lose weight faster than that?

Anyone who tries to lose more than about 2% of bodyweight per week is likely to eat so little that they experience ongoing hunger. The hunger means the metabolism is slowing down, and they are probably headed for a weight-loss plateau followed by a yo-yo weight re-gain.

---

[2] "Medically safe rate of weight loss for the treatment of obesity: a guideline based on risk of gallstone formation", Weinsier et al., February 1995, *The American Journal of Medicine*, National Institutes of Health pubmed, https://www.ncbi.nlm.nih.gov/pubmed/7847427

Metabolism vs. Calories

Weight loss cannot be achieved effectively by diet alone. Many other factors have substantial impact on the potential for success or failure. We will discuss these in greater detail later, but here is a summary:

Exercise and movement raise the daily caloric burn rate. They also use muscles and can prevent muscle loss. The typical dieter in our popular culture loses 1/3 pound of muscle for every pound of weight loss. That should be unacceptable. By doing the right exercises, dieters can change that to one pound of fat loss and no muscle loss for every pound of weight loss. This creates a much healthier and more attractive outcome. Also, a loss of muscle mass slows the metabolic rate, so it is wise to retain as much muscle as you can.

Sleep is also important. Too little or too much sleep is associated with obesity and numerous negative health outcomes. Having a good sleep strategy supports weight-loss efforts.

Alcohol consumption should be limited to one drink on any given day of beer, wine or liquor. Recent studies have shown that one drink or less is associated with the formation of "brown fat", which accelerates the metabolism. Do not average your daily alcohol consumption to arrive at one drink a day. Having no drinks today and two drinks tomorrow will only contribute to weight gain, not weight loss.

Having a purpose in life also helps with motivation, even if the purpose has nothing to do with weight loss. People who are purpose-driven are better able to stay on goal. Being able to pursue a life's mission is typically contingent on being healthier and fitter.

There are many good habits that are associated with sustained weight loss. Examples of good habits include watching less than 10 hours of television a week and planning your meals.

Pure calorie counting does not work

Our popular culture says "Eat less, move more." This cliché leads most people to self-impose hunger in their quest for weight loss.

Myth: Eat less than 1000 calories a day, and you will surely lose weight and keep it off.

Truth: To lose weight, you must consume fewer calories than you burn.

Our popular culture quickly takes a wrong turn in its relationship with calories. We have been taught that to lose weight, we mainly just need to count calories and do lots of exercise. The theory is that a) the more exercise you do, the more calories you will burn, and b) the fewer calories you consume while doing all that exercise, the more weight you will lose.

The flaw is this: What you eat and how you eat it has a dramatic impact on your endocrine system, satiety (or lack thereof), metabolic rate, health and energy levels. Traditional calorie counting almost always leads to a slowing metabolism and chronic hunger, which in turn leads to your body burning no more calories than you consume no matter how little you eat.

Have you ever quickly lost weight while counting calories and exercising? Millions have. That is exactly why so many people think that it works.

Did you keep the weight off without ever feeling hungry? That is the key. Millions of people who have lost weight with self-imposed hunger have ultimately lost the will to keep being hungry, so they gained the weight back just like my new client from yesterday.

Was your weight loss steady without a plateau? Calorie counting without the right approach to eating slows your metabolism down and can stop the weight loss after you have been losing for several weeks.

Most people who count calories quickly lose weight at first. After two to six weeks, the weight loss slows down, even though they are still sticking to the same caloric budget. A few weeks after that, the weight loss may stop. Meanwhile, hunger is building, and willpower is weakening. This is all because of hormonal changes happening as the body protects itself from starvation.

"What am I doing wrong?" I have been asked so many times. "I'm hardly eating anything, and my weight loss has stopped!"

This is the turning point when I get asked this question. This is when clients are finally ready to hear how to lose weight the right way.

Chemical reactions in your body

When I was a kid, I made a paper mache model of a mountain, and I installed a cup in the top of the mountain. This was supposed to be a replica of a volcano. I then put some vinegar with reddish-orange food coloring into the cup. To simulate a volcanic reaction, I added baking soda. Reddish-orange "lava" erupted out of the top of the mountain and flowed down the sides. That was great fun!

This was an example of a chemical reaction. It seemed strange because baking soda is used in various recipes, but it does not act that way in the recipes. Vinegar is used in salad dressings and on top of various foods, and it also does not act this way. But, when the two are mixed, boom, there is a big reaction.

Your body is very similar, even though the chemical reactions in it are not so violent. Your metabolic rate is the sum total of calories burned in chemical reactions in your body each day. Some of those reactions are for the production of hormones. Some are for lean tissue repair. Some are for the storage of energy. Some are for the expenditures of energy to fuel your movements (exercise), thinking, digestion, heart, brain activity, immune system, and so on.

Our normal brain functions typically burn approximately 26 calories per hour. Imagine how many calories are burned to produce white blood cells and fight disease. With the millions of viruses, bacteria and cancer cells in our bodies at any given time, I can only imagine that this must require a lot of energy.

Optimizing the burn rate

If the right nutrients are not available to the body throughout the day, the rate of these healthy chemical reactions will slow down. That means you need a great variety of different nutrients, and you need them frequently. This is why you need a balanced diet that includes nutrient-rich fruits and vegetables.

Now, imagine that you are counting calories, but you are eating junk food. Your metabolism will slow down. This will be partly because you will not be getting all the nutrients your body needs in each meal and partly because you will not be triggering the body's many satiety cues.

A major takeaway you should get from this book is how to trigger satiety. Avoiding hunger naturally boosts your metabolic rate, so you burn more calories.

Maintenance

"Will I have to be super disciplined after I make it to my weight goal?" my new client from yesterday asked me.

"That depends on what you mean by disciplined," I replied. "You can't binge for several weeks like you said you have in the past and expect the weight to stay off."

"I understand that," she said. "But will I have to maintain a strict diet?"

"That's certainly an option," I said. "You can continue to carefully follow my system, but the system is much less strict in maintenance..."

"Okay," she said. "I might be able to live with that."

"But another way to do it" I continued "is to keep the good habits you're going to develop like weighing yourself every day, exercising regularly, eating lots of fruits and vegetables, eating small amounts of lean proteins and Countable Carbs, keeping fat quantities low, and only occasionally splurging with your friends."

"Yeah. That sounds like more my style. I could live with that if I was never hungry."

"Good," I said. "And the beauty of weighing yourself every day is you find out if your weight is creeping back up before it gets out of control..."

"And I can go right back into weight-loss mode if that happens," she interrupted, "because I won't have a pent-up desire to binge."

"Exactly."

"It's a lot easier to lose three or four pounds than twenty or forty."

"You're getting it now," I affirmed.

"I can do that," she said.

"Good!" I said. "Let's get started."

Starvation Mode

Hunger is a big problem when it comes to weight loss. Less food undermines your weight-loss goals when you allow yourself to feel hungry a lot of the time. If your body registers hunger chronically, say for several hours a day over the course of several weeks, your endocrine system will transition into "starvation mode."

Being in starvation mode has a terrible impact on your body. Back in 1944 to 1945, a landmark study was conducted at the University of Minnesota.[3] While this research is very old, you will see from more recent studies referenced throughout this book the findings are still relevant today.

In the Minnesota Starvation Study, 36 single male participants were selected out of 200 volunteers because they were in good physical and mental health. After 24 weeks of a diet restricted to 1570 calories a day, their metabolism had slowed dramatically, they had lost 25% of their original body weight, and they became obsessed with food. They talked about food incessantly. They dreamed about food. They craved food. They withdrew socially, and their sex drives decreased substantially. They suffered from depression. Their heart rates slowed dramatically, their body temperatures dropped, and their respiration declined.

---

[3] "The Psychology of Hunger." Dr. David Baker and Natacha Keramidas, October 2013, American Psychological Association, https://www.apa.org/monitor/2013/10/hunger

At the end of the study, any participants who were allowed to binge did exactly that... for several weeks until they gained back more than the weight they lost.

Unintended consequences

Clearly, eating less in the way the participants in the Minnesota Starvation Study did was not a good way to lose weight. This was the textbook example of how to lose weight the wrong way. Even if my goal were to lose 25% of my original body weight, I would never knowingly do it in such a way as to dramatically slow my metabolism, supercharge my desire for food, cause me to feel depressed, suppress my sex drive, and make me want to withdraw socially.

Yet, that is exactly what people do all the time even now. They count calories or they fast intermittently, or they simply force themselves to eat less while using willpower to resist the resultant hunger. Weight loss becomes both an obsession and a torment.

"I'm determined to lose 50 more pounds," a client once told me. Actually, I have heard that from many clients.

"How much have you lost so far," I asked.

"Thirty pounds," she said.

"It sounds like you're doing great. Why do you need me?"

"I'm stuck. Losing weight was easy at first, but now the weight has stopped coming off."

"You came to the right place. How do you feel?"

"Discouraged. I've been trying so hard. I guarantee you I am only eating 900 calories a day." She sounded dejected.

Further discussion revealed she dreamed of the day when she could eat whatever she wanted to again, and she fantasized about bingeing. This is a very bad place to be in a weight-loss journey. And it is completely unnecessary. I am just glad she came to me when she did.

The wrong way to diet

The most significant aspect of the Minnesota Starvation study is that it showed us clearly what the consequences are of losing weight the wrong way, and it demonstrated what the wrong way looks like.

The funny thing is the 1570 calories a day allotted to the participants is not a terribly small amount of calories. According to a study conducted by the National Weight Control Registry (NWCR) in 1998[4], the average male who has successfully kept off a substantial amount of weight loss for several years is consuming 1685 calories a day to *maintain* the weight loss.

Why should you care about what the 10,000 participants in the NWCR do? I like to look at their habits because they have all lost at least 30 pounds and kept it off at least a year. The average NWCR participant has lost 66 pounds and kept it off 5 ½ years. They are all successful at losing weight and keeping it off.

So why is it that these NWCR men are able to maintain normal lives with 1685 calories a day when the Minnesota group was in semi-starvation with 1570 calories? Let's look at some differences between the right way and the wrong way to manage weight:

---

[4] "Persons successful at long-term weight loss and maintenance continue to consume a low-energy, low-fat diet." Shick et al., April 1998, *Journal of the American Dietetic Association,* National Institutes of Health pubmed, https://www.ncbi.nlm.nih.gov/pubmed/9550162?dopt=Abstract

The wrong way is to eat an unbalanced diet dominated by calorically-dense foods in small amounts. That is what the men in the Minnesota experiment did. They ate potatoes, cabbage, macaroni and whole wheat bread in "*meager*" quantities.[5] They ate very little protein and few nutrient-rich, low-caloric density foods.

The NWCR participants follow diets that at a minimum meet the RDA for various nutrients, and the foods in their diets tend to be of low-caloric density.[6] In other words, these successful NWCR participants eat nutritious foods that would tend to fill them up without a lot of calories, while the semi-starvation folks ate almost as many calories, but did not get nearly as full or have as many nutrients.

As to exercise, they were getting about the same amount. The NWCR participants average 60 minutes of exercise per day, seven days a week. About four hours of that was brisk walking, and three hours was challenging exercise. This is almost identical to the Minnesota men in amount of exercise; they were required to walk 22 miles a week and maintain an active lifestyle.

This impact of caloric density has been tested in other studies. According to Harvard Health Publishing of Harvard Medical School[7],

---

[5] "The Great Starvation Experiment, 1944-1945", The Mad Science Museum, https://archive.wphna.org/wp-content/uploads/2016/01/2005-Mad-Science-Museum-Ancel-Keys-Starvation.pdf
[6] "Provision of foods differing in energy density affects long-term weight loss." Rolls, et al., June 2005, *Obesity Research,* https://www.ncbi.nlm.nih.gov/pubmed/15976148
[7] "Eating Frequency and Weight Loss." July 2015, *Harvard Health Publishing of Harvard Medical School,* https://www.health.harvard.edu/diet-and-weight-lossweight-loss/eating-frequency-and-weight-loss

"Replacing high-calorie foods with healthier low-calorie ones can help decrease calories without limiting the total volume of food you eat. A 10-month study of 189 patients found they were able to lose weight by reducing calories from drinks and choosing foods with low energy density."

The Minnesota study participants ate only two times a day: at breakfast and at lunch. This is intermittent fasting, and it left them hungry and without food for large portions of each day. The NWCR participants lost weight in a variety of different ways.

According to the Harvard piece cited above,[7]

"Eating fewer than three times a day puts you at risk for overeating and choosing less healthy foods... There does appear to be an inverse association between weight and eating frequency. That is, the heavier a person is, the less often they eat." And, *"eating more than three times per day"* leads to a *"decrease in hunger and an increase in fullness, which can potentially prevent overeating. In fact, when people become very hungry the risk increases that they will choose unhealthy high-calorie foods, such as pizza and soda. This can lead to eating too much at one sitting."*

Higher volume leads to a faster metabolism

In the Minnesota study[5], when the semi-starvation period ended, some of the participants were allowed to eat without any restrictions, and they tended to overeat. However, the ones who ate the highest volumes of foods in the unrestricted period showed the sharpest increases in their metabolic rates. Those who remained much more restricted did not experience nearly the recovery of their metabolic rates.

This was an early clue that high volume eating speeds the metabolism. For them, it was bingeing, because the foods they were eating were high in caloric density. This was very similar to what my new client from yesterday says she has historically done after losing a lot of weight. That is the wrong way to eat.

We will see later in this book that eating a large amount of low-caloric density foods can help satisfy your hunger and speed your metabolism, but without making you fat. That right way to eat is exactly how NWCR participants typically do it.

Takeaways for Chapter 1

- **Open your mind to the possibility that you don't already know how to lose weight sustainably.**

- **Yo-yo weight loss always starts with hunger.**

- **Hunger for several hours a day leads eventually to food fantasies or cravings.**

- **Food fantasies and cravings lead to bingeing.**

- **Bingeing is eating large amounts of calorically-dense foods in a short period of time.**

- **When you've lost a lot of weight and been hungry a lot, one binge is never enough.**

- **Regardless of the marketing claims, if a weight loss plan makes you hungry, it is not sustainable.**

- **Your body has built-in mechanisms to make sure you don't stop eating until you've gotten all the nutrients you need. This is what creates hunger.**

- When you have triggered all the right mechanisms, your body tells you to stop eating. This is satiety.

- Your goal should be to achieve satiety without consuming as many calories as you burn.

- In every meal, eat a balanced diet that includes small amounts of calorically-dense protein and low-GI carbohydrates plus larger amounts of nutrient-rich, low-caloric density, low-GI whole fruits and veggies.

- Eat frequently throughout each day.

- Eat unlimited quantities of nutrient-rich, super low-caloric density foods.

- Eat enough volume to feel satisfied.

- Avoiding hunger naturally boosts your metabolic rate, so you burn more calories and prevent the urge to binge.

Chapter 2

Hunger is the Trigger

Avoid Starvation Mode

Before the Minnesota Starvation Study, the body's normal reactions to sustained hunger were little understood. Since then, numerous studies have verified the Minnesota participants' reactions were all part of an avoidable, but extremely common syndrome.

Now, the syndrome has many names in society and in the scientific community. The most common are "starvation mode," "persistent metabolic adaptation," and "adaptive thermogenesis." Some elements of the syndrome are as follows:

- Obsession with food

- Slowed resting metabolic rate

- Reduced sex drive

- Depression

The biological reason for starvation mode is clear; it is a coordinated adaptation of the body to preserve life in the face of a famine. Our ancient ancestors survived famines because their bodies were able to adapt in this way. The obsession with food drove them to do whatever they could to find food for survival. Their slowed metabolism allowed them to preserve their fat stores long enough to outlast the food shortages. Reduced sex drives were necessary because reproductive activities would have burned a lot of energy at a time when their bodies had no energy to spare. Cravings for calorically-dense foods to repeatedly binge on motivated them to eat the kinds of foods that would put lost weight back on their bodies.

In more recent years, evidence has shown various aspects of starvation mode do not occur independently of each other. Instead they all occur (or do not occur) as a package. For example, a 2010 study[8] conducted by Rosenbaum and Leibel concluded as follows:

---

[8] "Adaptive thermogenesis in humans." Rosenbaum and Leibel, October 2010, *International Journal of Obesity* (London), National Institutes of Health, https://www.ncbi.nlm.nih.gov/pmc/articles/PMC3673773/?fbclid=IwA R2A58oQAjNxfdKm1TC3Q3QalV6XIM37Rxr3u8emulSCCF2W_xiY hR6xk6c

"While weight reduction is difficult in and of itself, anyone who has ever lost weight will confirm that it is much harder to keep the weight off once it has been lost. The over 80% recidivism rate to pre-weight loss levels of body fatness after otherwise successful weight loss is due to the coordinate actions of metabolic, behavioral, neuroendocrine, and autonomic responses designed to maintain body energy stores (fat)…"

The study's authors point out that starvation mode (which they call *"adaptive thermogenesis"*) impacts *"both lean and obese individuals attempting to sustain reduced body weights"* by creating *"the ideal situation for weight regain."* They say a large number of *"interlocking systems"* in the human body actively defend obesity against the individual's best efforts to keep the weight off, and they point out these systems are primarily governed by hormones. The main hormone cited is leptin, which we will talk about extensively later.

Another study found that this syndrome did not improve over time. One study by Fothergill et al. tracked weight loss contestants for six years after "The Biggest Loser" competition[9] and found even after they had gained most or all of the lost weight back their metabolisms remained substantially slowed, their leptin levels remained substantially reduced, and their ghrelin levels remained substantially elevated.

Leptin is the primary satiety hormone. When it is released, your body tells you that you have eaten enough to be satisfied. Ghrelin is an appetite enhancement hormone. When you have a lot of it in your system, you will crave food.

---

[9] "Persistent metabolic adaptation 6 years after 'The 'Biggest Loser' competition" Fothergill et al., August 2016, *Obesity,* National Institutes of Health pubmed,
https://www.ncbi.nlm.nih.gov/pubmed/27136388

Condemnation

So to paraphrase these findings, if we lose a lot of weight based on methods the Biggest Losers used, or in the ways studied by Rosenbaum and Leibel, then we are condemned to a life obsessed with food. This obsession includes terrible cravings and dreams about food, an inability to satisfy our hunger, and a life-long slowed metabolism. That sounds awful, right? Losing weight without acknowledging these natural bodily responses to a substantial reduction in food consumption (i.e., starvation mode) will result in regaining the lost weight and a continued struggle with chronic hunger.

In effect, this is the predictable outcome of any weight-loss program that relies on hunger to cause the weight to come off. If you only focus on limiting your diet to a restricted caloric intake and you use willpower to fight your body's naturally occurring feelings of hunger, then you will almost certainly eventually put your body into some level of starvation mode.

Your Reprieve

The good news is you can lose weight without triggering hunger and all of those interlocking systems that defend obesity. There is actually an easier and healthier alternative path. This is indicated by the fact that Rosenbaum and Leibel could only cite *"over 80%"* of weight losers who gained it all back. It is also proven by the existence of the 10,000 participants in the National Weight Control Registry who have lost an average of 66 pounds and kept it off for an average of 5 ½ years.[10]

This book will guide you to sustained weight loss without hunger. In fact, hunger avoidance is the key to your potential success. If we

---

[10] The National Weight Control Registry, www.nwcr.ws

understand how leptin and ghrelin work, we can get ahead of those interlocking systems and prevent the body from going into starvation mode. Without hunger, there is no hormonal support for food fantasies, cravings or urges to binge. In fact, as we will discuss later, when you defeat hunger, you also boost your metabolic rate, thus undoing the damage that otherwise would have kept your metabolism slow for life.

Not used to eating this much

"The biggest problem I'm having is I'm not used to eating as much as you want me to eat," said one of my clients recently.

She was thrilled because the weight was melting away. She didn't understand why, because she was never hungry.

"I must really trust you, or I wouldn't be eating all this food!" she declared.

The proof she was on the right track when she said that a couple of months ago was she had already lost 10 pounds. And that was just the beginning.

"I'm down 25 pounds in 15 weeks, and I'm still never hungry," she told me a few days ago. "This is amazing! I've been telling all my friends about it."

Satiety

Satiety (pronounced suh-tee'-uh-dee) is the absence of hunger. When you are hungry, your metabolism is slow. The pairing of hunger and metabolic slowing is one of those interlocking systems that Rosenbaum and Leibel were talking about. But we can use the flip side of that system to our advantage--with <u>satiety</u>, your metabolism speeds up.

Metabolic slowdown can make weight loss nearly impossible. It is the cause of virtually every weight-loss plateau. Your first priority in losing weight must be to prevent metabolic slowdown.

Satiety is the key to breaking the slowdown. Satiety is naturally triggered in a variety of ways we will discuss. When you are the master of your own satiety, you can keep your metabolic rate up, and sustained weight loss will become relatively easy.

Satiety in action: the grapefruit studies

If you are scratching your head and wondering how you can eat as much as you want and still lose weight, fear not. I will be showing lots of evidence and plenty of scientific studies to prove this to you. But let's just get a quick glimpse now by looking at two different studies of grapefruit and weight loss:

Simply eating half of a fresh grapefruit before each meal three times a day with no other dietary changes has been shown to cause significant weight loss and improvements to insulin resistance in obese individuals.[11]

Fresh whole grapefruit is a good example of a low-GI, low-caloric density, anti-inflammatory, nutrient-rich food like most of the rest of the "Unlimiteds" (foods you can eat in unlimited quantities -- see Chapter 9). Grapefruit contains fiber to slow digestion, lower blood pressure, and keep you more regular. It also contains powerful antioxidants including Vitamin C, Vitamin A, lycopene (in red and

---

[11] "The effects of grapefruit on weight and insulin resistance: relationship to the metabolic syndrome." Fujioka et al., Spring 2006, *Journal of Medicinal Food*, National Institutes of Health pubmed, https://www.ncbi.nlm.nih.gov/pubmed/16579728

pink grapefruits), and flavanones. As a group, these nutrients help your body to fight cancer, reduce blood pressure and cholesterol, reduce risks of stroke and heart disease, protect against macular degeneration, and boost metabolic rates.

How you put grapefruit into your diet will have a major impact on whether it helps you to lose weight. In the study I just cited, it was consumed *before* each meal. That meant that it partially satisfied appetite before the participants decided how much to eat during their meals. I think we can safely assume they chose to eat less of the calorically-dense food- in their regular meals than they would have if they had not had the grapefruit first.

Another study did not show weight loss from eating grapefruit without any other dietary changes. [12] In this study, the grapefruit was eaten *with* the meals.

This is no small detail, because satiation is vital to both weight loss and boosting your metabolism. Eating filling, nutrient-rich, low-caloric density, low-Glycemic Load foods such as grapefruit before starting on the calorically dense foods partly satiated the first study's participants. Eating grapefruit during or especially at the end of a meal would make no difference in appetite and would therefore not impact how much of the calorically-dense food was consumed.

In other words, you won't feel like eating so much calorically-dense food if you already filled up on Unlimiteds. If you don't feel like eating as much, you may lose weight without any hunger.

Remember, these people who lost weight in the grapefruit study were not on a calorically-restricted diet. They were simply making

---

[12] "The effects of daily consumption of grapefruit on body weight, lipids, and blood pressure in healthy, overweight adults." Dow et al., July 2012, *Metabolism, Clinical and Experimental*, https://www.metabolismjournal.com/article/S0026-0495(11)00413-6/fulltext

the adjustment of eating a specific Unlimited before each meal. This small step can be seen as one piece of a much larger overall strategic approach to eating and life taught in this book: the "Eat As Much As You Want" system.

By the way, although grapefruit is a very healthy and nutritious food, I don't recommend that you eat it before every meal as happened in the study. To get all the nutrients your body needs for optimal function, variety is important. In fact, too much of any one food can create problems no matter what the food is. If you eat many different Unlimiteds, you will accomplish the satiety reflected in the grapefruit study, but you will also get the variety your body needs.

Takeaways for Chapter 2

- **When you are hungry, your metabolism has slowed down.**

- **Satiety speeds your metabolic rate.**

- **Unlimiteds are mostly low-GI, low-caloric density, anti-inflammatory, nutrient-rich foods.**

- **Eating Unlimiteds before other foods brings satiety with fewer calories.**

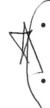

- **Making yourself hungry too often and for too long can put you into starvation mode.**

- **In starvation mode, you will crave the wrong foods, and your metabolism will be chronically slow.**

- **Chronic hunger and a slow metabolism make sustained weight loss nearly impossible.**

- Satiety and a faster metabolism make weight loss far easier.

Chapter 3

Caloric Restriction

Healthy Weight Loss Requires It

Ultimately, you will only lose weight if you burn more calories than you consume. Caloric restriction may be intentional or unintentional, difficult or easy. How challenging it is depends on whether you enable your body to gently take you to your goals, or you fight your body tooth and nail as it forces you away from your goals. Most people choose to fight their bodies, which is why yo-yo weight loss is so prevalent in our culture.

Caloric restriction substantially extends lives and prevents a host of metabolic, heart and brain diseases. It may or may not cause you to burn more calories than you consume. Obviously, if your metabolism slows down more than the amount of your restriction, you won't lose weight. So the goal of caloric restriction should be to keep the metabolism strong while reducing the number of calories consumed.

There are many approaches to caloric restriction. You can simply deny yourself certain foods, or eat smaller quantities of food, or skip meals, or fast, or count calories, or follow the Eat As Much As You Want system.

Hopefully, you are by now well aware that hunger and a slowing metabolism comprise one of the primary interlocking systems the human body uses to defend against weight loss. For our ancestors, this was helpful, because weight loss was a threat to survival. If they had not felt hunger when they lost weight, they would have starved to death.

We now live in a time of plenty. Obesity is the current threat to survival because it compromises health and longevity. But our bodies have not evolved in response to this modern reality. Our bodies still defend vigorously against weight loss, so we can only achieve sustainable losses if we learn to work with our bodies' existing interlocking systems. Our sense of hunger is the distillation of many bodily mechanisms working together to keep our weight up. This means we must vigorously defend against the onset of hunger.

Two of the most popular systems for caloric restriction are calorie counting and intermittent fasting. They both work for initial weight loss, but they both typically involve chronic hunger resulting in a well-documented history of very high dropout rates leading to yo-yo weight loss.

The Eat As Much As You Want system is much easier to sustain because it offers tremendous variety without hunger, metabolic slowdown or starvation mode.

Many clients have followed my advice to lose weight and keep it off. Some specifically came to me because they had reached a plateau following other programs. By making the changes I advise in this book, they were able to restart their weight loss and go on to reach their goals. Nutritious, balanced eating without hunger is the answer.

Myth vs. reality

Myths about how to lose weight and keep it off are now widely accepted in our popular culture. Here's one of the worst:

"Eat less. All you need is simple willpower."

This is false.

Simply eating less triggers all the body's weight defense mechanisms, resulting in chronic hunger. Willpower is no match for a constant unfulfilled desire for food. Food is readily available. Temptations lead to binges. This does not happen because of inadequate willpower.

Our survival instinct is extremely strong, and there is much more to it than a fear of heights or a reflexive scurry to get out of the way of an oncoming bus. It is also a complex network of responses to weight loss including a progression of sensations starting with mild hunger, then intense hunger, then cravings, fantasies and an insatiable urge to binge… repeatedly.

Danny Cahill, the winner of Season 8 of "The Biggest Loser" TV show, reported that after the show was over his metabolism had slowed by 800 calories a day, and he suffered from uncontrollable desires to binge even after he had gained back over 100 pounds of the lost weight.

> "His slow metabolism is part of the problem, and so are his food cravings. He opens a bag of chips, thinking he will have just a few. 'I'd eat five bites. Then I'd black out and eat the whole bag of chips and say, 'What did I do?'"[13]

The men in the Minnesota experiment intentionally ate a poor quality diet to mimic what would be available to starving Europeans during World War II.[5] Ironically, as food has become more readily available to nearly every American today, the quality of what we as a culture consume has declined, and how we choose to eat leaves us hungry even though we are eating too many calories.

Our natural survival instinct and hormonal system are wired for a bygone day when fast foods, processed foods and high-octane sweets were not so readily available. We have lost our way on nutrition and activity. Our ancestors moved more and ate differently. Today, chemical additives, low quality fats, and refined sugars are short-circuiting the natural processes that should be keeping us as slender as our forebears were in the 1950s and before.

Please don't make the mistake of comparing yourself to living relatives and concluding "Obesity runs in my family." All of your living relatives are subject to the same cultural temptations and

---

[13] "After 'The Biggest Loser', Their Bodies Fought to Regain Weight." Gina Kolata, May 2 2016, *The New York Times*, https://www.nytimes.com/2016/05/02/health/biggest-loser-weight-loss.html

influences as you are. Instead, look back at pictures of your ancestors taken in the early to mid 1900s. That is a better measure of your genetics.

Addictive junk food permeates our culture, and our propensity to integrate junk into our daily lives is killing us. Give your body needed nutrients and work naturally with the mechanisms that control metabolism and hunger. Do as your forebears did by filling your stomach with healthful foods that cure inflammation and truly satisfy hunger. Only then can you enlist your body's help to defeat obesity. Unless you make those changes, you must accept obesity or fight it in the face of an overwhelming survival instinct that defends it.

Calorie Counting

Calorie counting has been around for decades. Throughout most of the past 50 years, calorie counting has been the most popular way of losing weight.

Calorie counters believe they can use a formula to calculate how many calories they are burning ("Calories Burned"). They also believe that all they need to do to lose weight is to consume fewer calories than the formula says they burn.

Suppose the formula says we will each burn 1800 calories a day. If we consume 1300 calories a day, then we should burn 500 calories per day more than we eat. The 500-calorie difference is typically referred to as the "Caloric Deficit".

One pound of fat is 3500 calories. Seven days with a Caloric Deficit of 500 calories a day is a 3500 calories per week Caloric Deficit. If all of our weight loss is from fat, this math says we should lose one pound of fat per week.

The math is all very simple and straightforward. Unfortunately, the assumptions are severely flawed.

The calories burned formula

The first flaw is the assumption that the calories-burned formula will not change. The truth is the formula stops working after we have been counting calories for a few weeks. If caloric restriction makes us hungry, our metabolism will slow down and we won't burn as many calories.

Calorie counting only works if it incorporates the principles of the Eat As Much As You Want system. It must be done without hunger or it will break down.

While some calculations give us a good approximation of calories burned at the beginning of weight loss, over time our hormones dramatically change the number. Count on it, especially if our bodies go into starvation mode.

Fat loss

Another deception in the way the calorie-counting theory is presented is the explanation of how many calories are in a pound of fat. That implies that if we lose a pound, the loss all comes from fat. False again.

With most diet plans, especially those that do not include full-body resistance exercise, a pound of flesh burned off is about two-thirds of a pound of fat and one-third of a pound of muscle. The reduction in muscle is very difficult to gain back. And this loss of muscle results in even more slowing of the metabolic rate.

Chapters 7 and 18 are devoted to teaching you how to efficiently burn fat while retaining muscle. It is definitely possible to lose fat without losing muscle, but only with excellent nutrition and the right kinds of exercise. Calorie counting per se does not take into account nutritional completeness or balance, and it does not address exercise other than to look at how many calories are burned doing it.

Social media reinforces the fiction

This widely believed myth of the simplicity of weight loss has given birth to numerous simplistic slogans for weight loss that are commonly shared on social media today in response to questions such as "How can I reliably lose weight?" Here are a few such comments I have recently seen:

"Calories in versus calories out!!!"

"Eat less. Exercise more."

"Stop eating so much."

Here's an upbeat one:

"Keep your eyes on the prize."

These slogans encourage us to embrace the simplistic approach and to believe that all we have to do to lose weight is to cut calories using sheer willpower. It is sad to see that the vast majority of people who buy into these slogans lose weight for a little while, and then gain it all back.

Scientists have now accepted that simple calorie counting does not work. Starvation mode can stop weight loss dead in its tracks, according to a 2017 study by Benton and Young:[14]

---

[14] "Reducing Calorie Intake May Not Help You Lose Body Weight." Benton and Young, September 2017, *Perspectives on Psychological*

"[H]aving a reduction in calorie intake as the central plank of an antiobesity strategy fails to acknowledge the existence of physiological mechanisms that predispose to its failure... when a lower energy intake leads to hormonal changes that stimulate appetite (*Lean & Malkova, 2016*), reduces metabolic rate (*Dulloo & Jacquet, 1998*), and stimulates the consumption of more calorific foods (*Benton, 2005*). Although it may appear to be common sense to suggest that eating less will reduce the risk of putting on weight, this may not be the optimal approach."

Fortunately, further research studies have clarified that calories can in fact be reduced without triggering the interlocking mechanisms of the body that defend a higher weight.

Caloric restriction the right way versus the wrong way

"Medically supervised" diets are typically excessively low-calorie crash diets that initially cause rapid weight loss but dramatically slow the metabolism because of hyper-restriction of calories and inadequate nutrition throughout each day. This unhealthy approach can result in ongoing hunger and a weight-loss plateau that is likely to be followed by a yo-yo.

Instead, you should restrict calories by working with your body to stimulate metabolic hormones that stop your hunger. Done the right way, this will cause you to comfortably choose to stop eating before you have consumed as many calories as you are burning.

Set appropriate weekly weight-loss goals. Then make sensible changes to lifestyle and eating habits that lead to healthy weight loss.

Science, National Institutes of Health,
https://www.ncbi.nlm.nih.gov/pmc/articles/PMC5639963/

A new client came to me last year after being on a 500-calorie a day medically supervised plan. At first, she had lost weight rapidly following that plan, faster than 2% per week. Then her metabolism crashed and her weight stopped coming off.

If she had not come to me when she reached her plateau, her food cravings would likely have spiraled out of control, and she would have been caught in a yo-yo. Thankfully, she was receptive to my guidance. I advised her to substantially increase her food intake, to improve the balance, nutritional value and volume of foods she was eating, and to stop allowing herself to be hungry. She began to eat as I recommend in this book. Her weight loss resumed after she made these changes, and she continued to lose substantially more after that.

Now, she is stable at her goal weight and is in the maintenance phase of the Eat As Much As You Want system. She looks good and feels great.

I realize that it seems counterintuitive to say that to lose more weight you should eat more food and satisfy your hunger, so let's explore this concept further.

The speed of your metabolism is far more variable than people realize. If you throttle back your metabolic rate, you will pay major consequences including ongoing hunger, low energy, and stalled weight loss. When you can accelerate it by giving your body the nutrients it needs in the correct amounts throughout each day, you can lose weight without hunger while maintaining excellent energy levels throughout the day.

The first flaw we discussed in the calorie-counting theory was the invalid assumption that the amount of calories burned at rest each day stays the same. The typical calorie counter eats in such a way as to crash the metabolic rate. On the other hand, by changing the way you eat in the right way, you can actually increase the number of calories burned at rest instead of reducing it.

To be clear, I don't just advocate eating more. I advocate eating the right kinds of foods in the right balance to satisfy your appetite and accelerate your metabolism so that you burn more calories than you consume.

Intermittent Fasting

Intermittent fasting is a systematic approach to fasting. Proponents forego food for some portion of each day or for a couple of days per week. In my experience, before people start on intermittent fasting, they typically believe the following:

- The hunger of fasting will go away after awhile.

- It will be easy to just skip meals.

- They can be successful without changing how much they eat.

- They will instinctively eat fewer calories if they don't eat at all for part of each day.

- Even if they don't eat fewer calories, they will still lose weight.

- Intermittent fasting will encourage them to establish good eating habits

- Skipping breakfast is a sensible choice

Unfortunately, none of these beliefs are true. The biggest failing of intermittent fasting is that it causes a lot of hunger *every day.*

Intermittent fasting benefits mostly come from caloric restriction

In the interest of providing a balanced discussion on the subject of intermittent fasting, I will tell you that some people have made it work for them. There is no bigger fan of intermittent fasting than Mark P. Mattson, PhD. He has personally used it for more than 20 years. He and Rafael de Cabo, Ph.D. said

> *"Evidence is accumulating that eating in a 6-hour period and fasting for 18 hours can trigger a metabolic switch from glucose-based to ketone-based energy, with increased stress resistance, increased longevity, and a decreased incidence of diseases, including cancer and obesity."[15]*

The quote above is from Cabo's and Mattson's interpretations of results from numerous studies done by other people. However, a large percentage of the studies cited were either solely about caloric restriction or were about intermittent fasting used as a tool for caloric restriction.

Thus, many of the results Cabo and Mattson attribute to intermittent fasting were actually attributed by the scientists in the studies to caloric restriction. We already know that there are many ways to achieve caloric restriction.

It is indisputable that caloric restriction slows aging and increases lifespans in animals. And there is a huge number of other health benefits from caloric restriction for humans and animals alike. The Eat As Much As You Want system achieves caloric restriction without hunger.

---

[15] "Effects of Intermittent Fasting on Health, Aging, and Disease." Cabo and Mattson, December 26 2019, *The New England Journal of Medicine*, https://www.nejm.org/doi/full/10.1056/NEJMra1905136

Cabo and Mattson go on to argue that certain specific health benefits of intermittent fasting are beyond the levels that would be explained by caloric restriction alone, and they list many wonderful health benefits.

Almost all of these benefits they say were not due to caloric restriction may alternatively be achieved by eating nutrient-rich anti-inflammatory foods and consuming controlled amounts of "Countables" as is done in the Eat As Much As You Want system. Eating whole, natural, nutritious foods, keeping your blood sugar at healthy, relatively steady levels, and making appropriate lifestyle choices definitely confer a host of benefits that neither caloric restriction nor intermittent fasting provide. The balance of this book will cover many such benefits.

While Cabo and Mattson are highly respected, their views are in sharp disagreement with the mainstream scientific community. Now let's explore what the other scientists have found.

Intermittent fasting increases hunger and dropouts

A 2007 study [16] put healthy normal weight people on an intermittent fasting diet with sufficient calories to maintain weight on a *seven day "menu cycle of typical American foods"*. Participants experienced increasing hunger and desire to eat on fasting days. The hunger continued until the end of the study and resulted in an unusually high dropout rate. The study concluded disappointingly as follows:

---

[16] "A controlled trial of reduced meal frequency without caloric restriction in healthy, normal-weight, middle-aged adults." Stote et al., April 2007, *American Journal of Clinical Nutrition*, National Institutes of Health,
https://www.ncbi.nlm.nih.gov/pmc/articles/PMC2645638/

"The present findings suggest that, without a reduction in calorie intake, a reduced-meal-frequency diet does not afford major health benefits in humans."

Skipping meals is not easy

While it seems convenient not to plan as many meals, skipping meals as a long-term weight loss strategy is not easy, according to scientific findings.

In 2019, the *Harvard Heart Letter* commented on another study affirming that intermittent fasting spurs hunger, causes high dropout rates, creates an urge to overeat, and provides no health benefits beyond weight loss [17]:

> *"so there is a danger of indulging in unhealthy dietary habits on non-fasting days,' says Dr. [Frank Hu, chair of the department of nutrition at the Harvard T.H. Chan School of Public Health]. In addition, there's a strong biological push to overeat following fasting periods. Your appetite hormones and hunger center in your brain go into overdrive when you are deprived of food…"*

Not changing what you eat

The idea that you will lose weight without a change in how much or what kind of food you eat is quickly met with the reality of being famished by the time you are allowed to eat. This leads to poor food choices.

---

[17] "Not so fast: Pros and cons of the newest diet trend." July 31, 2019, Harvard Medical School, *Harvard Heart Letter*, https://www.health.harvard.edu/heart-health/not-so-fast-pros-and-cons-of-the-newest-diet-trend)

In fact, some marketers promoting intermittent fasting have misled people, according to the *Canadian Medical Association Journal*[18]

> *"...promoters of intermittent fasting will, perhaps unintentionally, encourage extreme behaviour, such as bingeing. This is reflected in the photos accompanying many recent new articles on 'the fast diet' or the '5:2 diet.' Often, they depict people eating heaps of high-calorie, high-fat foods, such as hamburgers, french fries and cake. The implication being that if you fast two days a week, you can devour as much junk as your gullet can swallow during the remaining five days.*

> *"Not so, say more moderate proponents of fasting. Their take on intermittent fasting: eat sensibly most of the time, eat nothing for an extended period every now and then, indulge only on occasion (perhaps once a week, say, on a designated 'cheat day')..."*

In short, what you eat and how much of it you eat matters even when intermittently fasting.

Our instincts urge us to overeat with intermittent fasting

Most people using intermittent fasting do not count calories. Instead, they use willpower to avoid overeating during the assigned eating periods. If they are successful at limiting their caloric intake adequately during the eating periods, then they will be successful at initial weight loss, just like the men in the Minnesota experiment who lost substantial amounts of weight. Sadly, animal studies suggest

---

[18] "Intermittent fasting: the science of going without." Roger Collier, June 11 2013, *Canadian Medical Association Journal*, National Institutes of Health, https://www.ncbi.nlm.nih.gov/pmc/articles/PMC3680567/

our instinctive response to intermittent fasting is to overeat whenever we are allowed.[18]

We must eat fewer calories than we burn to lose weight

A 2018 study[19] indicated that restricting eating to the first eight hours of the day can improve insulin sensitivity and blood pressure without increasing appetites over a five-week period, but the obese participants in this study **did not lose weight**. The participants who fasted every day ate the same number of calories as the participants who did not fast. Caloric restriction, not intermittent fasting, is what causes weight loss.

A 2018 study[20] found that longer-term commitment to intermittent fasting was *"equivalent but not superior to [calorie counting] for weight reduction and prevention of metabolic diseases."*

A 2017 study[21] found that *"[a]lternate-day fasting did not produce superior adherence, weight loss, weight maintenance, or cardioprotection vs daily calorie restriction."*

---

[19] "Early Time-Restricted Feeding Improves Insulin Sensitivity, Blood Pressure, and Oxidative Stress Even without Weight Loss in Men with Prediabetes." Sutton et al., June 5 2018, ScienceDirect, *Cell Metabolism*, https://www.sciencedirect.com/science/article/pii/S1550413118302535

[20] "Effects of intermittent and continuous calorie restriction on body weight and metabolism over 50 wk: a randomized controlled trial." Schubel et al., November 23 2018, American Society for Nutrition, *The American Journal of Clinical Nutrition*, https://academic.oup.com/ajcn/article/108/5/933/5201451

[21] "Effect of Alternate-Day Fasting on Weight Loss, Weight Maintenance, and Cardioprotection Among Metabolically Healthy Obese Adults: A Randomized Clinical Trial." Trepanowski et al., July

Most sustained weight losers don't skip breakfast

Skipping breakfast is not wise if your goal is to lose weight and keep it off. In a study of people who have sustained substantial weight loss for a year or more[22], 78% said they eat breakfast every day. This argues in favor of not fasting in the first part of the day.

My client with bad eating habits

You have already read quotes from various scientists saying intermittent fasting study participants have urges to eat unhealthy foods during their eating periods. I can attest to the truth of these statements. Fitness clients of mine sometimes follow their own weight management plans without consulting me. A few years ago, one client insisted intermittent fasting "always" works for him.

"I had doughnuts and chocolate chip cookies this morning!" he declared gleefully as he came into the workout one day.

He made such announcements frequently, and he would smile big at each disclosure because he believed he had found an easy path to weight loss. The result was that his self-reported eating habits during intermittent fasting periods were even worse than his already poor eating habits at other times. He seemed convinced that giving in to these urges was permissible.

"How are you doing on fruits and vegetables?" I asked one day.

---

1 2017, JAMA Internal Medicine, National Institutes of Health pubmed, https://www.ncbi.nlm.nih.gov/pubmed/28459931
[22] "Long-term weight loss and breakfast in subjects in the National Weight Control Registry", Wyatt et al., February 2002, *Obesity Research*, National Institutes of Health pubmed, https://www.ncbi.nlm.nih.gov/pubmed/11836452?dopt=Abstract

"Can't do it," he declared. "I tried it once, but then my stomach started hurting before I could finish all the good stuff like pasta, meats and cookies. By the time the pain went away, I was hungry, but it was my fasting period. I won't do that again."

The lure of intermittent fasting is that some people can lose a lot of weight quickly, which is the basis of the belief that intermittent fasting works.

"I've lost 15 pounds in three weeks!" he said upon arrival to a workout, grinning. "I bet no one loses weight that fast with the Eat As Much As You Want system!"

"Well, some do, but I don't encourage it," I replied. "You're more likely to keep it off if you lose weight more slowly."

He had no interest in hearing my point. He reveled in his ability to lose weight quickly, and it was clear he thought his approach was superior even though we both knew his history of many yo-yos.

"I'm very tired," he said after he had lost about 25 pounds. "I won't be in later this week. I have a doctor's appointment about this profound fatigue."

"It's normal to be tired when you don't eat for large parts of every day," I said.

"This has nothing to do with that," he said. "The doctors can't figure out what the problem is."

"Did you tell them that you're eating junk, then fasting the rest of the day?" I asked bluntly.

"No, but that's not why," he said. "I've read all the studies, and intermittent fasting is good for you."

He stopped coming in. Months later, his wife told me he had lost about 40 pounds before he quit both exercise and weight loss because he had no energy.

"Did he ever change his eating habits," I asked her.

"No, and he's put most of the weight back on now. I asked him to try the Eat As Much As You Want system, but he wouldn't."

"Well, good for you for trying!" I affirmed.

"Yeah," she sighed. "He said 'I can lose weight anytime I want.'"

He never returned to workouts. Since then, he has been fighting two different life-threatening illnesses associated with obesity and sugar intake. I am told he is as heavy now as he ever was before.

Conclusion

Calorie counting, intermittent fasting and self-denial are all declarations of war against your body's own survival mechanisms. When you drive your body into defending itself against weight loss, the mechanisms that allowed your ancient ancestors to survive will rise up to defeat you. Weight loss sustainability then becomes impossible.

Only the Eat As Much As You Want system is designed to use the body's own interlocking systems to cause it to naturally and willingly shed weight. Again, complete balanced nutrition and the elimination of hunger are the keys.

Takeaways for Chapter 3

- Unless you work with the body's interlocking systems that defend your excess weight, you must either accept obesity or fight it in the face of an overwhelming survival instinct that defends it.

- Caloric restriction will only yield weight loss if your metabolism does not slow down too much.

- Caloric restriction yields many great health benefits.

- Balanced, wholesome nutrition yields health benefits that caloric restriction and intermittent fasting alone cannot.

- Caloric restriction can lead to sustainable weight loss if you are consuming the right nutrients and avoiding hunger.

- Calorie counting, intermittent fasting, and willpower driven self-denial cause hunger.

- Calorie counting formulae rely on false assumptions that calories burned at rest will not change and that all weight loss is from fat.

- Our genetic propensity toward obesity or slenderness is better measured by what our ancestors looked like before 1950 than by what our relatives look like now.

- Intermittent fasting is associated with poor food choices.

- Intermittent fasting does not cause weight loss without caloric restriction.

- **Intermittent fasting is neither easier nor more effective than other forms of weight loss.**

- **Only the Eat As Much As You Want system provides caloric restriction without hunger.**

- **The Eat As Much As You Want system stands alone as the only system of weight loss that positively uses the interlocking systems that innately control weight instead of fighting against them**

- **Fighting your own body is a losing battle.**

Chapter 4

Don't Trick Your Body!

Keto is Unhealthy

As the obesity epidemic has grown, many diet fads have swept the country promising easy weight loss. Some of these misguided systems were said to trick your body into shedding pounds. Currently, a major fad is the low-carb, or "Keto" diet.

Millions of people have turned to "Keto" diets (aka ketogenic diets) to lose weight rapidly. They cut out carbohydrates and report great results. The media has lapped this up with glowing articles for several years now.

The public image of the Keto diet is great. The typical consumer thinks it is extremely healthy.

Just today, for example, I met a fellow alternative healthcare professional in connection with work. We exchanged pleasantries, then he asked what I spend my free time doing right now.

"I'm in the midst of editing a book I've written on healthy, sustainable weight loss and quality of life," I said.

"Cool," he said. "So I should cut out carbs, right?"

Truly, over the past several years, that has been an almost uniform assumption among casual acquaintances and new clients: To improve the healthiness of a diet, cut out carbs.

It is certainly ironic that this is the immediate assumption so many people make, because the exact opposite is true. Cutting out carbs is extremely unhealthy. If you had never heard of a Keto diet, what would you say to someone who tried to market this concept to you:

Marketer: "So you want to lose weight, live longer and have a healthier diet?"

You: "Yes, very much so."

Marketer: "Great! Quit eating beans, coarse grain breads, oranges, peaches, apples and avocados. Forget about having a balanced diet. In fact, try to avoid carbs almost completely."

You: "Really? What should I eat instead?"

54

Marketer: "Lots of fat. Animal proteins dripping with saturated fats like bacon and T-Bone steaks are very good for you."

You: "So it's a high-protein diet?"

Marketer: "That is evolving. Some say it's a high-fat diet. Moderate protein, cut out the carbs, and eat lots of fat."

I am amazed that some marketing geniuses were able to convince the masses of this preposterous assertion. And this myth has persisted in the general population for decades.

Keto, the real story

A big part of the popularity of the Keto diet is that it actually does cause weight loss, even though many people who have tried it say it is extremely difficult to maintain. There are multiple versions of this diet, and they include the Atkins diet and the South Beach diet. A *Harvard Health Blog*'s not-so-glowing description of the Keto diet in 2017[23] characterized these as "fad diets" that cause a process called ketosis to break down fat molecules in the body into ketone bodies that the body uses for energy in the absence of carbohydrates:

> *"Because it is so restrictive, it is really hard to follow over the long run... One of the main criticisms of this diet is that many people tend to eat too much protein and poor-quality fats from processed foods, with very few fruits and vegetables. Patients with kidney disease need to be*

---

[23] "Ketogenic diet: Is the ultimate low-carb diet good for you?" Marcos Campos, July 27 2017, Harvard Medical School, *Harvard Health Blog,* https://www.health.harvard.edu/blog/ketogenic-diet-is-the-ultimate-low-carb-diet-good-for-you-2017072712089

cautious because this diet could worsen their condition. Additionally, some patients may feel a little tired in the beginning, while some may have bad breath, nausea, vomiting, constipation, and sleep problems."

Further studies on the long-term impacts of a Keto diet have shown that it can shorten your life. A major 2018 study by Sara Seidelman et al.[24] found that the death rate among the 432,179 participants was greatest for people who consumed too much or too little carbohydrates. The ones who lived the longest ate balanced diets with somewhere in the range of 50 to 55% of their caloric intake coming from carbohydrates. By contrast, Keto experts recommend that only 5% to 10% of your dietary intake come from carbohydrates.

The Seidelman study found that when carbohydrate intake fell below 40% of total calories, death rates increased. At 5% to 10% from carbs, Keto is at the extreme end of the deprivation range. At that end of the range, death rates are substantially higher.

A 2019 study[25] by the South Australian Health & Medical Research Institute (SAHMRI) shed new light on why death rates are higher with high protein diets. Team Leader Professor Christopher Proud said that consuming high amounts of protein

"'speed[s] up protein synthesis within cells. The faster this process occurs the more errors are made…

---

[24] "Dietary carbohydrate intake and mortality: a prospective cohort study and meta-analysis." Sara Seidelman et al., September 2018, *Lancet Public Health,* National Institutes of Health pubmed, https://www.ncbi.nlm.nih.gov/pubmed/30122560

[25] "Study shows why high-protein diets are unhealthy." February 19 2019, *Medical Press,* https://medicalxpress.com/news/2019-02-high-protein-diets-unhealthy.html

"'The resulting build-up of faulty proteins within cells compromises health and shortens lifespan.'

"The research, which has been published in Current Biology, also reinforces established links between a low-protein, high-carbohydrate diet and longer, healthier lives – especially when it comes to brain health.

"'Carbohydrates get a lot of bad press, especially in relation to dieting, but the key is balance and knowing the difference between 'good' carbs and 'bad' carbs,' Professor Proud said.

"'Eating high-fibre carbohydrates like those found in fruit, vegetables and unprocessed grains and seeds will produce the healthiest benefits."

The practical reality of Keto

If you are only getting 5% to 10% of your caloric intake from carbs, then you are avoiding many of the good carbs that provide nutrients vital to good health. There are over 25,000 phytonutrients in plants, and many of them are needed to prevent inflammation and chronic disease. Simply taking multi-vitamins and other supplements is not an adequate solution. There are so many natural nutrients in fruits and vegetables, far more than you can get artificially, and they are best delivered from eating whole natural foods.

In recent years, some proponents of Keto diets such as marketers of the Atkins Diet have promoted the consumption of fibrous vegetables that are low in carbs but high in other nutrients, so that is some improvement. And they have especially emphasized cutting out high-GI carbs, which is another positive. However, it remains an extremely low-carb diet.

There is wide agreement that a Keto diet is difficult to stay on. Many people lose weight effectively for several weeks, but when it becomes especially difficult to stick with it, they quit. A few people proudly proclaim that they have been on Keto for years and have kept the weight off. Normally, maintaining a reduced weight is associated with greater health and longevity, but the Seidelman study implies that is not true with Keto.

Why? Maintaining a super low-carb diet shortens your life expectancy[24], and maintaining a high-protein diet causes flaws in protein synthesis.[25] This makes it all the more interesting that Dr. Robert Atkins, the inventor of the Atkins Diet, struggled so much in his later years with malfunctioning heart muscles.[26] Could that be because of flaws in protein synthesis? We'll never know.

Balanced Diet

Over and over through the years, my strong belief in the benefits of a balanced diet has been reinforced. Several years ago, a fitness client joined a weight loss contest I had organized. She attended a 30-minute nutrition talk I gave at the beginning, then opted to self-direct her own weight-loss efforts. Many contestants did that because it was less expensive than paying for coaching. She lost weight for several weeks until she hit a plateau. After a few more weeks, she made an appointment to see me for advice.

---

[26] "Just What Killed the Diet Doctor, and What Keeps the Issue Alive," N.r. Kleinfield, February 11 2004, *The New York Times*, https://www.nytimes.com/2004/02/11/nyregion/just-what-killed-the-diet-doctor-and-what-keeps-the-issue-alive.html

Plateau, Part One

"I've been really good!" she exclaimed in frustration. "I've followed your system, and it worked at first, but then I plateaued."

"I saw from the weigh-ins that you stopped losing weight," I acknowledged.

"Yes. No losses for the past three weeks. And I haven't changed what I've been doing one little bit."

"Tell me what you're doing," I prompted.

"I'm keeping under 1100 calories a day…" she said, "every day," she added for emphasis.

"Okay," I said, not wanting to dwell on the fact I don't advocate counting calories. "Are you avoiding hunger?"

"I'm trying to. I'm eating plenty of Unlimiteds, like you said to do, and I'm eating a balanced diet," she asserted. "You made a big deal about a balanced diet in your nutrition talk, and I heard you."

"But you still get hungry?" I asked.

"Yes, and tired. I start to get hungry mid-morning – about the same time that my energy drops. The energy stays low the rest of the day, especially mid-afternoon. And I don't really feel satisfied when I eat my lunch salad, even though my stomach is full. Other contestants I've spoken to aren't experiencing these problems. Do you think there's something wrong with me? Should I see a doctor?"

"Let's talk a little more before we decide," I responded. "You said you're eating a balanced diet. Tell me about that."

"Well, every day is about the same. I have my carbs for breakfast, then a big salad for lunch… That's mostly just lettuce, carrots, cukes, tomatoes, that sort of thing. That's all I have for the entire middle part of the day, but it fills me up."

"Uh huh," I acknowledged.

"Then I have my protein and some low-cal veggies at dinner."

"And that's it?" I asked.

"Yes, that's all I'm eating."

Let's pause for a moment in the story now. Can you figure out what is wrong with this picture? Do you know why she wasn't losing weight anymore? Try to think about it a little before you read further…

Plateau, part 2

Did you figure it out? If not, that's okay. You're still learning.

"Did I hear you correctly?" I asked. "Are you only eating three meals a day?"

"Yes. I know you said to have five, but I've always just done three, and it made it easier to divide up the proteins, carbs and salad logically this way."

"Okay, here's what is happening to you…" I began. "I know you believe you're eating a balanced diet…"

"I am!" she interrupted. "I'm getting carbs, protein and a variety of veggies, and I am drinking lots of water!"

"True," I agreed. "But your meals are not balanced. In the morning, you have a high carb diet with virtually no protein. In the evening, you have a high protein diet with virtually no carbs. Protein and carbs must be consumed at the same time for the protein to be utilized properly by the body. And when you get a lot of carbs all at once, especially certain breakfast foods, you get a sugar rush, then you end up low energy the rest of the day…"

"Ohhh," she said. A light was coming on in her head. "Wait! If that's true, why was I able to lose so much weight for the first three weeks?"

"Anytime someone starts a new diet where they're eating fewer calories than they were before, their body sheds weight fairly easily for a few weeks. It almost doesn't matter what the program is because it takes time for their metabolism to react to unbalanced eating. But once the body starts to react, bam! Their metabolism can crash and hunger pangs spike up. That seems to be what's happening with you, and it's why I stressed the importance of a balanced diet in my nutrition talk."

"So now my metabolism has crashed." She sighed.

"Yes," I agreed. "And it will keep getting worse if you don't make changes. For example, in the middle of the day, you have no carbs and no protein, so you have no real energy source to fuel your metabolism to give you energy for the rest of the day."

"That makes sense."

"So your metabolism perks up briefly for a sugar rush in the morning, then it crashes for the rest of the day. Does that resonate with you?"

"Yes, that's right," she agreed.

"What you need to do is more or less eat the same stuff you're eating, but spread the carbs, the protein and the veggies out throughout the day. Every meal should be balanced, not just your intake for the day."

"Oh," she said.

"Other than breakfast, the carbs should be low-Glycemic Index. That means they're foods that don't turn to blood sugar quickly. Do you understand?"

"Yes."

"Also, eat five meals instead of three. This will have you eating something every three to four hours."

"Why?"

"When you spread the food out and balance it at every meal, it will be much easier to avoid hunger, and it will stoke your metabolism," I explained. "Try it out and see."

"I will," she said.

"If you don't have time for an elaborate meal, there are plenty of meals you can do in five minutes," I said.

"Okay... So I really wasn't following your system after all, was I?"

"No, you weren't. Thank you for acknowledging that. But now you can!"

She did, and the weight started coming off again right away.

She smiled brightly at a weigh-in two weeks later. "This is amazing! Thank you so much!" She was four pounds down from the time of our conversation. "I am totally not hungry, and my energy is way up. This was so easy!"

"You're very welcome," I said.

These principles work consistently. You just have to do it to see.

High-Starch Diet

Several popular books tout benefits of eating mainly starches to lose weight. Proponents of this theory advocate potatoes and root vegetables similar to the diet that was followed by the men in the Minnesota Starvation Study.

There are some obvious drawbacks to such a diet. The first is that an extremely large percentage of our population is diabetic or pre-diabetic. Our digestive systems readily convert starches to blood sugar, so the result of eating a lot of starch is that it may cause frequent blood sugar spikes. Sugar is toxic to the body and can cause extreme harm to veins, lean tissues and eyes, so a healthy body will over-release insulin to quickly convert excess blood sugar to fat. An insulin resistant body will simply be harmed by the high blood sugar.

Sugar spikes in the blood stream feed your fat and tend to starve your muscles because muscles can only absorb blood sugar slowly while fat can absorb it rapidly. Type 2 diabetes, which is caused by insulin resistance, can develop as a direct result of prolonged periods of having frequent blood sugar spikes.

The 2018 Seidelman study[24] cited earlier did not just look at low carb diets. It looked at proportions of carbohydrates in all diets. The same higher death rate occurred for people who received more than 70% of their caloric intake from starches as for people who received less than 40%. Only the people with moderate carbohydrate intakes had the higher probability of greater longevity.

There are many peer-reviewed studies showing a high correlation between high- starch intake and excess weight. It causes obesity, high cholesterol, insulin resistance, high blood pressure and an unhealthy and abnormally high concentration of fats or lipids in the blood.[27] However, these problems come from high-GI foods, not from low or medium-Glycemic Index foods.[27]

Potatoes and whole wheat bread, two staples of both the Minnesota Starvation Study and of many popular high starch diets, are both hi-GI, high-Glycemic Load foods. Such foods spike your blood sugar, which leads to sugar crashes, low energy periods, and weight gain.

High starch diets focus on high-GI carbohydrates with lots of calories such as rice or potatoes. These cause weight gain if calories are not restricted and hunger if they are. If calories are unrestricted, your stomach will not feel full until you have eaten too many calories. Conversely, if you count calories while eating densely caloric carbohydrates, you can only eat tiny amounts of food before maxing out your caloric budget. This causes hunger, and it leads to starvation mode and a weight-loss plateau.

Fat-Free vs. Low-Fat Diet

A few decades ago, fat-free diets were extraordinarily popular, and there are still many people who strive to be fat free. This is also unhealthy.

---

[27] "High carbohydrate intake from starchy foods is positively associated with metabolic disorders: a Cohort Study from a Chinese population." Feng, R. et al., *Scientific Reports*, November 2015, National Institutes of Health pubmed, https://www.ncbi.nlm.nih.gov/pmc/articles/PMC4652281/

During the fat-free craze, many highly processed foods were developed as fat free substitutes for normally high fat foods. Instead of providing a healthy alternative to bad fats, these substituted sugar and other carbohydrates to deliver flavor. Thus, fat-free diets morphed unintentionally into high-starch, hi-GI diets for many people. We have already discussed why those do not work.

What does work is a low-fat, nutrient-rich, low-caloric density diet. Keep in mind that you should emphasize healthy fats and lean proteins for the little bit of fat included in your diet. In other words, avoid having high fat content in your foods, be especially vigilant about minimizing saturated and trans fats, and to the extent that you add any fat to a meal make sure it is a healthy fat. This is another subject we'll revisit in depth.

Why low fat?

Fats are by far the most highest-caloric density foods in existence. One gram of fat contains nine calories. One gram of alcohol contains seven calories. Carbohydrates and protein each contain four calories per gram. Whole foods containing carbohydrates and protein also have fiber and other nutrients as well as water, so they have far greater volume per calorie.

Let's do a comparison; think of one cup of olive oil, which would have 1,909 calories. To get 1,909 calories from raw spinach, you would need about 272 cups. To get 1,909 calories from blueberries, you would need about 23 cups.

Some fats are needed for good health. Thus, the fat-free diet has been discredited by scientists and largely dismissed by the general population now. Fat is a vital nutrient that plays a critical role in the functioning of the endocrine system. In short, you need a little fat for health, but more than just a little is too much if you are trying to lose weight.

Fats: truth versus myth

"I need fat, or I'll still be hungry after I eat!"

Have you ever heard someone say that? Substantial research has proven it to be untrue (Chapter 12).

The confusion is between palatability and satiety. Fat is extremely palatable, which is just another way of saying it tastes really good. However, that taste appeal causes us to want to eat more calories, not fewer. This is similar to the effect of refined sugar, which also spurs overeating because of enhanced palatability.

Here is another extremely common question: "What about good fats? Shouldn't I be eating those?"

Fat is truly misunderstood. Some years ago, a client came to me and said she did not understand why she was not losing weight. She said she was cooking with huge amounts of olive oil and coconut oil, so she believed the pounds should be melting away. Instead, she was gaining weight.

Clearly, she was taking in far too many calories from fats. In her mind, "good fat" meant weight loss, and the more she ate, the more weight she thought she would lose. That is not true, of course.

As Americans, we tend to think of everything in big numbers. If a little of something is good, then a lot of it must be great. The reality is that we need a little fat, and we are going to get some of that even if we are trying to avoid it. A fat-free diet is virtually impossible to achieve, and a mindful approach to eating can incorporate a small amount of good fat, which is all we need.

Takeaways for Chapter 4

- Low-carb diets are difficult to stay on and shorten life expectancy.

- High-carb, high-GI diets are associated with poor health, obesity, and shortened life.

- For a balanced diet to truly be effective, it must be balanced in every meal.

- A calorically-restricted, unbalanced diet will work for a few weeks, then your metabolism will crash, your hunger will spike, and you will likely feel tired.

- A small amount of fat is needed in your diet for good health.

- Even good fats must be consumed extremely sparingly to achieve healthy weight loss.

Chapter 5

Master Your Hormones

Accelerate Your Metabolism!

Our hormones can be our allies or they can be our enemies. Most people make enemies of their hormones during weight loss, and that is an unbeatable foe. To sustain weight loss, we must recruit our hormones to fight side by side with us against the common enemy of excess weight.

The same hormones that produce hunger and satiety also decelerate or accelerate our metabolic rates. When our hunger is high, our metabolism is slow. We constantly make choices to be hungry and have a slow metabolism or to be satiated and have a much faster metabolism.

I have worked successfully with many clients who came to me because their weight losses had plateaued while following popular diets. We immediately went to work on increasing their metabolic rates and reducing their hunger by increasing how much they were eating, improving their nutrient balances, and distributing the right nutrients throughout each day. Time and again, these adjustments resulted in a resumption of weight loss and an improvement in how my clients have felt.

What does your body want?

Believe it or not, your body actually wants to be at a normal, healthy weight. If you are not at a healthy weight, it is probably because your body's steering system is broken down. If your car's steering system were broken, would you get it fixed or just keep driving?

Nutrient-Rich, Low-Caloric Density

There is ample evidence that eating healthily without regard to calories can lead to positive outcomes including weight loss. In 2018, the *New York Times*[28] reported on the findings from a just published study in the Journal of the American Medical Association:

---

[28] "The Key to Weight Loss Is Diet Quality, Not Quantity, a New Study Finds." Anahad O-Connor, February 18 2018, *The New York Times,* https://www.nytimes.com/2018/02/20/well/eat/counting-calories-weight-loss-diet-dieting-low-carb-low-fat.html

"...people who cut back on added sugar, refined grains and highly processed foods while concentrating on eating plenty of vegetables and whole foods — without worrying about counting calories or limiting portion sizes — lost significant amounts of weight over the course of a year."

To be clear, the study did not say that calories do not matter. It's just that people in the study who ate nutritious foods chose to eat fewer calories without even thinking about it, because their hunger was satisfied.

A weight-loss diet focused on unlimited quantities of nutrient-rich, low-caloric density foods can work. Here's another similar study from 2007:

"Eating smart, not eating less, may be the key to losing weight. A year-long clinical trial by Penn State researchers shows that diets focusing on foods that are low in calorie density can promote healthy weight loss while helping people to control hunger.

"Foods that are high in water and low in fat -- such as fruits, vegetables, soup, lean meat, and low-fat dairy products -- are low in calorie density and provide few calories per bite.

"Eating a diet that is low in calorie density allows people to eat satisfying portions of food, and this may decrease feelings of hunger and deprivation while reducing calories" said Dr. Julia A. Ello-Martin, who conducted the study as part of her doctoral dissertation in the College of Health and Human Development at Penn State. Previously, little was known about the influence of diets low in calorie density on body weight...

"We have now shown that choosing foods that are low in calorie density helps in losing weight, without the restrictive messages of other weight loss diets," explained Ello-Martin,

whose findings appear in the June 2007 issue of the American Journal of Clinical Nutrition…"[29]

Confusion About Healthy Eating

The Mediterranean Diet ("MD") is widely praised as a healthy and effective way to lose weight, but it may be the most misunderstood popular diet plan in America. Many people try it and lose no weight, or they do lose weight but end up spurring chronic hunger and weight-loss plateaus. Many people have come to me for advice after they have hit a wall on this diet.

The actual permissible foods in the MD generally fit well with the Eat As Much As You Want system. The struggle that people typically have is how to balance the meals. The shortfall in this plan is that people do not realize that to make it work, they must accentuate unlimited quantities of low-caloric density, nutrient-rich foods.

Alcohol in moderation is okay with both the MD and my system. The main foods preferred within the MD are also foods preferred in my system. *Women's Health* published an article about the MD in which they listed out what is generally thought to be permissible to eat:

- *"**Fruits**: Any and all fresh fruits such as apples, oranges, pears, melon, grapes, berries, dates, figs, peaches, and grapefruit…*

- ***Vegetables**: Any and all fresh vegetables like tomatoes, spinach, broccoli, kale, mushrooms,*

---

[29] "Calorie Density Key To Losing Weight." June 8 2007, Penn State, *Science Daily*, https://www.sciencedaily.com/releases/2007/06/070608093819.htm

Brussels sprouts, cauliflower, cucumbers, peppers, summer squash, and onions. Don't forget about root vegetables like sweet potatoes, potatoes, turnips, and parsnips...

- ***Whole Grains****: Whole grains, plus bread and pasta made with whole-grain ingredients. This includes whole wheat, oats, barley, rye, quinoa, and brown rice.*

- ***Nuts and Seeds****: Whole nuts like almonds, walnuts, hazelnuts, cashews, and pistachios. Seeds such as sunflower seeds, pumpkin seeds, sesame seeds, and flaxseeds.*

- ***Legumes****: Black beans, kidney beans, pinto beans, peas, lentils, chickpeas, and fava beans.*

- ***Healthy Fats****: Extra virgin olive oil, avocados, avocado oil, walnut oil, olives.*

- ***Dairy****: Moderate amounts of dairy items like Greek yogurt, cheese, and milk.*

- ***Fish and Seafood****: Wild-caught fish and shellfish like salmon, sardines, mackerel, shrimp, tuna, trout, and clams.*

- ***Other Animal Protein****: Moderate amounts of poultry, pork, and other lean options. Save red meat for special occasions.*

- **Herbs and Spices**: *Garlic, oregano, basil, thyme, mint, sage, rosemary, cinnamon, nutmeg, and more."[30]*

There is nothing wrong with this list per se. And the author clarifies that frozen and canned fruits and vegetables are allowed as well if they have no other ingredients added and they are packed in either light juice or water. I agree with that.

However, while the foods listed tend to be very good choices, without appropriate guidance, most Americans choose to eat high-fat foods and densely caloric foods in abundance, and only have smaller portions of the low-caloric density foods that are necessary for satiety, weight loss and good health. What the Eat As Much As You Want system adds for the MD is the balance and guidance for actually putting these ingredients together into meals that satisfy, eliminate hunger, and provide weight loss. There will be much more on this subject in later chapters.

Throughout this book, I talk about the various principles of speeding your metabolism, increasing satiety, and filling up on nutrient-rich, low-Glycemic Index, low-caloric density foods. A simple list of foods without guidance regarding how to structure the meals is pointless.

Remember the client in Chapter 4 who had carbs in the morning, salad at lunch, and protein at dinner? There was nothing wrong with what she was eating. What was wrong was how the foods were paired and spread out throughout the day.

Americans tend to proportion meals much differently than the peoples of the Mediterranean. The MD will not work for optimal

---

[30] "The Mediterranean Diet Food List You've Been Waiting For." Christine Yu, May 23 2019, *Women's Health*, https://www.womenshealthmag.com/food/a27542959/mediterranean-diet-food-list/

health or weight loss if the proportions are done in the typical American style. People who have consulted with me have reported large intakes of olive oil and nuts, multiple glasses of wine on some days, large portions of bread dipped in olive oil, and pasta dishes. Those folks were gaining weight, not losing it.

Thus, for effective weight loss, simple lists of foods must be supplemented with guidance on how to satisfy appetites with the right mix and proportions of foods spread out across each day.

The Great Obesity Short-Circuit

We all know an epidemic of obesity has swept this country over the past 60 years. We also know 60 years is not enough time for our genes to have evolved us into a new, larger species. Why are we heavier?

We're eating a lot more calories. Why?

We're hungrier, and it takes more food to satisfy our appetites. Why?

Our innate appetite control centers have gone haywire due to inflammation. Why?

We're eating more processed foods with inflammatory chemicals, poor quality fats, and refined sugars. How does that give us bigger appetites?

It creates resistance to a variety of hormones that signal us to stop eating, especially "leptin".

Cruise ship

If you ever want to see hormonal systems in complete dysfunction, go on a cruise. Doug Parker, a fan of cruises, wrote

> *"Back in 2011, I managed to gain 11 pounds over the course of a seven-night sailing. On another cruise in 2016, I put on another seven pounds. The problem? Um… I like to eat."*[31]

Several years ago, I took a family cruise with my kids. I had heard that people typically gain a pound a day on these cruises, but I thought that must be an exaggeration. The promotional photos showed physically-fit people playing volleyball, dancing in a nightclub, and going on active shore trips.

"How can people do all those activities and gain so much weight?" I wondered.

Then we arrived at the ship. I don't know about other cruises, but adult passengers on this one were predominantly obese. Certainly nothing like the marketing shots.

The ship had a buffet-style dining area that was open long hours. All the food was included in the price of the cruise, so you could spend every waking moment eating if you had enough appetite.

"Look at all the food that lady has!" one of my kids exclaimed.

I had to shush him. He was too young to realize that was not an appropriate comment. The woman he had noticed weighed maybe 300 pounds and was carrying at least 4000 calories in the plates she was taking back to her table. The man she sat down with was even bigger, and he had his own massive supply of food.

---

[31] "The Truth About Cruise Weight Gain." Doug Parker, October 27 2017, CruiseRadio.net, https://cruiseradio.net/cruise-weight-gain/

We got in line at the sushi bar.

"Those look good," I said to my daughter as I pointed to some sashimi.

"It's all good, sweetie," said the woman behind me in line. My guess was she weighed about 250 pounds. "I come on these cruises to eat," she said. "Gain a ton every time, but it's worth every calorie."

This situation would have looked very different if the passengers had functioning endocrine systems. Their bodies had lost the ability to tell them not to be hungry. With all the hunger suppressing hormones circulating in their bodies, they should have had no desire to overeat. Yet there they were in a massive communal binge.

I don't blame them or judge them for their choices. Not at all. Their appetites were abnormally out of control due to inflammation. I suspect many of them would have made different choices before and during the cruise if they had known how to truly satisfy their appetites.

How do I know they had raging hunger suppressing hormones and inflammation? I am about to tell you.

Leptin resistance

Metabolic hormones are supposed to steer your weight. They should make you hungry when you need more calories for optimal health, and they should stop hunger when you have eaten enough. They worked for our ancestors, but they are not working for us.

Leptin is a key metabolic hormone that speeds up your metabolism and suppresses your appetite. When everything is working the way it is supposed to, if we have a lot of leptin in our bloodstreams, we should have fast-burning metabolism without hunger.

Here's how it's supposed to work: Your hypothalamus is a part of your brain that monitors leptin levels. If leptin is high, a healthy hypothalamus tells the rest of the brain you don't need any more food, and your metabolism speeds up.

It's very simple. It does this because leptin goes up when you gain more fat than normal, according to a 2006 study by Maskari and Alnaqdi.[32] The researchers reported that obese people tend to have more than three times as much circulating leptin as people who are normal weight on the Body Mass Index. So the vast majority of the people we saw on the cruise had extremely high leptin levels.

On the other hand, if leptin is low, the healthy hypothalamus tells the brain you need food right away, and your metabolism slows down. This is because leptin goes down when you lose fat.[32]

If your hypothalamus was healthy, you wouldn't be hungry if you were obese, because you would have so much leptin your hunger would cease and your metabolism would be very fast. The people on that cruise would not have been hungry at all if their endocrine systems were functioning properly.

However, we have an epidemic of hypothalamic inflammation that is causing leptin not to be perceived. With this inflammation, your hypothalamus thinks your leptin is low, so it tells your brain to make you feel hunger, and it tells your metabolism to slow down.

---

[32] "Correlation between Serum Leptin Levels, Body Mass Index and Obesity in Omanis." Maskari and Alnaqdi, December 2006, *Sultan Qaboos University Medical Journal*, National Institutes of Health, https://www.ncbi.nlm.nih.gov/pmc/articles/PMC3074914/

This condition is called "leptin resistance" according to a study of studies in 2016 by Stern et al.[33] If you are obese, and you are leptin resistant, your brain thinks leptin levels are super low even though they are three times as high as normal. That makes you hungry and it slows your metabolism, which sets you up to continue gaining weight.

Thus, the huge plates of calorific foods being consumed on that cruise were the result of appetites that were out of control because of inflammation. For good health, the passengers should have been avoiding calories, but they yearned for the calories because of hormonal dysfunction.

Leptin resistance is thought to stem primarily from a) inflammation in the hypothalamus that blocks its ability to register the presence of the hormone and b) poor gut health related primarily to sugar intake. Resolving that inflammation and gut health is the first major step in the battle to resolve obesity. As the inflammation is reduced, hunger abates and the metabolism speeds up.

Resolving resistance to metabolic hormones requires a multipronged strategy including exercise, anti-inflammatory foods, probiotics, elimination of refined sugar, limitation on alcohol to one drink a day, and improvement to your sleep.

Food sensitivities can also cause inflammation that may disrupt leptin sensitivity.[34] Avoid foods that you know cause inflammation or other problems for you. For example, if you are certain that eating

[33] "Adiponectin, Leptin, and Fatty Acids in the Maintenance of Metabolic Homeostasis Through Adipose Tissue Crosstalk." Stem et al., May 10 2016, *Cell Metabolism*, National Institutes of Health, https://www.ncbi.nlm.nih.gov/pmc/articles/PMC4864949/

[34] "How to Increase Leptin Sensitivity: 5 Strategies for Easier Fat Loss", UHN Staff, April 8 2019, *University Health News Daily*, https://universityhealthnews.com/daily/nutrition/how-to-increase-leptin-sensitivity-5-strategies-for-easier-fat-loss/

wheat causes your sinuses to flare up or promotes symptoms of irritable bowel syndrome (IBS), then the wheat may be causing inflammatory responses in your body that also lead to obesity.[35] However, scientists caution that, absent symptoms such as obesity or IBS, a gluten-free diet may actually be bad for you, so do not assume you should avoid a specific nutrient just because it causes inflammation in someone else.[35]

Anti-inflammatory foods are not enough

I gave you a simple explanation of leptin resistance, so it would be easier to understand. However, it is a little more complicated, so now I will explain why resolving inflammation is not enough. Leptin signals the hypothalamus in two ways, not one. The first is the absolute level of leptin in your bloodstream, which we just discussed. Next is any recent change in that level. The second signal is actually the more powerful of the two.

The existence of this second signal means that resolving inflammation does not completely solve the problem once a person is already overweight. When you lose a little or a lot of weight, you may hit a wall before you get to your goal. That wall is hunger and cravings and a slowed metabolism.

We'll look in more detail at what creates that wall, but the simple answer is that a sudden drop in circulating serum leptin slows the metabolism and increases hunger.

Fasting will rapidly reduce leptin disproportionately to body fat, and eating a large volume of food will increase it. Whenever fasting

---

[35] "Health Benefits and Adverse Effects of a Gluten-Free Diet in Non–Celiac Disease Patients." Niland and Cash, February 2018, *Gastroenterology & Hepetology*, National Institutes of Health, https://www.ncbi.nlm.nih.gov/pmc/articles/PMC5866307/

is involved, leptin can drop sharply without regard to weight loss, thus spiking hunger and slowing the metabolism.[36]

The same is true when you lose weight by reducing the volume of food you eat. This happens *after* leptin resistance has been at least partially addressed, because otherwise the hypothalamus would not be able to sense the drop.

The inevitable sudden drop in leptin that comes from choosing to make yourself hungry for the sake of weight loss can cause weight-loss plateaus while you are still overweight or obese. Stern et al.[33] said that many studies have shown that a reduction in leptin levels causes a metabolic slowdown, fat accumulation, obesity, and lethargy.

Thus, for optimal leptin management, our objective should be to keep the circulating leptin moderately high, avoid big fluctuations, and enhance leptin sensitivity. This is another reason why meals should be eaten frequently throughout the day.

We now know that hunger is not mitigated purely by caloric intake. For example, fat does not satiate. A 2005 National Weight Control Registry study found that reducing consumption of *"high-fat-dense food groups"* and increasing consumption of *"low-fat-dense food groups"* tended to reduce caloric intake, resulting in

"greater weight loss during obesity treatment and may assist with weight loss maintenance."[37]

---

[36] "Relation between circulating leptin concentrations and appetite during a prolonged, moderate energy deficit in women." Keim et al., October 1 1998, American Society for Nutrition, *The American Journal of Clinical Nutrition*, https://academic.oup.com/ajcn/article/68/4/794/4648627

[37] "Amount of food group variety consumed in the diet and long-term weight loss maintenance." Raynor et al., May 2005, The Weight Control and Diabetes Research Center, National Institutes of Health

Accordingly, some of the goals of the Eat As Much As You Want system are to enhance leptin sensitivity, increase leptin secretion, and satiate with fewer calories.

Metabolism Management

As you may recall, the same hormones that cause satiety spur your metabolism to speed up. If your hypothalamus was healthy and it perceived 100% of a normal amount of leptin, you would not be hungry and your metabolism would be faster. The people on the cruise had enough inflammation to prevent them from perceiving 100% of normal even though they had 300% of normal.

A little improvement in leptin sensitivity could bring them up to perceiving 100%, which would still be only a third of their actual leptin. That would be enough to satisfy their appetites and spur their metabolic rates. So your goal should be to improve sensitivity as you lose weight.

When you lose weight, your leptin will drop. However, if you keep fluctuations under control by what you eat and how often, and you continue to increase sensitivity, your brain will never know the leptin dropped. Your metabolism will continue to speed up, and you won't feel hunger.

The less hunger you feel and the faster your metabolism burns compared to your caloric intake, the more quickly and easily your body will burn fat.

---

pubmed,
https://www.ncbi.nlm.nih.gov/pubmed/15919842?dopt=Abstract

Without satiety triggers

Let's suppose now that you do not use your own built-in satiety triggers. Instead, you reduce inflammation purely by eating anti-inflammatory foods and you lose weight by cutting calories or intermittent fasting. You force yourself to be hungry at various parts of the day to stay within your caloric budget or because of fasting. Leptin levels will increase when you eat, and decrease during your hunger periods.

When you follow this pattern, even if your body's average leptin perception is at 100% of normal, it may swing wildly throughout the day. Whenever it swings down substantially below 100% of normal, you will probably have an urge to binge on super unhealthy, high-caloric density foods.

The moral of the story: Eat anti-inflammatory foods *and* avoid hunger.

Plateau Revisited

When you first start on a new diet, you can estimate your caloric burn the way we discussed in Chapter 3. However, that burn rate will not stay constant past the first two to six weeks of weight loss.

When a diet causes you to be hungry, it is slowing your metabolism down. At some point, it may be so slow you cannot consume quantities of food low enough to shed any more pounds. That is called a plateau. Avoid hunger, embrace balance and frequency, and you should be able to avoid plateaus.

Make your endocrine system happy, and it will reward you. Make it unhappy, and it will return the favor by making you miserable.

Takeaways for Chapter 5

- Hunger is satisfied with fewer calories when you consume healthy foods.

- Sticking to a list of healthy foods is not sufficient. It is vital to speed your metabolism and increase satiety by having the correct balance of foods and filling up on nutrient-rich, low-Glycemic Index, low-caloric density foods.

- Leptin is a key metabolic hormone that speeds up your metabolism and suppresses your appetite.

- It is the amount of leptin that your brain is able to perceive (perceived leptin) that matters, not how much there really is.

- With leptin resistance, you can have far more than the normal amount of leptin and still be hungry with a slow metabolism, because your brain doesn't know you have a lot of leptin.

- Obese people are almost all leptin resistant and average over three times as much circulating leptin as normal weight people.

- The brains of obese people typically perceive that circulating leptin is less than in normal weight people.

- A drop in perceived leptin increases hunger and slows the metabolism.

- Many diets such as calorie counting and intermittent fasting cause wild daily fluctuations in perceived leptin.

- Chronic hunger or cravings, slowed metabolic rates, and leptin resistance are leading causes of yo-yo weight loss and plateaus.

- Ant-inflammatory and fermented foods increase leptin sensitivity.

- Satiety triggers help prevent a) sudden declines in perceived leptin, b) increases in hunger and c) decreases in metabolic rates.

- Increases to perceived leptin speed up your metabolism, and decrease your hunger.

- The more your hunger diminishes, the less food you will want to eat.

- The faster your metabolism burns relative to your caloric intake, the more quickly and easily your body will burn fat.

- The Eat As Much As You Want system increases perceived leptin as you lose weight, so your hunger stays satisfied, and your metabolism speeds up.

Chapter 6

Satiety and What Causes it

Resolving the Obesity Epidemic

Your hormones regulate both appetite and metabolism. The body would keep you at a normal weight if your endocrine system were not dysfunctional. Obesity is caused by a regulatory system unable to do its job. This chapter will focus on how to use satiety to steer your body to normal weight.

Perceived leptin and actual leptin should be the same, but leptin resistance gets in the way of that. A healthy lifestyle and healthy eating habits can restore the regulatory system to normal. The obesity epidemic has caused 42.4% of American adults to be obese as of 2017 to 2018[38] and 71.6% to be either overweight or obese as of 2015 to 2016.[39] This is up from 22.3% and 54.9% respectively as of 1988 to 1994.[38]

Contrast that with the 1950s and 1960s, when the vast majority of American adults were in the normal range. Only about 10% of adults were obese in the 1950s[40] and severe obesity was virtually unheard of. In 1960 to 1962, only 0.9% of U.S. adults were severely obese,[41]

[38] "Prevalence of Obesity and Severe Obesity Among Adults: United States, 2017–2018", Hales et al., February 2020, *NCHS Data Brief No. 360*, Centers for Disease Control and Prevention, National Center for Health Statistics, https://www.cdc.gov/nchs/products/databriefs/db360.htm
[39] "Table 21. Selected health conditions and risk factors, by age: United States, selected years 1988–1994 through 2015–2016." 2018, United States Health Trend Tables, Centers for Disease Control and Prevention, National Center for Health Statistics, https://www.ncbi.nlm.nih.gov/books/NBK551099/table/ch3.tab21/?report=objectonly
[40] "How Much Have Obesity Rates Risen Since 1950?" Sara Police, *Livestrong.com*, https://www.livestrong.com/article/384722-how-much-have-obesity-rates-risen-since-1950/
[41] "Table 2: Age-adjusted prevalence of overweight, obesity, and extreme obesity among adults aged 20–74, by sex: United States, selected years 1960–1962 through 2011–2012." Fryar et al., *Prevalence of Overweight, Obesity, and Extreme Obesity Among*

according to the CDC. By 2017 to 2018, 9.2% had reached severe obesity,[38] a staggering 10-fold increase.

The Growth of Obesity

Survey Years	Severe Obesity (% of US adults)	Obesity (% of US adults)
1960 to 1962	0.9	13.4
1971 to 1974	1.3	14.5
1976 to 1980	1.4	15.0
1988 to 1994	3.0	23.2
1999 to 2000	5.0	30.9
2001 to 2002	5.4	31.2
2003 to 2004	5.1	32.9
2005 to 2006	6.2	35.1
2007 to 2008	6.0	34.3
2009 to 2010	6.6	36.1
2011 to 2012	6.6	35.3
2013 to 2014	7.7	37.8
2015 to 2016	7.7	39.7
2017 to 2018	9.2	42.4

All numbers in the table above and graph below are percentages of the U.S. adult population as determined by the CDC.[38,39,41]

What changed was lifestyles and eating habits. We spend more time sitting than people did in the 1950s, because we have television and computers that keep us sedentary. We also eat more

Adults: United States, 1960–1962 Through 2011–2012, September 2014, Centers for Disease Control and Prevention, https://www.cdc.gov/nchs/data/hestat/obesity_adult_11_12/obesity_adult_11_12.pdf

calories than people did in the 1950s. Not only do we eat larger portions, but we consume food that has been highly processed with chemical additives designed to give the food a higher shelf life and make it more palatable. These additives are foreign to the human body and cause inflammation. Increased inflammation decreases metabolic rates and desensitizes satiety triggers. This short-circuits our genetic set points and causes our de facto weight set points to move increasingly higher.

The Growth of Obesity
(% of US Adults)

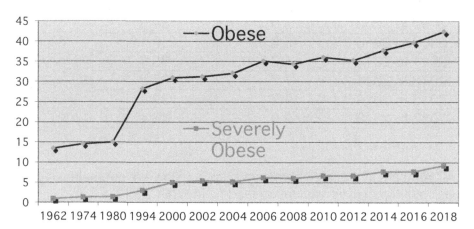

Set Point Theory

"Set point theory" is often badly misunderstood, as I will discuss, so I want to make sure you understand it fully. The theory says our bodies, given a healthy diet and a healthy lifestyle, would naturally take us to genetically pre-determined weights, or "set points." There is ample evidence that proves this is true, but it only works if we know how to help our endocrine systems.

Basic set point theory is built on four primary assertions:

1. Our bodies actively defend a specific weight by hormonal changes.

2. We will always tend to come back to our predetermined natural weight ("set point").

3. The body will cause us to be hungry and have a slow metabolism to regain weight if we go below the set point.

4. We will lack hunger and lose weight if we go above the set point.

For most of us, true genetic set points are in the "normal" range of the Body Mass Index, or BMI just as the large majority of adults in the 1950s were in the normal BMI range. BMI is a measure that has been used for over 100 years, and it is based solely on height versus weight. Its main drawback is it does not take into account musculature, bone density or skeletal size.

Don't assume that because you have been heavy for a long time your genetic set point is high. Or that because you have parents, cousins and siblings who are or were obese, your genetic set point is above normal weight. Remember, with obesity rates under 10% in the 1950s (compared with 42.4% now), it is clear that for 90% of us, if it were not for current cultural factors we would not be obese.

An exception to this rule is if you have a broad build or a lot of muscle, your BMI may say you are overweight even when you have little fat. When you reach a weight that does not include an excess amount of fat and does include healthy musculature, that may be your healthiest goal weight, rather than going purely by BMI. Nonetheless, BMI remains highly correlated with health and longevity.

The National Institutes of Health funded a BMI study of 1.5 million participants that was published in the New England Journal of Medicine on December 2, 2010. The statistics for overweight and obese individuals are startling.

> The "study looking at deaths from any cause found that... [o]verall for men and women combined, for every five unit increase in BMI, the researchers observed a 31 percent increase in risk of death."[42]

Thus, we should all want to get to our optimal weights. The Eat As Much As You Want system is all about taking you there.

Genetic versus de facto weight set points

The four primary assertions of set point theory only work if you do not have inflammation in your hypothalamus, and you do not suffer from leaky gut syndrome. These two conditions are equivalent to a thermostat in your house that does not turn on the air conditioner until your house's inside temperature reaches 210 degrees even though you have set the temperature to 70.

Leaky gut syndrome is generally associated with high sugar intake, which we'll talk more about later. Aside from obesity, some of the symptoms may include chronic diarrhea, constipation or bloating, nutritional deficiencies, fatigue, headaches, confusion,

---

[42] "NIH study identifies ideal body mass index; Overweight and obesity associated with increased risk of death." December 1 2010, National Institutes of Health, *News Releases*, https://www.nih.gov/news-events/news-releases/nih-study-identifies-ideal-body-mass-index

difficulty concentrating, skin problems (acne, rashes or eczema), and joint pain.

If you are seriously overweight or obese, and you still experience chronic hunger and urges to eat calorically dense foods, then the probability is very high that you have inflammation in your hypothalamus. Leptin levels tend to rise as your body fat increases, so this should reduce hunger and chronic food urges unless your hypothalamus is unable to perceive the leptin increases due to inflammation.

Getting to your true genetic weight set point

What we have today is weight set points gone haywire. When your perceived leptin is lower than your actual leptin, your weight set points increase. If you are obese, it may take more than three times as much leptin as normal for your brain to register that you have had enough to eat. If your brain cannot perceive 100% of normal leptin levels, then you will remain hungry, and your metabolism will remain slow. If your leptin resistance progressively grows worse, your leptin levels may need to be four times or more the normal amounts before your hunger is satisfied, which means you would be eating your way to morbid obesity.

The average adult weight is far above normal BMI now because leptin resistance and lifestyle choices have driven up our de facto weight set points. The typical American on a diet still eats saturated fats, refined sugars, bleached flours, and processed foods. Intermittent fasters and calorie counters frequently choose such food. Meal delivery diet plan systems often include highly processed foods with lots of chemical additives. These choices support the inflammation and gut dysfunction to guarantee a return to obesity.

The result of poor diet and inadequate exercise is that our de facto set points keep getting pushed increasingly higher, and our bodies vigorously defend these ever-higher set points regardless of our true genetic weight set points. The outrageous appetites of some of the cruise ship passengers would not have been possible if their de facto set points had not been pushed so high.

The Eat As Much As You Want system is the antidote to this obesity syndrome; it helps us to realign our de facto set points with our genetic ones.

By the way, even if you look back at pictures of ancestors from the 1950s or before, and they were overweight, consider whether they had healthy or unhealthy lifestyles. Just as now there are many people who have inappropriate eating habits, there were people in the 1940s and 1950s with unhealthy eating habits and life styles.

There were not as many unhealthy options then, and it was not as easy to find a sedentary job, but such lifestyles did exist. Did they eat lots of pasta and sweets, for example? Did their jobs require a lot of sitting? Many of the under 10% who were obese back then may have been able to lose the extra weight if they had known about the principles shared in this book.

Steering your set points to take you to normal weight

Once you understand set point theory and become skilled at steering your set points, you can get to a normal weight without hunger and without a plateau. And you can stay there, because the hunger will not return. Your repaired endocrine system will do the heavy lifting.

Set point theory operates the same whether or not you have a healthy endocrine system, such as our predecessors had in the 1950s. The only difference is that if your endocrine system becomes dysfunctional, your set points go up, which leads to obesity. To understand the theory in the context of the obesity epidemic, we need to update it based on new factors. Failure to address these new factors is what has pushed obesity rates ever higher since that decade. When we address these three factors, we can bring our set points back down to normal weights:

- Perceived, not actual, hormonal levels determine set points.

- Set points rely on satiety as their guide.

- Satiety is determined by many factors, not just calories.

Satiety vs. Perceived Hormonal Levels

Metabolic hormones spur your metabolism to be faster. That includes Leptin, of course, but also some others such as ghrelin, insulin, testosterone, estrogen, and human growth hormone. However, if the hormone detectors in your body are clogged up by inflammation, there is dysfunction that leads to a slowed metabolism and storage of fat.

When metabolic hormones can only be partially perceived by your body's detectors, the stimulation that the hormones are supposed to give becomes similarly partial. Thus, in the case of leptin, your metabolism slows and your hunger increases when the leptin cannot be fully detected.

The natural systems that your ancestors' bodies used to keep their weight normal are not fully available to anyone whose detectors are inflamed due to consuming processed foods, sitting more than they did, and various other lifestyle habits we of this generation typically follow. Only if we improve the sensitivity of our metabolic hormone detectors can our bodies begin to regulate naturally toward a more normal weight.

Set points rely on satiety as their guide

Self-regulatory systems within the body are built around internal signaling that you have or have not had enough to eat. Getting enough to eat of the right nutrients in the right volume should increase leptin, which should create a signal of satiety to the brain.

If the brain falsely perceives leptin levels as too low (as with the cruise ship passengers), that translates to hunger and also to a slowed metabolism. If inflammation distorts the brain's perception, and the hypothalamus only sees a small portion of the leptin, then the brain will slow your metabolism down and make you feel hungry even though your fat is accumulating to higher and higher levels.

Satiety Not Just from Calories

Many people believe that greater volume of food equals more calories and greater satiety. This is untrue. A cup of oil is obviously far more calories than two cups of raw spinach, for example.

Satiety is achieved not by calories alone but by a combination of factors including achieving fullness, chewing, hydration, the avoidance of highly processed foods, and reaching instinctive targets for low-GI carbohydrates and proteins. Fat, salt, and refined sugar does not satiate. Instead, these foods enhance palatability, which encourages excessive caloric consumption. When people binge, it is because an instinctive switch has been flipped in their brains, and they automatically gravitate toward high-caloric density, highly-palatable foods such as chips, junk food, cakes, ice cream, breads, potatoes, and pizza, and they eat far more calories than they burn. That leads to excessive weight gain, more inflammation, and reinforcement of leptin resistance. This becomes a vicious cycle.

Hunger or the lack thereof is the primary way that your endocrine system is wired to control your weight. Knowing this, you can learn

Jim Frith

to steer your endocrine system to direct your body to lose weight down to a normal weight without you being hungry. This is done by a) enhancing leptin sensitivity by reducing inflammation, b) utilizing satiety triggers, to reduce fluctuations in leptin, and c) boosting metabolic rates through a combination of healthy nutrition, exercise, and hunger avoidance. All of this works together strategically to sustainably keep your hunger satisfied, speed your metabolism, and reduce your desire to consume additional calories. I will teach you how to accomplish all of these objectives.

Perils of a "Set Point Journey"

There is a small but growing group of people who talk about their set point journeys. If you are overweight or obese, I urge you not to follow their example. They are not following a sensible path on Set Point Theory.

More famous fans of the set point journey concept have typically started out as people who have obsessively lost weight to the point of becoming emaciated. They have looked at the Minnesota starvation study and have concluded that bingeing is their way out of starvation mode.

Specifically, there were men in the Minnesota starvation study in starvation mode who were allowed to binge and gain weight tremendously. After extreme weight gain, they finally settled down to normal eating. Over the course of the year that followed the end of that weight gain, they lost much of the excess fat again. They had beaten starvation mode, and their appetites reduced enough to take them back to just a little heavier than when they started the experiment.[43]

---

[43] "Is there evidence for a set point that regulates human body weight?" Müller et al., August 9 2010, *F1000 Reports|Medicine,*

This last fact is the part that set point journey fans say is the cure for starvation mode. They argue that weight should be controlled through use of the set point, but their dietary approach is extraordinarily flawed. They advocate that if you have lost weight to the point of going into starvation mode, you should eat ad libitum (or even binge) for a period of months until you no longer feel like eating, because you will have gained so much weight. At that point, they argue that you should shift to a healthy diet and continue to eat your fill, but that you will naturally lose weight down to your set point.

However, there are serious problems with this:

- It ignores that foods available for bingeing today are different from those available in the 1940s to the men in the Minnesota experiment.

- It ignores that bingeing on highly processed foods – today's typical binge foods of choice -- can and probably will lead to leptin resistance.

- It assumes that everyone in starvation mode is severely underweight. The truth is that many people with leptin resistance are still overweight or obese when they hit starvation mode.

- Breaking plateaus and starvation mode can be achieved through healthy eating. If someone truly needs to gain weight, consuming greater quantities of healthy Countables along with smaller proportions of Must Haves (anti-inflammatory foods) can cause weight gain without creating leptin resistance.

- Binge eating causes fat gain with little muscle gain. Healthy increases in weight should be done slowly, allowing for

National Institutes of Health,
https://www.ncbi.nlm.nih.gov/pmc/articles/PMC2990627/

muscle growth and minimizing the risk of triggering metabolic syndrome (i.e. diabetes, obesity, high cholesterol, and high blood pressure).

- If a person starts out underweight, weight gain can be stopped with no hunger at normal weight using appropriate satiety cues. There is no good reason to overshoot normal weight by ongoing bingeing. Wild weight fluctuations are unhealthy.

Bingeing is not the answer

Chronic dieters often binge, then immediately return to starving themselves to try to lose weight. Set point journey fans correctly note this binge and starve pattern only serves to reinforce starvation mode. I could not agree more.

However, set point journey fans use this rationale as a justification for continuous binge eating over a long period of time, which is very unhealthy. Major weight fluctuation up and down is hard on the body in a number of ways, especially if you have a heart condition. [44]

Also, if you are overweight or obese, any weight gained is a challenge to lose if you do not take the correct approach. It is far healthier and easier to get where you want to go if you break starvation mode without gaining weight above normal. That should be common sense. That is the way we do it with the Eat As Much As You Want system.

Conversely, repeatedly going into starvation mode in a binge, starve, binge, starve cycle only serves to increase the urge to binge

---

[44] "Body-Weight Fluctuations and Outcomes in Coronary Disease." Bangalore et al., April 6 2017, *The New England Journal of Medicine*, https://www.nejm.org/doi/full/10.1056/NEJMoa1606148

the next time and to slow down the metabolism even more. Losing weight can become increasingly difficult every time you yo-yo. Even if you manage to lose the weight each time, it becomes harder and harder to keep the weight off. This becomes a downward spiral into the abyss of non-sustainability, and the highest weight you reach in each yo-yo weight cycle tends to get heavier and heavier.

Years ago, I ran frequent weight-loss contests in an effort to encourage and teach my clients. Points were awarded based on hitting a weekly target loss of 0.5 to 2% of bodyweight. Any loss greater than 2% of the prior week's weight gained no points. Additional points were awarded based on percentage of inches lost over the course of the contest. My intent was to make a game of the weight loss process so that clients would establish good habits and learn how to lose weight naturally and sustainably. I feel good that I helped a lot of people.

Unfortunately, not everyone adopted the spirit of learning about healthy weight loss. One year, a team of obese women did well in one particular contest ending in November, but they were nowhere near their final goals by the end. These were women who thought they "knew what to do", and they did not follow my advice on weight loss. Meanwhile, they were intensely competitive and got caught up in an unbridled desire to win. So they forced themselves to be hungry.

One of them constantly talked about inappropriate foods such as cakes and desserts that she yearned to eat. Yet they leaned on each other to keep their motivation up to do well in that first contest. They did not win it, but they did place.

Their unwillingness to accept guidance and their disregard for healthy habits took me completely by surprise. Their competitiveness at the expense of good health was illogical to me. I had intentionally set the prize money to be much less than they were paying to participate, so their motivation was not money.

Jim Frith

After the end of that first contest, still reeling from the food fantasies that had emerged during their self-imposed hunger period, they got together and decided it would be easier to lose weight the next time if they gained a lot of weight in the two months before the next contest. Their theory: Recently gained weight would be easy to lose. This twisted rationale gave them permission in their own minds to go crazy on eating during the holidays. Hunger and food fantasies definitely cloud judgment.

In a two-month period, these four women each gained between 20 and 25 pounds by continuously bingeing on junk food, holiday feasts, and holiday treats. When they joined the next contest, they had acquired horrible eating habits, and had no less appetite than when the previous contest had ended. Instead of easily winning the next contest as they had envisioned, they struggled terribly and were among the poorest performers in the competition.

To this day, I remain flabbergasted that *anyone* would approach my contests the way they did. Yet, based on things they told me along the way, they truly believed that bingeing for a couple of months would make it easier to reach their ultimate weight goals. Like the Set Point Journeyers, they had concluded that they would overcome their food fantasies and let go of weight faster if they first went through a long period of continuous bingeing.

The new contest started in January and ended in April. Come April, none of them had yet returned to their ending weights from the previous contest.

Their struggles continued. The one who had been most vocal about food fantasies went back to bingeing and reached a new personal record on her weight. Her teammates tried, but even a year later none of them lost all of the weight they had gained.

My point in telling you about this is that recently gained weight is no easier to lose than weight you have had for a long time. Binge eating is self-destructive, and it can cause inflammation of your endocrine system that is difficult to undo, especially if you do not follow my system.

I don't push. I offer my knowledge and experience to those who will listen. But I allowed these women to continue as fitness clients and to participate in the contests on their own terms despite their lack of interest in being guided. After that contest, I changed eligibility rules for later contests so no one could join who weighed more than their end weight from a previous contest.

I did this because I did not want contestants who had the wrong motivations for joining, and I did not want misguided yo-yo weight loss to be a temptation to anyone. The point is to learn good habits and sustain the losses.

If you are overweight or obese, I strongly recommend against weight gain to get out of starvation mode. I have ample experience working with clients who were able to end hunger and weight-loss plateaus by eating the right way, using satiety triggers, and establishing the right habits. This has led to continued weight loss time and again. By understanding and implementing what truly creates satiety, we can move the body out of starvation mode and directly back into weight loss.

Menopause and Perimenopause

"I have no willpower against hunger," said the woman on the phone four months ago. "But I want to lose weight."

"I can help you with that," I replied.

"A friend told me you have a system that doesn't require me to be hungry. I haven't been able to keep weight off for decades now, because I hate being hungry all the time."

"Your friend told you right."

"But I'm 69 years old, and I've been in menopause for a long time now. So my metabolism is shot."

"No problem," I assured her. "The system has worked for lots of women in menopause. In fact, it works extremely well."

She lives locally, so she made an appointment and came to see me.

"You're a genius!" she exclaimed two weeks later. "I've lost five pounds already, and I'm never hungry. My only challenge is I'm not used to eating as much food as you want me to eat. But I'm doing it, and it's working."

In July, a couple months later, she sent the following email:

"Still doing well on my diet and am down 25 pounds. The daily log really helps me see my pattern. I tend to bounce up and down for two or three weeks and then I'll drop as much as a pound in a very short time, then the pattern starts again. I don't care how my body works as long as I continue to lose weight. It's coming off slowly in my mind but in a healthy way, whether I like it or not. I think 25 pounds in 3 months is pretty significant. I hope by November I may have doubled that. See you on Monday!!"

She lost another four pounds in one month since that email despite falling off substantially on exercise.

"I lost another four pounds in the last month," she said in her latest email. "29lbs down now, but I know I'm not exercising enough." She fell off on exercise quite a lot since the first email. "I'm lazy, I guess."

"Good job on sticking with the nutrition part of the system and on logging," I praised. "Do try to pick up on exercise, though. It will pay you big dividends and make continued weight loss much easier."

This is real world, and we don't always do the things we know we should, but the system is very resilient. She is still amazed that this is working without hunger despite the fact that she is in menopause. Willpower is much more achievable when you are never hungry.

"Feeling very good," she said at the end of the latest email. "Thanks for checking in. I know you're right about exercise. I'll pick up my pace."

For women, hormonal swings associated with menopause and perimenopause are strategically addressed in the Eat As Much As You Want system. The decline of estrogen is especially impactful, because it can lead to a slowing of the metabolism, a reduction in protections against joint pain and other pains all over the body, diminishment of sexual function, depression, loss of bone mass, loss of muscle mass, and increasing LDL cholesterol.

Hormonal swings typically associated with perimenopause and menopause are ameliorated by enhancing hormone signaling, improving satiety, and boosting the metabolism. A balanced, healthy low-caloric density diet rich in fiber and bone health minerals such as calcium help to keep LDL cholesterol at healthy levels. Adequate protein is important too, along with appropriate exercise for the preservation of muscle tissue. Anti-inflammatory foods are especially important in reducing joint pain and other widespread body pains. Exercise, omega 3 fatty acids, healthy sleep strategies, and the avoidance of starvation mode during weight loss are vital components in the battles to reduce or avoid depression and potential loss of sexual desire.

Hot flashes are impacted by frequency of meals and by steadiness of blood sugar. Having more frequent meals with emphasis on low-GI foods that will sustain steadier blood glucose levels between meals is consistent with research findings on how to reduce the frequency of hot flashes (HF):

> *"HF frequency increased as length of time between meals increased (r = .242, p = .05). As time from last food intake increased, the number of HF experienced also increased... menopausal HFs were most often observed when blood glucose was lower..."*[45]

Depression associated with perimenopause and menopause is made worse by refined sugar consumption[46]. Kicking a sugar addiction is an important step toward achieving a sense of wellbeing.

Bone density loss associated with perimenopause and menopause is made worse by consumption of processed foods[47].

In short, following the Eat As Much As You Want system helps reduce the symptoms and side effects of perimenopause and menopause.

---

[45] "The Effect of Dietary Intake on Hot Flashes in Menopausal Women." Dormire and Howharn, October 22 2009, *Journal of Obstetric, Gynocologic & Neonatal Nursing*, National Institutes of Health, https://www.ncbi.nlm.nih.gov/pmc/articles/PMC2765999/
[46] "High glycemic index diet as a risk factor for depression: analyses From the Women's Health Initiative." Gangwisch et al., June 24 2015, *Journal of Clinical Nutrition*, National Institutes of Health pubmed, https://pubmed.ncbi.nlm.nih.gov/26109579/
[47] "Dietary patterns, bone resorption and bone mineral density in early post-menopausal Scottish women", Hardcastle et al., March 2011, *European Journal of Clinical Nutrition*, National Institutes of Health pubmed, https://pubmed.ncbi.nlm.nih.gov/21179049/

Satiety and Metabolic Rate Triggers

To put the next bit of research into perspective, remember that we have already learned that leptin not only reduces appetite, but it also speeds up the metabolic rate. Ghrelin, on the other hand, increases appetite and slows down the metabolic rate. So we should strive to have our bodies increase leptin, decrease leptin resistance, and decrease ghrelin.

A full stomach can speed your metabolism

A 2006 review of various studies by Klok et al.[48] indicated that the stomach immediately responds to food intake by releasing appetite suppressant and metabolic enhancement hormones. The study's authors said up until that time, leptin had been thought to only be a long-term player in metabolism and hunger, fluctuating with the amount of fat in the body. However, more recent findings pointed to leptin also being released by the stomach in response to meal size.

Klok et al.[48] also cite ghrelin as primarily a hormone released by the stomach in response to how empty it is. Ghrelin levels go up before a meal and down as your stomach fills up. Ghrelin stimulates appetite, so it makes you hungry when your stomach is empty. A high volume of food intake (meal size) causes satiety, because ghrelin goes down and leptin goes up when the stomach is full.

Klok et al.[48] go on to state that changes in leptin levels happen much faster in response to hunger (fasting) than would be indicated by the change in the amount of fat in a person's body. They

---

[48] "The role of leptin and ghrelin in the regulation of food intake and body weight in humans: a review." Klok et al., August 24 2006, *Obesity Reviews*, World Obesity, Wiley Online Library, https://onlinelibrary.wiley.com/doi/full/10.1111/j.1467-789X.2006.00270.x

conclude that it is the body's perception of starving due to an extended period of insufficient food that initiates the hormonal change, not solely the amount of fat the person is carrying.

This study shows that weight gain or loss and number of calories consumed are not accurate measures of the changes in leptin. Instead, hunger is a very strong indication that leptin has dropped, which means your metabolism has slowed. Fortunately, we can help keep this from happening by eating sufficient volume in meals to trigger the stomach to reduce ghrelin and secrete leptin.

Chewing adds to the sense of satiety

For the past few decades, there has been a great amount of hype around juicing and smoothies and meal replacement shakes. There are three big problems with this way of getting your nutrients.

First, juicing often reduces the quantity of pulp and fiber that you get out of the ingredients. Pulp and fiber are important for satiety and weight loss because they help a) fill you up, b) slow down the digestive process and c) keep you satisfied for longer.

Second, juicing typically reduces volume. Whole fruits and vegetables, for example are reduced to a fraction of their original volume when they are juiced. We now know that volume is a big part of satiety.

Third, juicing, smoothies and meal replacement shakes do not require any chewing. Numerous studies have shown that chewing is vital to maximize satiety. In 2015, a review of numerous scientific studies concluded there is *"a significant effect of chewing on satiation or satiety using self-report measures"*, and *"chewing reduced food intake"*, and *"increasing the number of chews per bite increased relevant gut hormones"*, which in turn enhanced satiety.[49]

To enhance satiety, these studies show that most of our food intake should be from whole foods that require chewing. Heavy reliance on smoothies, juices or meal replacement shakes is likely to lead to greater hunger and its accompanying metabolic slowdowns.

Optimize health

Do not limit your eating to super low-caloric density foods. That would not be a balanced diet. A balanced diet is necessary for optimal health.

Your body carries on a great many functions all the time. It is manufacturing blood cells, fighting diseases, healing lean tissues, building muscle, digesting foods, circulating blood, thinking, breathing, filtering impurities, creating hormones, restoring muscle energy, burning muscle energy, and too many other tasks to list here.

To have a fast-burning metabolism, you must adequately provide for all of your body's needs. Unless you give the body what it needs nutritionally, it will not be able to do all of these tasks efficiently. Unless you stress your body through exercise, and rest your body through sleep, many of these functions will not happen, or they will happen less optimally. When the body's functions are disrupted, your metabolism slows down.

This does not mean you have to provide your body with an excessive number of calories. Calories are purely contained in four

---

[49] "Effects of chewing on appetite, food intake and gut hormones: A systematic review and meta-analysis." Miquel Kergoat et al., November, 2015, *Physiology & Behavior*, National Institutes of Health pubmed, https://www.ncbi.nlm.nih.gov/pubmed/26188140

macronutrients: carbohydrates, proteins, fats, and alcohol. Unless you are consuming one of those four, you are not getting calories. Each macronutrient plays a unique role, as will be discussed in detail later. Balance is vital.

Many nutrients do not have calories, but they serve as catalysts for the critical chemical reactions that keep your body healthy. These include micronutrients (vitamins and minerals), and phytonutrients (nutrients from plants.) There are over 25,000 phytonutrients, so you should be eating a wide variety of foods from plants to get the nutrients that will help optimize health.

Keep your metabolism burning as strongly as your genetics allow

All of us have different genes. It is undeniable that our genetics wield a large influence over how fast we burn calories. And it is also clear that if we do not get the nutrients our bodies need, or if we introduce inflammation, then our metabolism will slow down.

Think back to that fake volcano I built when I was a kid. How many calories do you suppose were in the vinegar and baking soda that created that big reaction? The answer: Almost none. Baking soda has essentially no calories, and vinegar has very few. So imagine how many processes are taking place in your body that are using calories which are supported by nutrients that have no calories. It is vital that you give the body what it needs!

Most of the time, our hormones dictate how the calories we consume are used. Are the calories used rapidly, or are they placed in fat reserves for when they may be needed later? This is partly dependent on whether your body is in a normal state or in starvation mode. Make it a priority to break or avoid starvation mode.

The research and my own experience working with clients have clearly demonstrated an undeniable fact: Healthy, appropriately balanced consumption of high-quality foods, coupled with healthy lifestyle habits, works to bring the de facto weight set point in line with the genetic set point to create weight loss that stays gone.

Takeaways for Chapter 6

- **Everyone has a weight set point that the body will defend.**

- **The defenses of your weight set point are satiety and a faster metabolism when you are above your set point or hunger and a slower metabolism when you are below it.**

- **Absent leptin resistance, the vast majority of people have weight set points in the normal range according to the BMI.**

- **Leptin resistance pushes your weight set point artificially higher, often to obesity and beyond.**

- **Eating the right way and exercising can lower your weight set point back to normal weight.**

- **Sudden drops in perceived leptin will make you hungry and slow your metabolism.**

- **When your weight set point is in the normal range, and perceived leptin is held steady, you will not be hungry, and your metabolism will remain faster.**

- **Bingeing is never a good way to manage weight.**

- **Satiety triggers and healthy nutrition break weight-loss plateaus.**

- The Eat As Much As You Want system aids with symptoms and side effects of menopause and perimenopause, and it is effective for weight loss in menopausal and perimenopausal women.

- Chewing your food and filling your stomach with low-caloric density foods boosts satiety and metabolic rate.

- Complete nutrition with the right balance of low-Glycemic Index carbs, protein, low-caloric density foods, and a broad spectrum of micronutrients and phytonutrients will speed up your metabolism and enhance satiety to move you toward your normal weight set point.

Chapter 7

Move

Sitting is the New Smoking

Too much sitting causes muscle loss, fat gain and poor health. Whatever you do, find a way to get up frequently.

Exercise can be fun. Seriously. Choose activities you like. Sample different activities until you find some you enjoy. Becoming active will make you stronger and healthier and happier, even though you may not think so at first. You mainly need to get in the habit of exercise and make it a regular part of your life for it to work for you. You will live much longer and have a far higher quality of life if you exercise regularly.

Remember that whether or not you count calories, the only way to lose weight is to burn more than you consume. There is no magic to this, only science. Your health and strength will diminish and your metabolism will slow down if you do not exercise. That is a given.

Eat to feel satiated, end starvation mode, and give your body the healthy nutrition it needs. And exercise. Only with exercise will you retain your muscle mass and push the calories you burn to a higher number than the calories you consume.

It's not necessary to start out with a lot of exercise, but an immediate shift is needed from little or none to some. Once you get started, you can build from there.

Self-regulation only works if you are active

With adequate exercise, if you eat the right way, then your body will tell you when you have had enough to eat. Eating a balanced diet with plenty of low-caloric density, low-Glycemic Load, nutrient-rich foods will empower your body's hormones to give you a faster metabolism and avoid hunger. My goal is to continue to equip your body to regulate itself successfully toward being healthier and more slender.

When you get up and move, that does more than just burn calories. You also will feel more invigorated and awake throughout the day if you are exercising regularly. This makes you more alert and productive, and increases your metabolic rate.

However, if you sit all day and make no effort to get up and move around, then you are far more likely to become or remain obese and to suffer from metabolism-related chronic diseases, according to numerous studies. For example, in a 2013 study[50] of 63,048 Australian males age 45 to 65, the conclusions were as follows:

> "[E]ven when age was held constant, ... [i]ndependent of physical activity, BMI, and additional covariates, sitting time was significantly associated with diabetes and overall chronic disease..."

On the other hand if you exercise regularly, not only are you much more likely to have a high-quality life, you are also much more likely to live a long life. A 2015 study looked at 661,137 people from ages 21 to 98 with a median age of 62. Those who did the minimum recommended amount of exercise 75 vigorous-intensity or 150 moderate-intensity minutes per week were 31% more likely to be alive 14.2 years later.[51] People who did three times that amount were 39% more likely to be alive.

---

[50] "Chronic disease and sitting time in middle-aged Australian males: findings from the 45 and Up Study." George et al., February 8 2013, *International Journal of Behavioral Nutrition and Physical Activity*, National Institutes of Health,
https://www.ncbi.nlm.nih.gov/pmc/articles/PMC3571940/
[51] "Leisure time physical activity and mortality: a detailed pooled analysis of the dose-response relationship", Arem et al., June 2015, *Journal of the American Medical Association Internal Medicine*, National Institutes of Health pubmed,
https://pubmed.ncbi.nlm.nih.gov/25844730/

Start Slowly

To tip the scale in favor of better health and burning more calories than you consume, you must exercise regularly. I am not asking you to do crazy amounts of exercise like they did in public weight-loss contests such as "The Biggest Loser." That is not sustainable. But I am asking you to be mindful of moving as much as you can *every day.*

Start out slowly in any exercise plan you choose. You do not have to push yourself extremely hard, especially at first. Len Kravitz, Ph.D., a professor and exercise scientist at the University of New Mexico, says that getting up from your seat and moving around for three minutes during every 30 minutes of otherwise continuous sitting can easily burn from 300 to 400 additional calories per day. 350 extra calories burned per day, five days a week, can potentially translate into burning one-half pound of extra fat each week.

What kind of movement you do during these three-minute periods is up to you. It should be something that works for you, whether it be taking a brisk walk, doing squats, or just shifting back and forth from one foot to another or generally fidgeting while standing up. Dr. Kravitz says "Brisk is better," and he encourages all of us to walk faster. The key is to get up and move around anytime you can.

When I started exercising regularly

In my mid-thirties, I was terribly out of shape. It would not be until several years later that I started regularly working out my entire body. Really, I did not yet understand what harm would befall my body if I did not start exercising soon. I only knew that my job was very stressful, I felt tense a lot of the time, and I easily got out of breath if I did anything active.

One Saturday afternoon, a friend showed up at my apartment door dressed in Spandex®.

"Why are you all dressed in Spandex®?" I asked her, puzzled.

Keep in mind, she was a woman of larger proportions, and I did not imagine her to be athletic, so her outfit was all the more mysterious.

"I ran here," she replied.

"You ran here?!" I was perplexed. "How far?

"Five miles."

"Five miles?! I can't run five miles. How do you even do that?"

My reaction may seem strange to you, but my world was truly rocked. Suddenly, I realized how far gone my own fitness had become. This seemingly out-of-shape woman could do what I did not see myself capable of doing.

"Just run slowly," she advised. "Work your way up to five miles, then begin to pick up your pace."

I was challenged. The next day, I went running – very slowly – and I found that I was able to last for five miles. It was hard, but I did it. More importantly, I physically felt the stress melt away as I ran. I was hooked! Over time, following her advice, I was able to pick up the pace.

This changed my life. It led me much later to a career in fitness. But it also taught me that wherever you are in your life with respect to fitness, you can improve it by easing into exercise slowly. For me, it was five miles, but it will be different for everyone.

I have advised many clients to start out much more slowly, depending on their level of health and fitness. For example, I would not have been able to finish anywhere near that first five miles if I had been obese at the time. Yes, I was overweight. But we all can make strides forward from wherever we are. Maybe you start by walking around the block, then build from there.

Find the challenge level you can manage, then work your way up. Your body will thank you. Mine did.

Baby Steps

Once you have implemented some added movement such as Dr. Kravitz recommends, and you are comfortable with this new habit of movement, you may decide that you are ready to take it to the next level.

The average participant in the National Weight Control Registry gets about an hour a day of exercise (including walking) seven days a week. Remember, all of these folks have lost large amounts of weight and kept it off for a long time. Their average loss is 66 pounds that has stayed off for 5 ½ years.[52]

Don't feel like you have to rush to get to their level too quickly. You might start with 15 or 20 minutes of walking a day. After a few weeks of that, maybe you can join a gym and go there once or twice a week. Baby steps are fine in improving the amount of movement you do. Pat yourself on the back every time you move more than you used to.

Fit the workouts into your schedule, and enter them into your calendar. Treat them the same way you would a doctor's

---

[52] "NWCR Facts." The National Weight Control Registry, http://www.nwcr.ws/Research/default.htm

appointment or a work-related appointment. Make sure you do them no matter what, even when you are traveling.

There is no specific timeline for getting to seven hours a week. It might take you six, 12 or even 24 months to get there. However long it may take you is completely up to you. Set seven hours a week as the goal you will eventually reach, and give yourself a timeline you are comfortable with to get there. This is life changing, so just keep moving forward toward your goal of a better life.

What does seven hours a week look like?

First, remember that you do not have to start doing seven hours a week immediately. This is a *future* goal. Part of their seven hours average weekly total is three hours a week of challenging exercise. If you are getting less exercise than this, then try to gradually increase what you are currently doing.

Seven hours a week of exercise seems like a huge amount, but it isn't as difficult as it sounds. Let's break it down. Walk briskly for 15 minutes every morning, then 15 minutes again every evening. Then, twice a day, walk for five minutes. This could be on your lunch break and during a coffee break. That adds up to 40 minutes a day, which is four hours and 40 minutes a week. If you miss some of the walking on some days, that is fine, because all you really need is four hours. If you miss the 15 minutes in the morning, walk for 30 in the evening.

Next, find some online exercise videos, or join a tennis club or a gym, or buy a bike or take up jogging. Whatever type of challenging exercise you settle on, work your way up to doing it three times a week for an hour each time. What is challenging is subjective -- if it feels challenging to you, then it is challenging. As time goes by, and you become more fit, you will be able to work harder during your workouts in order to feel challenged.

Between the 40 minutes a day of total walking and three hours a week of challenging exercise, you will reach your goal of seven hours a week, even if you miss one whole day of walking.

"I don't have time for all that!"

I have heard this protest too many times to count. If you decide not to make the time, you will not be alone. The vast majority of American adults do not get enough exercise. However, you will live a lot longer and have a tremendously higher quality of life if you make exercise a priority.

Many people I've known have put other priorities ahead of exercise, and they have aged far faster than they could have imagined. I am 63, and I feel younger than most 50-year-olds and can do more than a many 25-year-olds. I tell you this as a way of relating that every minute I have put into exercise has given me countless extra minutes of quality life.

Lots of people use work as their excuse for skipping exercise. They say they are too busy. In truth, advancement and productivity and mental acuity are higher when you have been regularly exercising, so you are more likely to do well financially if you exercise regularly.

Along the same lines, exercise is a great stress reliever. Does it really make sense to put all of your energy into earning money so you can build up a retirement nest egg if by the time you retire you are going to be too unhealthy to enjoy it? The best retirement investment you will ever make is the time you spend exercising.

Make It Fun

Don't get caught up in thinking there is some specific type of exercise you have to do even if you are not comfortable with it. Find something you can stick with. It could be a group fitness class like aerobics or Zumba®, or it could be swimming or jogging or weight lifting or bicycling or tennis or pickleball or any number of other kinds of exercise. You can even do vigorous gardening, brisk shopping mall walking (with breaks to look at stuff you are interested in), dancing, sightseeing, museum touring, apple picking (in season), festival going and any other fun activity you can think of to keep you on your feet and moving.

Fun is the key. There is even a trend now in the fitness industry to incorporate games and fun into small group fitness classes. For the past several years, high intensity interval training (HIIT) has gained enormously in popularity. Many studies have shown it to be highly effective in enhancing fitness levels and burning calories more quickly than continuous aerobic exercise. Consistency is the key to success here so pick an exercise program or method you enjoy enough to keep doing.

If you know of a small-group training program near you, and you are interested in joining in, find out if they do HIIT and if they play any games or do fun activities within the workouts. Fun and games build much greater enthusiasm for returning time and again to exercise. Heart rates and exertion levels tend to be higher during the games than at any other part of the workouts. The competitions may only comprise a small portion of each workout, but they spur laughter, camaraderie and conversation in the midst of a challenging workout. Fun is definitely here to stay as a part of sustainable exercise strategies.

Exactly what your workout looks like at first is not nearly as important as the fact that you are exercising. You choose. Doing any specific type of exercise is not vital when you are just getting started.

The key is to do something that you feel good about and will continue doing.

Your main goal should be to establish a habit of exercise. For it to be a habit, it should be something you like doing. Exercise is an acquired taste, so do not rush to judgment, but do look for something that you think you will like.

Go easy at first

I recommend that you go very easy with your workouts the first few weeks and gradually build the intensity. Your goal should be to feel as good when you finish as when you started. Your fitness progresses during recovery from the workouts, not during the workouts themselves, so make sure that you do not push yourself so hard that your body is too sore to do the next workout.

One or two workouts will not make you fit or healthy. It is the habit of exercise that will carry you to your goals. So when you reach your goal of doing three challenging workouts a week, make it a priority to do them every week even if you feel the need to lower your challenge level sometimes. Doing the exercise faithfully and regularly is FAR more important than pushing the limits of how hard you can workout.

Workout Recovery

As you begin to do challenging workouts, you may find that you are sore after a workout. There are ways to alleviate that.

The soreness from a workout is called "delayed onset muscle soreness" because it usually does not set in until a day or two after your workout. It comes from lactic acid and other natural chemicals that seep out of your muscle cells after you exercise. Because you are exercising harder than you have in a very long time, your vascular system is not used to carrying away and processing lactic acid in such volume all at once. So the lactic acid stays around the muscle tissues too long and irritates them.

Over a period of weeks, you will grow more capillaries and improve the blood flow to your muscles, but at first you should take precautions to minimize the soreness and speed recovery. The faster you recover between workouts, the better and stronger you will feel.

Here are some things you can do to speed recovery and minimize soreness:

1. Stretch immediately following the workout.

Your muscles are most malleable when your body temperature is elevated and you have been using them, so the perfect time to stretch is right when you finish the workout. This not only improves range of motion, but it opens the cell walls and allows for better nutrient exchange and more rapid movement of lactic acid away from the muscle tissues and into the bloodstream. From there, it will go to the liver to be re-processed.

2. Walk or stand for at least 15 minutes right after you stretch.

If walking is not practical, try to remain standing. Resist the temptation to sit immediately after your workout, because that slows circulation and traps the lactic acid locally. Walking improves circulation and allows the body to do a better job of moving the lactic acid out of the local area.

3. Eat a meal within 30 minutes after your workout.

That magic 30-minute window is when you can eat and accelerate recovery by efficiently providing glucose and amino acids to the muscle cells while they are most receptive to absorbing them. Unless you are insulin resistant, consume a *very* small amount of healthy high-Glycemic Index carbohydrates with the meal, such as mango, watermelon or pineapple. You can even eat these while on your walk!

By the way, don't confuse eating whole natural high-GI carbs with taking in sugary "sports" supplements. Such supplements are super calorically dense, lacking in natural nutrients, and the epitome of highly processed foods. Remember that sugar and processed foods are a huge source of inflammation. Think *anti*-inflammation!

4. Rub your muscles a couple of hours after the workout and just before bed.

Don't wait until the next day when the muscles are already sore. Do it soon enough to get the lactic acid out of there before the muscles become irritated.

Always remember that most fitness gains happen during recovery, not during the workout. The workout spurs the body to have a need for recovery. It is in this recovery period when the body prepares itself to handle the challenges of the next workout and of life in general. Anything you can do to make recovery speedier and better will improve how fast your body adapts and becomes stronger, more capable, and more fit.

After you have the habit of exercise

Once you have established the habit of regular exercise, you may wish to tweak some of what you are doing. When you start feeling healthier and stronger, your eyes may be opened to the possibilities of continuous improvement and challenge. After years feeling trapped in a body you did not like, it can feel miraculous to experience a body that looks and functions better than you had thought possible.

At this point, it may become appealing to you to make exercise as effective as it possibly can be. Maybe you will want a greater challenge, or maybe you will want to understand how to burn calories most efficiently or how to make your body as functional and strong as possible as you do the activities of your daily life.

I discuss all of this plus what kinds of exercise I most highly recommend in Chapter 18, "Optimize Exercise." If you are already fairly fit, this is essential information and I encourage you to read it as soon as possible, because it also covers the subject of how to retain or gain muscle while focusing your weight loss on fat.

Movement Goals

Following is a quick cheat sheet to set goals for yourself to increase the amount you move:

Movement during previously sitting times. Set a goal to make the amount of consecutive time sitting as short as possible. Aim for being up at least three minutes out of every 30.This could be walking to get a drink of water, going up and down the stairs, or just shifting back and forth from one foot to the other.

Moderate Exercise. This includes brisk walking, and it should eventually reach at least four hours a week. Shoot for getting to this level sometime in the next six months to a year, gradually increasing between now and then.

Challenging Exercise. Set a goal to increase the amount of challenging exercise you are getting. Work toward eventually getting three hours a week of challenging exercise. You might give yourself a timeline for getting there. Don't beat yourself up if you are not getting the full three hours a week in the first few months. Remember, *any* increase in challenging exercise over time is good. Pat yourself on the back for any forward progress.

Do not lose sight of your ultimate goal on this habit, even if it is challenging to get there in the first few months. Remember, the amount of movement and exercise you do will make a huge difference in your ability to lose weight, keep it off, and feel so much better in the process.

TV Watching. The average American spends 28 hours a week watching TV. The average National Weight Control Registry participant spends 10.[53] This is a huge difference. Time spent watching TV is mostly seated. Keep track of how much time you are sitting in front of the TV. Log it each day and set a goal to reduce that time. For the purposes of this log, do not count the time you are up and moving. If you really want to see a program that will put your time over your goal amount, then get up and move while you watch it.

Main goal: Reduce longest continuous time sitting each day.

Steps per Day

I am often asked about setting goals for steps per day. I am including this section, because so many people track their steps using fitness watches or phone apps. More steps are generally better than fewer steps, if you have the time and ability to take them.

We can look at this question based on a goal of improved health or weight loss or both. Walking is an important part of an overall fitness plan, but it should not be the entire plan. Generally, I recommend that you set a steps goal that you feel is personally

---

[53] "Television viewing and long-term weight maintenance: results from the National Weight Control Registry." Raynor et al, October 2006, *Obesity*, National Institutes of Health pubmed, https://www.ncbi.nlm.nih.gov/pubmed/17062812

achievable in the short run within the Movement Goals recommendations stated above, then build up from there.

The more steps you take, the greater your likely life span. In a 2019 study[54], women averaging 72 years old were tracked for one week. The ones who walked an average of at least 4400 steps a day were significantly more likely to be alive 4.3 years later than those walking 2700 steps a day. Life expectancy continued to improve with greater numbers of steps per day until 7500 steps. At least in this study, walking more than 7500 steps a day did not change the near term mortality outcome.

Many people in the fitness industry have promoted the idea of taking 10,000 steps a day. That is a great idea. However, according to a 2017 study[55], the average number of steps per day per person averages substantially less than 10,000 steps a day all over the world. This study used activity data from smartphones of 717,527 people over an average 95 day period in 111 different countries.

Here are some of the results:

---

[54] "Association of Step Volume and Intensity With All-Cause Mortality in Older Women." I-Min Lee et al., May 29, 2019, *JAMA Internal Medicine*, https://jamanetwork.com/journals/jamainternalmedicine/article-abstract/2734709

[55] "Large-scale physical activity data reveal worldwide activity inequality." Althoff et al., 2017, *Springer Nature*, http://activityinequality.stanford.edu/docs/activity-inequality-althoffetal-nature.pdf

Country	Average steps per day
Hong Kong	6,880
China	6,189
United Kingdom	5,444
Germany	5,205
France	5,141
Australia	4,491
Canada	4,819
United States	4,774
India	4,297
Indonesia	3,513

10,000 steps per day is around twice the average number of steps taken by the Althoff et al. study participants.[55] 10,000 is in fact an arbitrary number, but it may be a worthwhile target for some people, especially for non-senior adults who can realistically walk that much. *Livestrong* provides a calculation of the burn potential:

> "10,000 steps would equate to approximately five miles per day and approximately 425 calories burned for a 120-pound person; 525 calories burned for a 160-pound person; and 625 calories burned for a 200-pound person."[56]

---

[56] "How Many Steps Per Day to Lose Weight?" Dena McDowell, October 17, 2019, *Livestrong.com*,

10,000 steps a day translates to burning about a pound a week of bodyweight for a 160-pound person as compared with someone who is not walking at all. Of course, if they were not walking at all, they would face a myriad of other problems.

It is indisputable that walking burns calories. And it should definitely be one of your goals to walk more than you did when you were gaining weight. However 10,000 steps a day is not a magic number. According to statistics provided by *Healthline*, 10,000 steps may be too few if you are a male teenager and more than you can feasibly do if you are a female over 70:

> *"There appears to be a significant difference in the average number of steps taken by females and males. From childhood through adulthood, males tend to walk more. As children and teens, they walk an average of 12,000 to 16,000 steps per day. Young females, on the other hand, get 10,000 to 12,000.*
>
> *This trend continues into adulthood, at least in the United States. A 2010 study looked at pedometer data for just over 1,000 adults. Overall, males took an average of 5,340 steps per day, compared to 4,912 for females."[57]*

The number of steps you take per day is a good reference point as you establish new exercise habits. Just don't become fixated on some magic number. Instead, establish a habit of regular exercise and frequent movement in accordance with the guidance laid out in the Movement Goals section above. Many weight loss apps help you to set age and gender appropriate steps goals.

---

https://www.livestrong.com/article/171629-how-many-steps-per-day-to-lose-weight/
[57] "How Many Steps Do People Take Per Day on Average?" *Healthline*, https://www.healthline.com/health/average-steps-per-day

Your success will hinge first and foremost on establishing a habit of exercise, whatever that looks like. Once exercise becomes habit, look at ways to do more. If your long-term goals are to burn calories, lose weight, and be healthier, think about the factors that will lead to these goals: more movement, more muscle tissues involved in your movements, and greater challenge. Chapter 18 will discuss optimal exercise patterns in much greater detail.

Takeaways for Chapter 7

- Better health and sustained weight loss are feasible with exercise and good nutrition.

- Start slowly. Start moving, and gradually increase your movement and exercise.

- The habit of exercise is much more important than the amount or intensity of what you do at first. Start out easy!

- Start with exercise and movement that you enjoy.

- Set a goal to eventually exercise seven days a week totaling 60 minutes a day including brisk walking. This could be way out in the future.

- Stretch and eat right after exercise. Feel good between workouts.

- Good health is alluring. Don't be surprised if you wake up one day yearning to challenge yourself even more.

- Get up for at least three minutes for every 30 minutes you are sitting.

- **Set a goal for doing some challenging exercise.**

- **Try to watch no more than 10 hours of TV per week.**

- **Set an age and gender appropriate target for steps per day.**

Chapter 8

Logging

Plan it. Log it.

Keeping a record of what you have done substantially improves your odds of success in your quest for sustained weight loss. Do not cheat yourself by failing to record your behavior. Those records empower you to control the strategic direction of your quest and to make adjustments when and where needed.

Many studies link frequent self-monitoring with significantly greater likelihood of success in weight loss. The more often, for example, you log your weight, the more likely you are to lose weight and to keep it off. The more often you log meals and exercise, the more likely you are to be successful in eating right and exercising sufficiently to make a difference and, again, to lose weight successfully.

"...there was ample evidence for the consistent and significant positive relationship between self-monitoring diet, physical activity or weight and successful outcomes related to weight management."[58]

This is a matter of mindfulness. When you pay close attention to what you are doing, and you keep a record of it, you become aware of your behavior and what should be changing. You also take personal responsibility for outcomes when you see how your patterns of eating and exercise translate to specific results.

Logging May Have Saved My Life

Back in 2008, when I was 40 pounds overweight, my blood pressure went through the roof. I knew I had to do something, or my health would decline rapidly. I did not want to be a candidate for a heart attack!

Extensive reading on diet, exercise, health and fitness taught me the importance of a balanced diet. I also learned about important phytonutrients (nutrients from plants) and their impact on health and

---

[58] "Self-Monitoring in Weight Loss: A Systematic Review of the Literature", Burk et al., January, 2011, *Journal of the Academy of Nutrition and Dietetics*, https://www.ncbi.nlm.nih.gov/pmc/articles/PMC3268700/

metabolism. I had formulas for calculating calories burned. And my fitness training textbooks had information on how many calories were contained in various whole foods.

I had also learned in my research that blood sugar crashes would slow the metabolism, and that the body needed proteins to be paired with carbs for optimal lean tissue repair and growth.

I began to write down exactly what and how much I ate at every meal. I calculated calories, and I stayed within my budget. I did not have the benefit of many of the more recent studies on balancing meals optimally, but my National Federation of Professional Trainers textbooks did tell me that I should have around 60% of my intake from carbohydrates, 20% to 30% from protein, and not more than 20% from fat. These numbers were not far off from optimal, as we'll see in later chapters, so I strove to stay close to these percentages in every meal.

What I did not want was to be hungry. I have to admit that this was purely pain avoidance. I hated hunger to the point of equating it with pain. I didn't yet know that hunger and metabolic speed were so completely connected.

I paid attention to what meals satisfied my appetite and still met all of the requirements on calories, carb-protein-fat balance and phytonutrient content. I quickly found that I could stop hunger by eating plenty of certain foods without going over my caloric budget. These foods happen to be many of the same ones that are now Unlimiteds.

None of this would have been possible if I had not been faithfully logging all of my meals and my weight each day. That's the beauty of writing it all down or of logging it electronically. The logs reveal patterns, either good or bad, and they kept me on track.

The logs revealed what satisfied my appetite. They revealed that when my appetite was most thoroughly satisfied, I could lose weight steadily without the discomfort of hunger. At that time, I was relieved that my weight loss was just as fast when my hunger was satisfied as it was when I allowed myself to be hungry.

It wasn't until much later that I began to notice that people I knew who had stopped being able to lose weight had been regularly making themselves hungry or eating unbalanced meals during the weeks before. Again, logs told the tale.

Log Your Weight Every Day

Self-weighing frequency has specifically been identified as most effective when it is done at least daily, and those who begin to weigh themselves less frequently after they have reached their goals are more likely to yo-yo. Those who weigh themselves least frequently regain the most weight.[59] This data comes from a study of National Weight Control Registry participants, a group that has been successful at losing weight and keeping it off.

> "At baseline, 36.2% of participants reported weighing themselves at least once per day, and more frequent weighing was associated with lower BMI and higher scores on… restraint… Weight gain at 1-year follow-up was significantly greater for participants whose self-weighing frequency decreased… compared with those whose frequency increased… or remained the same... Participants who decreased their frequency of self-weighing were more

---

[59] "Consistent self-monitoring of weight: a key component of successful weight loss maintenance." Butryn et al., December 2007, *Obesity*, National Institutes of Health pubmed, https://www.ncbi.nlm.nih.gov/pubmed/18198319?ordinalpos=2&itool=EntrezSystem2.PEntrez.Pubmed.Pubmed_ResultsPanel.Pubmed_RVDocSum

likely to report increases in their percentage of caloric intake from fat…

"Consistent self-weighing may help individuals maintain their successful weight loss by allowing them to catch weight gains before they escalate and make behavior changes to prevent additional weight gain. While change in self-weighing frequency is a marker for changes in other parameters of weight control, decreasing self-weighing frequency is also independently associated with greater weight gain."

Plan Your Meals

Planning your meals, even if you are not trying to lose weight, is associated with less incidence of excess weight. A 2017 study in France included 40,554 participants and looked at whether or not they were planning their meals at least a few days ahead.

"Our results highlighted that individuals planning their meals were more likely to have a better dietary quality, including a higher adherence with nutritional guidelines as well as an increased food variety. Additionally, meal planning was associated with lower odds of being obese in men and women..."[60]

The evidence is clear; frequently logging and planning makes you much more likely to be successful, not only in taking the weight off, but also keeping it off.

---

[60] "Meal planning is associated with food variety, diet quality and body weight status in a large sample of French adults." Ducrot et al., February 2, 2017, *International Journal of Behavioral Nutrition and Physical Activity*, National Institutes of Health, https://www.ncbi.nlm.nih.gov/pmc/articles/PMC5288891/

If you really pay attention to what you are doing and what you are putting into your mouth, then you begin to control the outcomes.

You can log with a pen and paper, but most people prefer the convenience and analytical tools associated with electronic apps. If you choose to use an app, make sure it provides you with guidance on balancing your meals appropriately, including the right kinds of foods, and keeping track of lifestyle issues such as sleep, exercise, and television watching. When you have a tool that makes it easy to plan the right kinds of meals, and to log the right kinds of activities, you are well on the way to achieving success in reaching your goals and staying there.

Be sure that *everything* you eat gets into the plan and the log. Many people overlook fats such as olive oil and butter, but these are by far the highest caloric density foods you will eat. A very small amount of fats equals a large amount of calories. You need some of these in your diet, but it is vital that they be planned and logged.

Starting Out: Pictures & Measurements

Another form of self-monitoring is visual. Before you make any changes to your diet or your exercise, take some pictures of yourself. You do not need to look your best. You just need to look the way you look. Just take the pictures or have someone take them for you. These will be a valuable reminder later of how far you have come.

Also, take measurements. Ideally, you should measure six places on your body. Every measurement should be at an easily duplicated landmark position as follows:

- Right arm where it meets the shoulder
- Chest at your nipples

- Waist at your navel

- Hips at their widest point

- Right thigh at the gluteal fold

After you get started, return to measure these same spots once a week. If you are working out with vigor and gain muscle weight, you may see a change in your measurements before you see the scale move much. This is because muscle weighs more by volume than fat does, and an increase in muscle weight may offset a loss of fat. Losing more inches than pounds is a sign you have gained muscle weight and lost fat.

It is wonderful when that happens, because you look better, you feel better, and your clothes fit you better.

Understanding Odd Weight Shifts

Forewarned is forearmed. Equip yourself with knowledge, so you can interpret certain events appropriately. This will help prevent discouragement.

1. No weight loss in first two weeks. During the first couple of weeks that you are working out harder than you have in a long, long time, there is a good chance you will not lose weight, even if you have been eating correctly. Do not be surprised if you step on the scale, and the weight has increased or stayed the same. The good news is you have probably lost fat.

If that happens, you can take your measurements, and see if there is any improvement. If there is improvement, then you know you have lost fat. Why? When you increase the intensity of your exercises, muscles cry out for nutrients. The nutrients go into the muscles approximately the ratio of three parts water for one part nutrients. This makes the muscles heavier, and that extra weight will offset fat loss, leaving the scale unchanged or up.

Take heart, though. This kind of water weight does not make you look or feel bloated. It makes you look better and more fit. After the first couple of weeks, the muscles will have about all the water weight they are going to gain, so in the third week is when you will probably see your fat losses begin to show up on the scale.

2. Weight loss on vacation. Suppose you have been working out steadily and losing weight, then you take a vacation and do not exercise for a week. Your vacation diet is bad. You expect your weight to go up by a couple of pounds during your week off, but when you step on the scale after the vacation, do not be surprised to see that you actually lost weight.

This is *definitely* not a good excuse to stop exercising and eating right. This happens because when you stop exercising, your muscles lose that extra water weight they gained from grabbing more nutrients. During your vacation, fat increases and muscle weight goes down. This is nothing to celebrate.

3. Weight gain after being good again. If you experienced #2, you will almost certainly experience this one. A week after you return to working out and eating right, when you step on the scale, you are likely to have gained weight again. Once again, your muscles will have taken in more nutrients with water, and now the fat you gained during the vacation is showing up on the scale. Take heart: If you continue to exercise and work out, the weight will start coming off again.

4. Pre-menstrual weight gain. Ladies, do not be disheartened just because you gain weight just before your period starts. Or, if your weight stays the same even though you have been eating right and exercising. That is normal due to menstrual bloating. Just stay with your good habits of eating right, exercising regularly, and the

140

next week you should see two weeks' worth of weight loss show up on the scale.

Takeaways for Chapter 8

- **Keeping records make you more likely to be successful.**

- **Take your picture at the start of your weight-loss journey.**

- **Log your weight every day.**

- **Plan and log your meals.**

- **Log measurements weekly.**

- **Log sleep, television watching, and exercise.**

- **Sometimes your weight will shift in predictable ways depending on circumstances. Understanding these shifts helps put them in perspective.**

Chapter 9

Unlimiteds

You Are Smarter than a Mouse

If given the right foods, mice instinctively eat the right quantity for good health. Like them, with the right foods, you will simply stop eating because you're not hungry anymore.

When mice are given as much as they want of the wrong kinds of foods, they eat too many calories and gain weight. When they are given the right kinds of foods, they choose to stop with much fewer calories, which causes them to live longer and to be healthier, according to a 2014 study by Solon-Biet et al. [61]

The Eat As Much As You Want system guides you to the right foods. In this chapter, we will look at the foods you can eat in unlimited quantities. Your own body will tell you when you have had enough.

Think about your own experiences with eating. Were you ever offered food when you had recently eaten a well-balanced, healthy meal, and you just did not want anything more? Filling up with balanced nutrition helps you to feel that way.

On the other hand, how have you felt after eating a dessert, or maybe Chinese food with white rice? Or Thanksgiving dinner? Has there ever been a time when you ate sugary or high-starch meals, and you were full, but you still wanted more to eat? Then, a short while later, you felt sleepy or lethargic?

Thanksgiving Crash

When I was a boy, I loved Thanksgiving! I was the seventh of eight kids. On any other day, I often had to eat fast to get enough food before it ran out at the table. My sisters seemed happy with one or two helpings, but I needed three or I would leave the table hungry.

---

[61] "The Ratio of Macronutrients, Not Caloric Intake, Dictates Cardiometabolic Health, Aging, and Longevity in Ad Libitum-Fed Mice." Solon-Biet et al., March 4 2014, *Cell Metabolism*, https://www.sciencedirect.com/science/article/pii/S1550413114000655

My mom had never adjusted her quantities to get beyond having an average of maybe one and a half helpings per person at every meal. That meant I had to eat fast enough to get my third helping before half of my sisters got to their second helping. Every meal felt like a fight for survival.

At Thanksgiving, however, there was always an abundance of food. We all helped with food preparation, and the quantities were enormous. There were always leftovers to last for several days afterwards.

I would pile my plate with turkey, dressing, gravy, rice, sweet potatoes, beans, cranberry sauce and rolls. I would eat that, then pile my plate again. Then came pumpkin pie, pecan pie and ice cream.

I had no clue about hi-Glycemic Index or high-Glycemic Load foods, but I was eating massive quantities of them. Thirty minutes after the meal ended, I couldn't keep my eyes open. I would lie down and drift off for a deep sleep. When I awoke, I would feel very droopy for another hour or so. American folklore is that the drowsiness is caused by tryptophan in the turkey. Think again.

Why the crash?

That massive blood sugar overload had forced my body to defensively purge my blood of blood sugar. If it had not, the sugar would have caused severe damage to my lean tissues.

Hi-GI means high-Glycemic Index, which is a measure of how quickly foods you eat turn to blood sugar in your blood stream. Examples include potatoes, table sugar, and white bread. High-Glycemic Load foods are foods such as rice, pies, ice cream and sweet potatoes that put a lot of blood sugar into your blood stream in a short time. Eating such foods, as I did every Thanksgiving, causes a blood sugar spike followed by a crash.

These are natural hormonal responses to how you eat. When you fill up with fruits, vegetables and a well-balanced meal, you will typically choose to eat less than may be available. If the balanced meal is made up of the right kinds of foods, you will be satisfied with fewer calories than you are burning. On the other hand, in my boyhood Thanksgivings I ate far more calories than I could reasonably burn that day.

This book teaches you to navigate these same mechanisms in the body to stay satisfied and to maintain a high level of energy. The sleepiness and lethargy I felt after my Thanksgiving meals made me not want to move or burn calories. You may have episodes of sleepiness every mid-afternoon if you make a habit of eating a lot of bread or rice or potatoes or sweets at lunch. Frequent nutrient-rich, balanced meals can keep you satisfied and help you to optimize your metabolic rate.

Optimize satiety and usable energy

The opposite of my boyhood Thanksgivings is to eat nutrient-rich, low-GI foods that have few calories relative to a given volume of food. This fills you up without overloading your bloodstream with sugar. That means afternoons without feeling droopy, and satiety without too many calories.

In the 2014 Solon-Biet study, mice were fed the same basic food and they were allowed to eat as much as they wanted. However, some of the mice were given foods that were bulked up with non-digestible cellulose, which meant they had to eat more to get the same amount of calories. The end result was they chose to eat fewer calories.[61]

Unlimiteds are to you what the bulked-up foods were to the mice. They are good, healthy foods, and you can choose to eat only the ones you like, but they fill you up and satisfy your appetite without giving you too many calories. So, when you eat Unlimiteds, you choose to stop eating before you have consumed too many calories. However, Unlimiteds do more for you than the bulked-up foods did for the mice, because they are tasty and packed with life-extending, health-enhancing micronutrients.

This 2014 study[61] taught us something else that echoes what we already learned in Chapter 4: The mice who were fed high-protein, low carbohydrate diets did not live as long as the mice who ate balanced diets with sufficient protein and higher amounts of carbohydrates. To be clear, the carbohydrates in these diets were not sweets.

Let's go back to the well-balanced, healthy-meal example. Would you have said "No thank you" if what was offered was your favorite dessert? Refined sugars and high fat content foods offer palatability that is often difficult to say no to. When we expose ourselves to the wrong choices, we may choose to eat additional food even when we are already full. And if we are hungry to begin with, we are especially vulnerable to making bad choices.

The goal, then, is to plan ahead and to stock up on the foods we should be eating to satisfy our appetites. Then, if we are presented with temptations, we will be in a much better position to resist.

With the Eat As Much As You Want system, satiety is primarily achieved using a combination of Unlimiteds, Countables and frequent eating. The Unlimiteds do some of the work of filling you up and satisfying your appetite, but frequency and Countables also play very important roles. The ad libitum fed mice from the 2014 study ate until they reached their target intakes of protein and carbohydrates, so satiety will not be reached without the Countables. You need both, and you need the Countables in the right balance, but this current chapter focuses primarily on Unlimiteds.

Recap of the Book So Far

Before moving on, let's review, what we have learned so far.

1. **Avoid hunger.** The less time spent hungry each day, the better. Your metabolism slows down dramatically when you allow yourself to endure long periods of hunger. Over a longer period of time, these temporary metabolic slowdowns morph into chronic hunger and a chronically slow metabolism in a condition called starvation mode.

2. **Avoid starvation mode.** Consume a balanced diet of nutrient-rich, low-caloric density, low-GI foods. Chew your foods well. Fill up with these foods to satisfy hunger, to spur the release of hormones that will increase the metabolic rate, and to give your body all of the nutrients it needs to fuel a wide variety of healthy biological processes.

3. **Listen to your body** when you judge how much to eat of the Unlimiteds. Satisfy your hunger, but do not overeat. Even when consuming Unlimiteds, eat a variety of foods you like, not just a few you like the most. Include green vegetables, berries, citrus, probiotics and others. Greater variety yields greater satiety, better health, and a faster metabolism

4. **Eliminate any addiction to sugar** (see Chapter 11). Your body cannot guide you appropriately if it is blinded by the tastes and urges associated with refined sugars and hi-GI processed foods.

5. **Eat whole natural foods** and avoid highly processed foods as much as possible.

6. When you **plan and log meals**, include everything you eat or drink, without exception, even if it's just an extra pat of butter, a tablespoon of oil, or a bite of muffin or pastry.

7. **Self-monitor** your behaviors. This includes logging meals, workouts, moderate exercise such as standing, walking, or our favorite activities, as well as sleep and watching television. The better you keep up with all of these, the more likely you are to be successful.

Starting your sustained weight-loss journey

Immediately after taking pictures and measurements, it's important to begin to eat more of certain foods. Yes, that is not a typo; I meant to say "more".

The major failure of so many diet plans is that they start with deprivation, which leads the body into the starvation mode. To avoid starvation mode, we must eat enough to stay satisfied, and we must chew our food adequately.

Thus, identify foods you like that will fill you up without a lot of calories, keep you satisfied, and provide high nutritional value. That is the role of Unlimiteds, especially Must Haves. Whenever possible, choose foods that are whole and that require chewing. Stock up on Unlimiteds and get rid of processed, unnatural foods, especially ones with lots of chemical additives.

Must Haves

Must Haves are foods so valuable in the quest to reach your goals we must have at least a serving of one of them with every meal. These are Unlimiteds, meaning you can eat as much as you want of any of them. However, Must Haves combine the best qualities of nutrient-richness, low-caloric density, low-GI and satiety potential into a single food.

Within this umbrella Must Haves category, there are various smaller lists as follows: Appetite Suppressors, Sweet Super Foods, Anti–Agers, and Burn Boosters. For guidance on how to combine these high-value, filling foods with Countables to make great, satisfying meals, see Chapter 21.

Disease-fighting qualities of Must Haves

The foods found in the Must Haves lists help to support our immune systems and to battle certain kinds of cancer. A 2007 study[62] found

"High intake of cruciferous vegetables has been associated with lower risk of lung and colorectal cancer in some epidemiological studies…"

A 2016 study[63] found

"Dietary patterns, including regular consumption of particular foods such as berries as well as bioactive compounds, may confer specific molecular and cellular protection in addition to the overall epidemiologically observed benefits of plant food consumption (lower rates of obesity and chronic disease risk), further enhancing health. Mounting evidence reports a variety of health benefits of berry fruits that are usually attributed to their non-nutritive bioactive compounds, mainly phenolic substances such as flavonoids or anthocyanins. Although it is still unclear which

---

[62] "Cruciferous Vegetables and Human Cancer Risk: Epidemiologic Evidence and Mechanistic Basis." Higdon et al., March 2007, *Pharmacological Research*, National Institutes of Health, https://www.ncbi.nlm.nih.gov/pmc/articles/PMC2737735/
[63] "Protective Role of Dietary Berries in Cancer." Kristo et al., October 19 2016, *Antioxidants*, National Institutes of Health pubmed, https://www.ncbi.nlm.nih.gov/pmc/articles/PMC5187535/

particular constituents are responsible for the extended health benefits, it appears that whole berry consumption generally confers some anti-oxidant and anti-inflammatory protection to humans and animals."

This same 2016 study goes on to detail how foods such as whole berries help prevent, slow down or reverse cancer and other serious diseases.

Stone fruits, such as peaches, nectarines and plums (as well as other fruits such as apples, pears, strawberries and citrus) are listed among those that protect specifically against esophageal cancer according to a study that included 490,802 participants[64].

The studies cited above are just a fraction of the many studies that have shown that the fruits and vegetables in the Must Haves lists protect our bodies from many kinds of cancer and other health problems.

Appetite Suppressors

Appetite Suppressors -- the first Must Haves list -- are cruciferous vegetables. We may eat these in unlimited quantities. They are so important to weight loss and good health that I strongly recommend that you consume at least one serving from this specific list every day:

Arugula
Broccoli
Broccoli raab
Brussels sprouts

---

[64] "Fruit and vegetable intake and esophageal cancer in a large prospective cohort study." Freedman et al., December 15 2007, National Institutes of Health pubmed, https://www.ncbi.nlm.nih.gov/pubmed/17691111

Cabbage
Cabbage savoy
Cauliflower
Chinese cabbage
Collards
Garden cress
Horseradish
Kale
Kohlrabi
Mustard greens
Mustard spinach (or tendergreen)
Radishes
Rutabagas
Spinach
Turnips
Turnip greens
Wasabi
Watercress

Sweet Super Foods

Sweet Super Foods is the next Must Haves list. The foods in this list are also powerful tools in the battle against obesity, because once you have kicked the sugar habit, they will taste very sweet. Thus, they are great for a recovering sweet tooth.

Despite their inherent sweetness, they are low-GI, nutrient-rich, low-caloric density, high-satiety foods. Thus, you can eat them in unlimited quantities; in fact, it is recommended that you have a serving from any of the Appetite Suppressors, Sweet Super Foods, and Anti-Agers lists in at least three different meals every day.

Keep in mind, however, that these should be eaten whole or sliced and preferably raw or frozen. They should not be juiced, dried or sweetened. Juicing eliminates chewing, reduces satiety, and raises GI. Drying and sweetening both raise GI and reduce satiety, and drying reduces bulk. Here are the Sweet Super Foods:

Apricots
Blackberries
Blueberries
Cherries, sweet or sour
Cranberries
Elderberries
Grapefruit
Mulberries
Nectarines
Peaches
Plums
Raspberries
Strawberries

Anti-Agers

Anti-Agers is the third Must Haves list. These are similar in nutritional values to Sweet Super Foods, but in some cases are not as sweet. Some may help you to live longer and speed your metabolism by giving your body vital nutrients and antioxidants, or by helping the good microbes in your gut to reproduce:

Alfalfa sprouts
Apples
Beet greens
Beets
Citrus including Tangerines, Oranges, and Lemons
Cocoa powder, unsweetened
Crabapples
Eggplant
Prickly pears
Probiotic fermented red beets and cabbage
Rhubarb

Sauerkraut
Seaweed
Shallots
Swiss chard
Tomatoes
Turnips

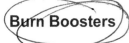

Burn Boosters

Burn Boosters is the fourth and final Must Haves list. These fill you up while rounding out your phytonutrient intake. By helping to complete a broad spectrum of micronutrients that your body needs to function ideally each day, Burn Boosters help your metabolism to burn faster and your body to become healthier. Again, you can eat as much as you want!

Artichokes
Asparagus
Acorn squash
Bamboo shoots
Bean sprouts
Butternut squash
Carambola or starfruit
Carrots
Celeriac
Celery
Chicory roots and greens
Chinese water chestnuts
Chives
Cilantro
Cowpeas leafy tips
Crookneck and straightneck summer squash
Cucumbers
Endive
Fennel bulb
Grape leaves

Green chilis
Hearts of palm
Hubbard squash
Jalapeños
Leeks
Lettuces, including Romaine, green leaf, red leaf, bibb, boston and spring mix
Lotus root
Mushrooms, including white, portabella, brown, Italian, crimini, chanterelle, maitake, shiitake, morel, straw, enoki, oyster,
Okra
Onions
Parsley
Pasta sauce
Peppers, red hot chili, banana, ancho, green hot chili, serrano,
Picante sauce
Pickled cabbage
Podded peas such as sugar snap peas and snow peas
Pumpkin
Radicchio
Scallop summer squash
Snap beans, green or yellow
Spaghetti squash
Spring onions and scallions
Sweet peppers, including red, green and yellow
Taro leaves and shoots
Tomato sauce
Vegetable broth
Zucchini

Other Unlimiteds

In addition to the Must Haves, there are Unlimited Beverages and Spices and Herbs.

Unlimited Beverages

It is vital that you get enough water each day. Water is a major catalyst to a faster burning metabolism[65], and it is a major component of satiety[29].

For example, a 2018 study[66]

> "found that pre-meal water consumption, indeed, reduced energy intake among the non-obese young adults. An acute reduction in energy intake following water ingestion was observed."

It is generally recommended that women consume at least 96 ounces of water each day and men consume at least 120 ounces. This water can come from all sources, including foods and beverages. If you are not certain how to count water in your foods, some apps count it for you, in part because high-water-content foods satisfy your appetite more effectively than drier foods. Certain beverages are more appropriate than others, because they provide water without many calories. In certain cases, unlimited beverages may have other positive health benefits besides hydration.

I do not advocate the use of artificially-sweetened low-calorie or no-calorie beverages, because they tend to have many chemicals that are foreign to the body. However, there are many such drinks on the Unlimited Beverages list for the simple reason that 53% of

---

[65] "Water-induced thermogenesis", Boschmann et al., December 2003, *Journal of Clinical Endocrinology and Metabolism*, National Institutes of Health pubmed, https://pubmed.ncbi.nlm.nih.gov/14671205/
[66] "Effect of Pre-meal Water Consumption on Energy Intake and Satiety in Non-obese Young Adults", Ji Na Jeong, October 2018, *Clinical Nutrition Research*, National Institutes of Health, https://www.ncbi.nlm.nih.gov/pmc/articles/PMC6209729/

National Weight Control participants in a study reported regular use of low- to no-calorie sweetened beverages.[67]

There has historically been some controversy regarding whether artificial sweeteners are bad for you. According to the Cancer Council,

> *"Early animal studies showed varied results about the safety of aspartame. There was a large controversy regarding the approval of aspartame in the US. In 1981, the head of the FDA was fired, allegedly after refusing to approve the legalisation of aspartame. His successor legalised it and later accepted a job offer with Searle, the company which owned aspartame…*
>
> *"There have been cases in which sufferers of birth defects, brain cancer, Alzheimer's disease, multiple sclerosis and seizures have attributed their condition to aspartame consumption. These claims are anecdotal and not based on scientific evidence."[68]*

In this same research piece the Council cites a lot of research that indicates the initial studies were flawed. In particular, the dosages given to animals were extremely high. The Council concludes as follows:

---

[67] "Low/no calorie sweetened beverage consumption in the National Weight Control Registry." Catanacci et al., October 2014, *Obesity*, National Institutes of Health pubmed,
https://www.ncbi.nlm.nih.gov/pubmed/25044563
[68] "Cancer myth: Sweeteners and Cancer." July 2015, Cancer Council WA,
https://www.cancerwa.asn.au/resources/cancermyths/sweeteners-myth/

"Despite public concern, there is no evidence that artificial sweeteners cause cancer, or unsafe in the doses typically consumed."[68]

They do however recommend that concerned parents choose whole fruits and vegetables for their children instead of artificial sweeteners *"to prevent overweight and obesity and lead to a reduction in risk for many chronic diseases and cancer."* I found this to be a curiously odd way to end an article about the safety of artificial sweeteners.

It is also unclear whether carbonated beverages (especially colas) and coffee may be linked to osteoporosis. The research on this is conflicting.

"Colas and coffee appear to have some effect on women's bone density and could lead to osteoporosis. But tea — even the kind with caffeine — and other sodas do not. And men are not affected at all by these beverages."[69]

Caffeine and coffee are similarly extremely controversial, with many studies showing numerous health benefits to the consumption of both. Among those cited is weight loss. Because of this, I am not prepared to recommend against them.

Accordingly, all of these beverages are included in the Unlimited Beverages category, because they hydrate you, they are more palatable for many people than plain water, and they have very few calories. However, I recommend you use your own judgment about which ones you will choose to regularly drink.

---

[69] "Sodas, Tea and Coffee: Which Can Make Your Bones Brittle?" December 7 2016, Cleveland Clinic, Rheumatology and Immunology, https://health.clevelandclinic.org/sodas-tea-coffee-can-make-bones-brittle/

What is important to remember is (a) you need to get plenty of water each day, (b) your water can come from your food and your drinks, and (c) you should avoid beverages that contain a lot of calories. Here are the Unlimited Beverages:

Water:

Naturally sparkling water
Non-carbonated water with natural fruit flavors sweetened with low calorie sweetener
Water, tap, bottled or filtered

Tea:

Black tea
Brewed unsweetened tea
Decaffeinated unsweetened tea
Green tea
Herb tea
Instant artificially sweetened zero calorie tea
Instant unsweetened tea

Coffee:

Brewed coffee with chicory (black)
Brewed espresso coffee
Instant coffee with chicory (black)
Regular and decaffeinated and half caffeinated brewed coffee (black)
Regular and decaffeinated and half caffeinated instant coffee (black)

Soda:

Club soda
Zero calorie colas
Zero calorie soft drinks

Juice Drink:

Fortified low calorie fruit juice beverage
Vegetable and fruit juice drink, low calorie with artificial sweetener
V8 Splash Juice Drinks: Diet Fruit Medley, Diet Strawberry Kiwi, Diet Berry Blend, or Diet Tropical Blend

Cocoa:

Cocoa mix powder with artificial sweetener prepared with water

Energy drink:

Sugar free energy drinks

Electrolyte drink:

Gatorade G2, low calorie
Powerade Zero, calorie free
Propel Zero

Spices and herbs

Palatability is a major part of satiety and enjoyment. It is important to actually like the foods that are healthiest to eat, and that means we should strive to make them taste good. This common-sense principle was confirmed in a 2015 study[70] that found that

> "animals (including humans) learn to eat in response to sensory cues, by forming associations between the early experience of a food's sensory characteristic and the post-ingestive effects of nutrient delivery... This learned integration of pre-ingestive and post ingestive signals can be expressed as increased liking for nutrient-rich foods and explicit beliefs about a food's potential satiating power, which in turn modify food selection and intake."

In other words, we naturally choose to eat nutrient-rich foods only if they taste good to us and satisfy us. Sometimes we need to spice up bland foods and make them taste better. Fortunately, there are many spices, sauces and dressings that have few or no calories. Using these in dishes can help to make the experience of eating nutritious, low-caloric density foods a pleasure.

The benefits of herbs and spices go beyond good taste and palatability. They can be extraordinarily healthful, providing a wide array of valuable phytonutrients. A 2019 study[71] concluded the following:

> "Spices and herbs have been in use for centuries both for culinary and medicinal purposes. Spices not only enhance the flavor, aroma, and color of food and beverages, but they can also protect from acute and chronic diseases. More Americans are considering the use of spices and herbs for

---

[70] "Sensory influences on food intake control: moving beyond palatability." McCrickerd and Forde, December 11 2015, *Obesity Reviews*, World Obesity, Wiley Online Library, https://onlinelibrary.wiley.com/doi/full/10.1111/obr.12340
[71] "Health Benefits of Culinary Herbs and Spices." TA Jiang, March 1 2019, *Journal of AOAC International*, National Institutes of Health pubmed, https://www.ncbi.nlm.nih.gov/pubmed/30651162

medicinal and therapeutic/remedy use, especially for various chronic conditions. There is now ample evidence that spices and herbs possess antioxidant, anti-inflammatory, antitumorigenic, anticarcinogenic, and glucose- and cholesterol-lowering activities as well as properties that affect cognition and mood."

The goals of the Eat As Much As You Want system are greater than mere weight loss. Enhancement of health, longevity, and quality of life is just as important. Spices and herbs can help with all of these pursuits. Some of the items on the Spices and Herbs list are simply calorie-free items that enhance flavor. Others are extremely healthful. Some have significant calories in higher quantities but have such potent flavor that it would be very unusual to consume large amounts. You can choose which to use and which not to use. None of the items on this list are mandatory:

Bouillon

Beef broth cubes, dry
Beef broth powder
Better than Bouillon Mushroom Base
Better than Bouillon Vegetable Base
Bone broth
Chicken bouillon, dry
Chicken broth
Chicken broth cubes, dry
Consomme with gelatin, dry mix
Organic Better Than Bouillon Reduced Sodium Vegetable Base
Vegetarian Better Than Boullion No Beef Base
Vegetarian Better Than Bouillon No Chicken Base

Condiment

Dijon mustard

~~Hamburger pickle relish~~
~~Hot mustard sauce~~
~~Sweet pickle relish~~
Yellow mustard

Fruit or extract

Imitation vanilla extract, alcohol
Imitation vanilla extract, no alcohol
Lemon juice
Lime juice
Orange peel
Raw lemon
Raw lime
Ripe olives, canned
Vanilla extract

Leavening agents

Baking powder
Baking soda
Cream of tartar

Pepper

Black pepper
Chili peppers
Crushed red pepper flakes
Freeze dried sweet red peppers
Red or cayenne pepper
Trader Joe's Lemon Pepper Seasoning Blend
White pepper

Salad Dressings

Balsamic Vinegar
Champagne vinegar
Cider vinegar
Distilled vinegar
Maple Grove Farms of Vermont Fat Free Greek Dressing
Red wine vinegar
Rice wine vinegar
Walden Farms Sesame Calorie Free Dressings
White wine vinegar

Sauce

Bragg Liquid Coconut Aminos All Purpose Seasoning
Cocktail sauce
Hot sauce
PACE Tequila Lime salsa
Pepper sauce
Pico de gallo
Salsa, ready-to-serve
TABASCO
Triple pepper salsa
Worcestershire

Spice, dry

Anise seed
Baharat, Middle Eastern Seasoning
Basil
Bay leaf
Cacao powder
Cajun seasoning
Caraway seed
Cardamom

Celery seed
Chervil
Chili dry seasoning mix
Chili powder
Cocoa powder
Coriander leaf
Coriander seed
Cumin seed
Curry powder
Dehydrated onion
Dill seed
Dill weed
Fennel seed
Fenugreek seed
Fines Herbes
Freeze dried shallots
Garlic powder
Ground allspice
Ground cinnamon
Ground cloves
Ground ginger
Ground mace
Ground mustard seed
Ground nutmeg
Ground sage
Ground savory
Ground turmeric
Harissa powder
Herbes De Provence
Italian seasoning
Louisiana Fish Fry Products Cajun Seasoning
Marjoram
McCormick Gourmet Collection Blends Greek Seasoning
Old Bay Seasoning
Onion powder
Oregano
Paprika

Parsley
Poppy seed
Poultry seasoning
Pumpkin pie spice
Rosemary
Saffron
Salt
Seasoning mix, dry, sazon, coriander & annatto
Spearmint
Taco seasoning mix
Tarragon
Thyme

Spice, wet or fresh

Capers
Fresh basil
Fresh dill weed
Fresh lemon grass (citronella)
Fresh rosemary
Fresh thyme
Peppermint leaves
Raw chives
Raw garlic
Raw ginger root
Spearmint leaves

Sweetener

Aspartame
Erythritol
Pectin
Saccharine
Stevia liquid
Stevia powder

Takeaways for Chapter 9

- Eat well-balanced, healthy meals.

- Eat as much as you want of Unlimiteds.

- Avoid hi-GI and high-Glycemic Load foods.

- If you eat the right foods in the right balance, you will be satisfied with fewer calories than you burn.

- Must Haves satiate and fight cancer and other diseases.

- Have some Must Haves with every meal.

- Have at least one serving of Appetite Suppressors every day.

- Have at least one serving of Appetite Suppressors, Sweet Super Foods, and/or Anti-Agers during three meals a day.

- Consume at least 96 ounces of water each day if female and at least 120 ounces if male, including the water in your food and beverages. (Some apps count this for you.)

Chapter 10

Frequency

Where will your calories go?

Will your body use them to store fat? This may be what you are choosing now. Wouldn't it be better for your calories to maintain a feeling of high energy and to build and repair lean tissues? What and how often you eat has a major impact on how the calories are used.

Eat the right kinds of foods every three to four hours to dramatically shift how your calories are used. This keeps you energetic between meals and cause less energy to go to fat. When you feel energetic, you are more likely to be active and burn more calories. Eating frequent balanced meals that include small amounts of natural proteins with each meal makes amino acids (the building blocks of protein) more continuously available in your blood stream. When amino acids are available, they can be used to build and repair lean tissues, which boosts your metabolic rate.

Frequent eating does not need to be difficult. Meals can be extremely simple and take only a few minutes, or they can be leisurely. That is completely up to you. We'll talk more later about guidance for meal planning.

To help your body utilize nutrients effectively, make sure to have sufficient carbohydrates and protein in each meal in accordance with your Countable Ranges (Chapter 24). Natural proteins and low-GI carbohydrates help with satiety. They also help with muscle retention.

Retaining or building muscle is extremely important in the quest for sustained weight loss. Muscle mass helps with overall health and vitality and strength, but it also burns calories. The greater your muscle mass, all other things being equal, the more calories you will burn each day. In this chapter, we will discuss how meal frequency impacts muscle retention and fat burning.

Steady blood sugar

The more steadily sugar (glucose) is introduced in small quantities into our bloodstreams, the more usable energy we have throughout each day. Feeling more energetic makes us more productive and more inclined to be active. The more immediately available energy we have throughout each day, the more calories we are likely to burn.

Our digestive systems break down different foods at different rates. Carbohydrates that put blood glucose into the bloodstream extremely rapidly (hi-GI foods) include refined sugars, white rice, potato and bleached flour products such as white bread. These foods can spike your blood sugar. Your body reacts quickly to sugar spikes by releasing extra insulin. If you are not insulin resistant, insulin will direct your body to quickly convert the blood sugar to fat. Then, your energy level crashes, and you feel drowsy.

Natural starches and sugars enter the blood at varying rates. Glycemic load is a measure of how much total sugar goes into your bloodstream over a period of time from 100 grams of any given food. The Eat As Much As You Want system's Unlimiteds and the recommended Countables mostly have low-GI, low-glycemic load foods. These are low-caloric density foods that contain calories that turn to glucose slowly in digestion, so the bloodstream will not be overloaded with a sudden influx of sugar.

When the foods you eat convert very slowly to blood sugar, this keeps blood sugar levels steadier, which prevents so much of it from being stored as fat. Steadier blood sugar levels are what give you that feeling of having more usable energy. If you are insulin resistant, steady blood sugar levels are especially important, because elevated blood sugar can cause severe damage to lean tissues.

Your goal is to burn fat, not store it. If you feel energetic because of steady blood sugar, you'll want to move, and you'll burn more calories. If you feel lethargic due to a blood sugar spike and crash, you'll want to nap, and you won't burn many calories.

Protein: building block or glucose and uric acid

Protein is also a vital nutrient. Any protein your body uses to build and repair lean tissues does not break down into calories. Moreover, the more lean tissues you have, the more calories your body burns while at rest.

For good health and vitality, strive to at least retain the muscles you already have by getting regular exercise. Exercise is not enough, though. You also have to eat slowly-digesting proteins throughout the day, so the proteins can be used as building blocks for lean tissue repair and growth. Most proteins from whole foods digest slowly and enter the bloodstream as amino acids. However, once amino acids get into the bloodstream, they break down rapidly if they are not used right away. If they break down, they become glucose and uric acid. At that point, they cannot be used as building blocks. Consuming small amounts of protein at all your meals throughout the day makes it possible for your body to use more of it for repair and growth.

Other than immediately following a workout, cells in lean tissues only invite amino acids in for repair and growth when their insulin receptor sites are open. This means there must be a modest amount of insulin circulating, and the necessary insulin levels only happen in healthy bodies when there is adequate blood sugar circulating as well. *Frequent correctly-balanced meals -- including low-GI and low-GL carbohydrates, along with the right amounts of complex proteins -- can provide both amino acids and blood glucose at the same time and in the correct proportions to support the efficient use by muscle cells of amino acids as building blocks.*

My Fitness Journey

I am stronger and have a better-looking physique than I did before I learned how to eat right, and that was decades ago. In late 2004, I was as weak as a kitten and unable to do a single pull up. Just two years later, I was doing multiple sets of pull-ups with a 40-pound weight hanging from me.

One afternoon, I was at a warehouse with a co-worker who was very muscular with impressively large biceps. We were killing time waiting for someone, and he spied a long steel bar. On a lark he put it on a nearby scale and found that it weighed 50 pounds. Then, with a twinkle in his eye, he started to do single-arm curls with it as he looked at me. He struggled.

"The length of this thing makes this a lot harder," he said. "You should give it a try."

There was no question in my mind that he had done more curls than I would ever be able to do with that bar. This was a guy who lifted weights regularly and took protein supplements to bulk up. All I had been doing was eating a balanced diet of whole foods five times a day and exercising regularly including running and a variety of exercises in all different planes of motion.

I picked the weight up after he had done all he could. I was shocked to find I could actually do more reps than he had, even though my biceps were much smaller.

This was direct evidence that eating right and providing my body with high quality foods and the right kinds of exercise had helped my body to synthesize higher quality muscle fibers and made my body function better. I could never bench press as much as he or do any number of other weight lifting feats that he could do, but in a real world situation of bearing a heavy and unstable load with my arms, my little biceps were more capable than his massive ones.

Make Better Muscles

Years later, studies would come out that explained my experience that day with my co-worker. He was consuming a huge amount of protein, but the quantity of protein consumed in a day is not the only factor that dictates how well your muscles will recover from a workout. Eating protein more frequently in smaller amounts allows your digestive tract to release small amounts of amino acids into the bloodstream at any one time. This increases the proportion of amino acids that can be absorbed by the muscles and other lean tissues before they break down.

Studies have shown the importance of evenly distributing protein throughout the day across multiple meals for optimal muscle repair and development. This 2014 study[72] looked at even distribution across three meals a day instead of concentrating protein into the evening meal:

> *"[C]onsuming a moderate amount of high-quality protein 3 times a day stimulates muscle protein synthesis to a greater extent than the common practice of skewing protein consumption toward the evening meal. Specifically, 24-h muscle protein synthesis was ~25% greater when protein intake was evenly distributed..."*

A 2018 study[73] went even further. They found that the body is only capable of absorbing a small amount of protein at a time, so to maximize the body's ability to use amino acids for lean tissue growth and repair, we should be eating a minimum of four meals a day.

The authors of this same study[73] also said

---

[72] "Dietary Protein Distribution Positively Influences 24-h Muscle Protein Synthesis in Healthy Adults." Mamerow et al., June 2014, *The Journal of Nutrition*, National Institutes of Health pubmed, https://www.ncbi.nlm.nih.gov/pmc/articles/PMC4018950/
[73] "How much protein can the body use in a single meal for muscle-building? Implications for daily protein distribution." Schoenfeld and Aragon, February 27 2018, *Journal of the International Society of Sports Nutrition*, National Institutes of Health pubmed, https://www.ncbi.nlm.nih.gov/pubmed/29497353

"Consumption of slower-acting protein sources, particularly when consumed in combination with other macronutrients, would delay absorption and thus conceivably enhance the utilization of the constituent amino acids."

Put another way, slow-digesting proteins consumed along with slow-digesting carbohydrates enhance the body's ability to use the proteins for lean-tissue growth and repair.

Note that I substituted "carbohydrates" for "other macronutrients" in my paraphrase. Robert Cruder, a former student at University of Missouri-Columbia, explained this nicely[74],:

"Protein DOES require significant energy to digest but more importantly the deposition of temporary lean tissue requires… as much as 10 times… the energy content of the amino acids being assembled. On a high-carb diet, that is easily available from glucose. On a low-carb diet energy is supplied far more slowly from fats and ketone bodies. That may prevent muscle from utilizing all the available amino acids and allow them to just become glucose."

Thus, high-quality carbs are needed in your diet so your body can efficiently use proteins as building blocks for lean tissue repair. This further supports the points made in Chapter 4 about appropriate consumption of carbohydrates.

Amino acids don't last

There is a common misunderstanding about protein. Many people mistakenly think amino acids just circulate about until the

---

[74] https://www.quora.com/How-long-does-consumed-protein-stay-on-your-system-to-be-used-for-muscle-repair-growth-Is-there-any-protein-poll-which-would-stock-this-protein-for-use-when-needed-like-with-fat-energy

body uses them for muscle growth. That is incorrect. Others think that amino acids go into the bloodstream and circulate for many hours. That is also incorrect. The truth is amino acids only circulate in the bloodstream extremely briefly. For that reason, it is important to send the amino acids into the bloodstream slowly in a constant trickle spread throughout the day.

Evenly-distributed protein intake from natural sources spread over multiple meals a day helps to optimize the use of amino acids for lean tissue repair and growth. Natural sources include soy, meat, fish, eggs, and poultry, but not supplements such as protein drinks and powders. Natural proteins are much more complex, so they tend to break down very slowly as they move from the stomach to the intestines. They also digest slowly in the small intestine, where they break down into amino acids and small peptides.

The entire process is so gradual that nearly 100% of them get absorbed into the lining of the intestine and from there into the bloodstream, and the amino acids enter the bloodstream in a slow trickle that is spread over the time of digestion.

If it were not for this slow trickle, most of the amino acids would become unusable for muscle repair and growth. According to Cruder,

"Blood from the intestine passes through the liver before entering general circulation. Some fraction of amino acids are converted into glucose on that pass. The proportion is somewhat sensitive to the existing level of liver glycogen but common estimates are that HALF of the amino acids might be lost at that point…

"The remaining amino acids enter general circulation and are available to muscles… Whatever is not taken up by muscle circulates back to the liver where it is converted into glucose. It is reasonable to assume that the liver destroys HALF on each pass and that each pass requires only minutes… [74]*"*

Thus, the more evenly distributed the protein intake during the day, and the more complex the protein is, the more effective the body can be at using the amino acids. Keep in mind, however, that you also must create a demand for the protein, because muscles will only ask for amino acids if they are needed. See Chapter 18 for the exercise principles that will create that demand and spur the resulting retention or growth of muscle tissue.

Get your protein from whole foods

Despite his big muscles, my co-worker had been getting a lot of his protein from supplements. This was a mistake. A better approach would have been to vary his protein sources more and to emphasize complex natural proteins that do not digest quickly. Cruder[74] points out protein supplements that move out of the stomach too quickly are relatively useless for lean tissue repair or muscle development. Specifically, whey isolate and hydrolyzed whey are broken down and go into the bloodstream far faster than natural proteins, leading to their conversion by the liver to glucose instead of their use as building blocks:

> *"Proteins which ARE absorbed but which reach the bloodstream more rapidly than muscle can utilize them are again destroyed within minutes."*

Livestrong.com explains[75] that one of the reasons a refined supplement may be faster to digest (and thus, according to Cruder, less available to muscles) is the fact that it is probably in a simpler form than a protein coming from whole food:

---

[75] "How Quickly Does Protein Metabolize." Lauren Armstrong, Reviewed by Lindsey Elizabeth Pfau, MS, RD, CSSD, LD/N, October 17 2019, *LiveStrong.com*, https://www.livestrong.com/article/550839-how-quickly-does-protein-metabolize/

"[T]here are multiple factors that can affect the protein digestion time. One of those factors is the composition of the consumed protein.

"The simplest forms of protein are strings of amino acids held together by peptide bonds. Foods that we consume contain proteins in their most complex form, where the strings of amino acids within the protein are raveled up. They need to be unraveled, and broken apart, in order for the intestines to absorb the individual amino acids and transfer them into the bloodstream.

"The acids within the stomach help to unfold all of the raveled amino acid chains, allowing digestive enzymes produced by the stomach's wall to work on breaking the peptide bonds apart. The easier it is to reach the amino acids, the quicker the protein can be processed.

"Therefore, protein with a composition that is less-complex has quicker digestive rates. Whey protein, found in milk, is an example of a quick-digesting protein. Its absorption rate has been estimated at approximately 10 grams per hour, compared to a cooked egg that has an absorption rate of approximately 3 grams per hour, according to the Journal of the International Society of Sports Nutrition…"

In case you might think that the comparison above is between milk and egg, think again. Whey protein is only a small part of the total protein in milk. Casein, the main protein in milk, makes up about 82% of the total milk protein.[76] Casein digests more slowly than whey. Thus, milk has a combination of faster and more slowly digesting proteins that naturally spreads out the release of amino acids into your bloodstream.

---

[76] "Milk Protein", Milk Facts,
http://www.milkfacts.info/Milk%20Composition/Protein.htm

Jim Frith

When you are getting most of your protein from whey, you are always getting it from a supplement. Thus, the complex proteins found in whole foods are far more effective in helping you to retain or build high quality muscle fibers than the proteins found in supplements.

Other supplements such as pea protein isolate are similarly fast to be absorbed into the bloodstream after consumption. Promoters of pea protein talk about how nearly complete it is, which is good. But they also tout the fact that it is highly absorbable into the bloodstream and as beneficial as whey protein isolate as if this is a good thing. This marketing strategy plays on the fact that most people do not know that fast absorption undermines the body's ability to use the protein for lean tissue repair. Bragging about it implies that this is a favorable characteristic when in fact it is not.

Eat Five Times a Day

Eating frequently is counter-intuitive. Most people think they will lose weight faster and better if they only eat when they are hungry. This is wrong!

Eating while hungry will likely cause us to eat much more, because hunger slows the satiation response in the brain. In other words, it takes more food to satisfy us. Hunger also triggers cravings for sugar and fat, breaks down our willpower to make good food choices, and slows down our metabolism. This is a huge booby trap that leads many people back to the yo-yo.

Eating frequent, nutritionally-balanced meals allows our brains to register satiety quickly and to stay satisfied longer. Fewer calories will be needed to keep our bodies nourished and satisfied with such meals, and they help us to have faster metabolisms.

Takeaways for Chapter 10

- Consume a balance of protein, slow-digesting carbohydrates, and nutrient-rich low-caloric density foods every three to four hours.

- Get your proteins from whole foods such as chicken, fish or dairy, because they break down more slowly and build a higher quality of muscle fiber.

- Slow-digesting carbohydrates put sugar into your bloodstream more steadily, which supports higher usable energy and higher quality protein synthesis.

- Balanced, nutrient-rich meals every three to four hours provide a broad spectrum of nutrients just when our bodies need them throughout the day.

- A steady supply of complete nutrients in your bloodstream speeds your metabolism and makes you stronger and healthier.

- A fast, healthy metabolism will help you to lose weight and to keep it off without hunger or cravings.

Chapter 11

Kick the Sugar Habit

Refined Sugar is Like Heroin

Neither one exists in nature. They're both addictive. They're toxic. Our bodies are not built to handle them in high concentrations. Excessive regular use of either of them can lead to body systems shutting down and to the destruction of lean tissues.

Common Sense

Refined sugar tastes really good. In fact, it tastes so good that it encourages you to consume more calories than you should. And it dulls your taste for the natural sweetness of healthy, whole foods. The more frequently you eat refined sugar, the more frequently you will crave more of it.

Refined sugar is highly inflammatory, so if it is consumed frequently over a long time, it frequently leads to type 2 diabetes. The damage I have seen in multiple people from long-term refined-sugar use includes blindness, missing teeth, amputations, edema, spider veins, lack of mobility and overall poor health.

Do this first

The first step toward a healthy body -- or toward sustainable weight loss -- is to kick the refined sugar habit. Don't try to start a weight-loss diet and kick sugar at the same time. Deal with the addiction first. If your body is in open rebellion against you because of your sugar addiction, that will undermine your other efforts to lose weight and keep it off.

It's just a minor indulgence, right?

I've been there! I've gone through periods of my life when I regularly craved sugar. In our popular culture, we joke about sugar addiction, then we rave about businesses that sell sweets "to die for," or a cookie recipe or a favorite sweet dessert. The whole thing is very alluring. Our culture glorifies sugar.

Some very well-meaning people love to bake sweets and pastries to distribute to the elderly and shut-ins. Church socials feature big spreads of sweets, and congregants sometimes compete to bake the most enticing recipes. It all seems so innocent.

I was married for 26 years to a fantastic cook who regularly made baked goods for her friends, family, and community members. Eyes would light up when she entered a room carrying her creations such as cakes and cinnamon rolls drenched in sugar glaze. I was the biggest fan of all of her cooking. Yet, despite my efforts to resist those temptations, when I indulged, I could physically feel the sugar rush surging through my arteries and into my brain.

At times, I would think of my grandmother. When I was a boy, we would visit her in the mountains of Pennsylvania, and I loved to stand in her kitchen to watch her bake rhubarb pies and her ever-popular "1-2-3-4 pineapple upside down cake". Those sugar rushes from my wife's cooking brought me back to the pure delights of tasting Grandma Frith's gooey glazed sugary tops of the finished cakes.

But my kitchen conversations with Grandma were sometimes a challenge. She was a strong, commanding woman who could issue clear instructions as if they were orders. She told me where to go to find, identify, and pick rhubarb for her. But she also seemed to stumble over remembering answers to questions she had already asked me.

Unfortunately, refined sugar is not a minor indulgence; it is a major health hazard. In addition to causing obesity and diabetes, regular refined-sugar intake is linked to heart disease, depression, cancer, impaired cognitive function, and dementia. It is highly addictive. Despite being seen as an energy source, a spike in blood sugar leads to a drop in energy shortly afterwards. It can cause tiredness, drowsiness, anxiety, irritability, and mood swings.

My memories of those visits to Grandma's house also recalled the hushed conversations among adults in her living room while she worked in the kitchen. My parents and my aunt and uncle were very concerned about her.

"Why is Grandma becoming so forgetful?" I asked.

"She has a circulation problem," I was told.

Little was known about the causes of dementia at that time. In retrospect, it is obvious they had not connected her sweet tooth with any part of her memory issues. We can never fully know what caused it, but her slight forgetfulness soon progressed to full-blown dementia. My childless aunt and uncle moved her to Virginia to live with them for the last 20 years of her life.

She became gaunt and frail, and she regressed to her childhood. She became stuck in the 4th grade, talking about events of her day as a fourth grader as if they were current. The responsibility for caring for her robbed my aunt and uncle of freedom and destroyed their health.

How is sugar regulated in your Body?

A hormone called insulin regulates blood sugar to keep it at healthy levels in your bloodstream. However, your bloodstream is only able to hold about 80 to 100 calories of blood sugar (glucose) at a time. Significantly more for a sustained amount of time causes terrible damage to your lean tissues. When you eat foods that cause your blood sugar to rise, your pancreas over-releases insulin to quickly purge it. The only place that sugar can go quickly from blood is to fat. Suddenly, you will have newly-stored fat, and your blood sugar will be low. This process is exactly what my body was going through on my boyhood Thanksgivings.

Marketers who sell candy bars and call them "energy bars" can legally make that claim, because any food that has calories in it is delivering energy. However, when that "energy" comes in the form of a sugar high, it will soon lead to a sugar crash.

Those are short-term effects of high sugar intake, but what about the long term? Over a period of years, if you regularly eat too much refined sugar and other hi-GI foods, your body is likely to develop insulin resistance, or type 2 diabetes. When this happens, blood sugar levels can go out of control.

What's so bad about sugar?

Sustained high blood sugar is highly toxic to your body. The damage to your body can be severe. I have known many people with diabetes who have lost body parts due to sugar damage: toes, fingers, eyes, feet, and legs. High blood sugar can kill you.

I once had a client come to me when he was in his seventies. Just walking around his yard and up and down his driveway was a huge challenge for him. He had too much weight around his middle, and he had a "circulation problem". He spent his days sitting a lot, and hardly got up from his chair. He had type 2 diabetes.

"I'm next," he told me.

"Next for what?" I asked.

"All of my brothers and sisters have lost limbs because of high sugar," he said. "I'm the only one who still has both feet."

"Are you still eating sugar?" I asked.

"I love sugar," he answered. "I can't give it up."

"If you don't want the same outcome as your siblings, you need to give it up. And you need to start getting more exercise."

Sadly, his heart was not in it. He did not want to hear any advice that included giving up sugar. He stopped coming. A couple of months later I called him to encourage him to return. He told me the little toe on one of his feet had been amputated to save the rest of his foot. He had scraped it, then it became infected and it would not heal because of the diabetes.

"Have you stopped eating sugar?" I asked.

"I can't. It's my main pleasure in life."

This made me very sad. Worse, there are many other sugar addiction stories I could tell. I have seen in the eyes of too many people that sugar is powerfully addictive.

Cigarette smoking is similar to that. I had a client who really wanted to get healthy, and she said she desperately wanted to quit cigarette smoking.

"It's a very nasty habit," she told me. "But I can't quit. I know that about myself."

She had emphysema, and she came to workouts towing an oxygen tank on a little cart behind her. Her loving neighbors who had referred her to me said her house was always smoky and littered with cigarette butts and ashtrays.

Unfortunately, her attempts at regaining her health were too little too late. After several months of her coming see me with tank in tow, she finally emailed to say she no longer had the strength to leave her house. Her neighbors, still coming to see me, reported that she had continued to chain-smoke despite her awful condition. A few months later, she died. Once again, I was deeply saddened.

Sugar, cigarettes and heroin. They are all addictive. They are all potentially highly damaging and can even be fatal. Of the three, sugar is the most insidious, because it is socially accepted and even encouraged, few people recognize how bad it can be for you, and there is little social support for kicking the addiction.

But you can beat the addiction if you decide to. I am going to tell you how in just a moment.

Addiction Compromises Judgment

When you are addicted to something that interferes with your ability to think clearly, that makes combating the addiction even more difficult. A lot of people who have asked to be my clients have told me the one place they draw the line is they will not give up sugar. They want a magic bullet that allows them to lose weight and get into shape while continuing to regularly consume sugar.

Acknowledge that sugar is a problem you need to solve. If you cannot see that it is harming you or holding you back from attaining your goals, you will not permanently achieve them. While you are still able to deny its impact, it has probably not caused you to have full-blown dementia or to lose a limb. But it may be affecting your judgment at the same time that it is causing inflammation that supports obesity.

Sugar clouds your mind. Mice that were fed a high-fat or high-sugar diet by researchers at Oregon State University were unable to navigate mazes as well as mice who did not have the high-fat or high-sugar diets:[77]

"In this research, after just four weeks on a high-fat or a high-sugar diet, the performance of mice on various tests of mental and physical function began to drop, compared to animals on a normal diet. One of the most pronounced changes was in what researchers call cognitive flexibility.

"'The impairment of cognitive flexibility in this study was pretty strong,' [said Kathy Magnusson, a professor in the OSU College of Veterinary Medicine and principal investigator with the Linus Pauling Institute.] 'Think about

---

[77] "Fat, sugar cause bacterial changes that may relate to loss of cognitive function." Oregon State University, June 22 2015, https://today.oregonstate.edu/archives/2015/jun/fat-sugar-cause-bacterial-changes-may-relate-loss-cognitive-function

driving home on a route that's very familiar to you, something you're used to doing. Then one day that road is closed and you suddenly have to find a new way home.'

"A person with high levels of cognitive flexibility would immediately adapt to the change, determine the next best route home, and remember to use the same route the following morning, all with little problem. With impaired flexibility, it might be a long, slow, and stressful way home."

In a 2018 study by Zheng et al., diabetes was associated with acceleration in cognitive decline.[78] These findings were echoed by another 2018 study, this one by Lee et al.:

"[C]hronic exposure to diabetic environment with high fat/high sugar diets and physical/mental stress can cause hyperglycemia, one of the main characteristics of insulin resistance, metabolic syndrome, and diabetes...

"Cognitive impairment is often accompanied by progression of diabetes. The association between diabetes and dementia is supported by findings from several epidemiological studies... Once dementia is diagnosed and pathological changes become evident, it is difficult to reverse its progression."[79]

My point is that kicking a sugar addiction is extremely important, not only for weight loss, but also for intelligence, cognition, good

---

[78] "HbA$_{1c}$, diabetes and cognitive decline: the English Longitudinal Study of Ageing." Zheng et al., April 2018, *Diabetologia*, https://link.springer.com/article/10.1007/s00125-017-4541-7

[79] "Diabetes and Alzheimer's Disease: Mechanisms and Nutritional Aspects." Lee et al., October 23 2018, *Clinical Nutrition Research*, National Institutes of Health, https://www.ncbi.nlm.nih.gov/pmc/articles/PMC6209735/

health, quality of life, and longevity. No matter what diet plan you follow, a sugar addiction can derail all of your best intentions.

Take your time. This process will probably take at least three weeks if you are really going to kick the sugar habit for good. From then on, it will take strong discipline not to backslide. Sugar is so highly addictive that a single episode of eating a lot of it can send you right back into the abyss of addiction that you worked so hard to end.

It's worth it to beat sugar. You are now forewarned about the pitfalls.

How to Stop the Addiction:

You can definitely do this! Build a foundation for your weight-loss and health-enhancement efforts. Before you start trying to "diet" with planned meals or caloric restriction, first focus completely on eliminating refined sugars with these 10 steps:

Step 1. Reflect on how sugar has impacted you in the past and how it could impact you in the future.

Think about any of the following that has occurred after consuming a significant amount of sugar: bouts of depression, anxiety, irritability, mood swings, tiredness or drowsiness. Do you want to have more consistent energy and emotional stability?

Are you insulin resistant, or do you have heart disease? If so, think about the dire consequences of uncontrolled high blood sugar. If not, has anyone in your family suffered from either of these conditions? What happened to them? Are you concerned enough about this for yourself to take steps to avoid it?

I remain amazed that the client I told you about knew that all of his siblings had lost limbs due to type 2 diabetes and continued sugar consumption, yet he could not bring himself to give up sugar.

Has anyone in your family had Alzheimer's or dementia? Is that something you would like to avoid? This has been my most powerful motivation to avoid sugar. I do not want to repeat Grandma's experience or to be a burden on other family members.

Are you tired of being overweight? Are you concerned about the long-term health consequences of that? Are you able to connect the dots between chronic sugar addiction and extra weight? I have coached a large number of people through weight loss, and the ones who have struggled the most and had the least success are the ones who would not give up sugar.

If you are male, are you concerned about a future of erectile dysfunction (ED)?

> *"Studies of ED suggest that its prevalence in men with diabetes ranges from 35–75% versus 26% in general population. The onset of ED also occurs 10–15 years earlier in men with diabetes than it does in sex-matched counterparts without diabetes."[80]*

Please think very carefully about the answers to these questions, and write about them. Keep what you have written, whether on paper or in your computer, in an easily accessible place. Refer to often, especially whenever you get tempted to relapse.

---

[80] "Diabetes and Erectile Dysfunction." Chu and Edelman, January 2001, *Clinical Diabetes*, https://clinical.diabetesjournals.org/content/19/1/45

Step 2. Begin to eat more sweet Unlimiteds. Specifically, eat plenty of the foods that are nutrient rich and naturally sweet, and have a low-caloric density and low-GI. Some of these include blueberries, raspberries, strawberries, cherries, plums, oranges, apples, grapefruits, clementines, peaches and nectarines. These fruits are good for you, and they can satisfy your sweet tooth without spiking your blood sugar.

Two great examples of healthy, delicious Unlimiteds are tangerines and grapefruit. For example, Tangerines (also known as mandarin oranges or clementines) are super sweet and delicious. They are packed with high-value phytonutrients including Vitamin C and A, fiber and flavonoids. Yet, with a moderate GI, the sugars in tangerines will turn to blood sugar slowly. This makes tangerines of great value to anyone who is attempting to break a refined sugar habit, because they can eat tangerines instead of giving into the temptation of unhealthy sugary foods. Grapefruit has more Vitamin C and A and flavonoids by volume than tangerines and a super low GI, so grapefruits and tangerines each hold an important place in a healthy diet. If tart flavors appeal to you, then by all means fill up on grapefruit.

Be sure to eat your fruits whole, not juiced, if you are trying to lose weight, because they will satisfy your appetite better that way. Also, choose raw over canned. Raw tangerines, for example, have a lower GI (42 versus 47.) Citrus of various kinds has potent, wonderful flavor that lends it to use in many dishes -- both cooked and raw -- so add sections to a salad or to a veggie dish, and let the flavors merge and explode!

Step 3. Fill up on other Unlimiteds and recommended Countables while eating frequently enough that you are not hungry (i.e., five times a day.) Steps 2 and 3 are perhaps the most important ones, because they prevent hunger.

Step 4. Educate yourself about where your sugar is coming from. Processed foods are a huge source of sugars, so you should look at food labels before you buy them. Know the names of sugars. They may be called by any number of names ending in "ose", but that is an imperfect way of identifying what to avoid. For example, lactose, which is in milk, actually takes a long time to digest, so it is low-GI and okay to have unless you are lactose intolerant. Fructose, which occurs naturally in whole natural fruits, is moderate-GI, and is similarly okay to have if consumed in whole fruits.

However, sucrose, dextrose, and "high fructose" are high-GI sugars, so avoid them when you can or consume them only in very small quantities. Other ingredients to avoid or severely limit are table sugar, cane sugar, corn syrup, fruit juice concentrate, brown sugar, molasses, corn sugar, honey, raw sugar, turbinado sugar, and maltodextrin. Think seriously about beginning to cut back on processed foods in favor of whole, natural foods.

Step 5. Find alternatives to sugar. Cloves and cinnamon are great in coffee. Oregano, thyme, basil, rosemary and garlic are great in tomato sauces. Stevia and monk fruit extract are examples of calorie-free herbal sweeteners. Cardamom mixed with coffee gives an interesting Middle Eastern twist to the flavor. Cocoa powder, cacao powder, vanilla extract, and Chai tea blend are other possibilities, especially in combination with an herbal sweetener.

I don't encourage you to make a habit of eating or drinking artificial sweeteners such as saccharin, sucralose, and aspartame, because they can disrupt your ability to taste the sweetness and wholesome flavors of whole foods, and there is some controversy about whether they may be unhealthy. Some people report that artificial sweeteners spur sugar cravings for them. The following gives me even greater pause:

> "Recent evidence from Suez et al.. suggests that consumption of all types of artificial sweeteners is actually more likely to induce glucose intolerance than consumption of pure glucose and sucrose… The evidence seems to suggest that, contrary to popular belief, artificial sweeteners

may actually be unhealthier to consume than natural sugars."[81]

Despite this serious controversy, I do not object to artificial sweeteners for the purpose of facilitating weight loss if you feel you must, because 53% of participants surveyed in the National Weight Control Registry regularly drink low/no calorie sweetened beverages.[67] I leave it to you to decide whether elimination of artificial sweeteners from your diet is a worthwhile goal.

Step 6. If you are not insulin resistant, **consider when it might be okay to have up to about 100 calories of a healthy sweet.** A little high-GI food within 30 minutes of a workout can accelerate recovery if it is in combination with some protein.

If you are not insulin resistant, then as you wean yourself from a refined sugar habit, replace the refined sugars after workouts with healthy, high-GI foods such as red grapes, mango, watermelon, or pineapple. The sooner you can make that transition, the better.

On the other hand, if you *are* insulin resistant, then you should avoid high-GI foods all the time, because your body will not handle the increase in blood sugar appropriately.

Step 7. Cut back or eliminate your consumption of foods that turn rapidly to blood sugar after you eat them. Many of these do not contain sugar, so you will not find sugars on labels for these foods. Examples are potatoes, corn, gluten-free pastas, white rice and breads containing bleached flour. Replace these foods with others that are low-GI such as quinoa, wild rice, and coarse-grained breads.

---

[81] "Influence of diet on the gut microbiome and implications for human health." Singh et al., April 8 2017, *Journal of Translational Medicine*, National Institutes of Health, https://www.ncbi.nlm.nih.gov/pmc/articles/PMC5385025/

Step 8. Eat foods containing probiotics. There has been a tremendous amount of research in recent years on the beneficial impact of the trillions of microorganisms dwelling in our digestive tracts.

A recent study found that simple sugars in your diet "silence" the colonization of good bacteria in the gut,[82] (which makes the case for kicking the sugar addiction all the stronger).

Probiotics have a positive impact on the gut that specifically helps with health, increases leptin, suppresses appetite, and improves glucose metabolism. Gut health, which is helped by probiotics, is vital to overall good health:

> *"Changes in present-day society such as diets with more sugar, salt, and saturated fat, bad habits and unhealthy lifestyles contribute to the likelihood of the involvement of the microbiota in inflammatory diseases, which contribute to global epidemics of obesity, depression, and mental health concerns.*
>
> *"Ingestion of vibrant probiotics, especially those contained in fermented foods, is found to cause significant positive improvements in balancing intestinal permeability and barrier function. Our guts control and deal with every aspect of our health. How we digest our food and even the food sensitivities we have is linked with our mood, behavior, energy, weight, food cravings, hormone balance, immunity, and overall wellness."[83]*

---

[82] "Dietary sugar silences a colonization factor in a mammalian gut symbiont." Townsend et al., January 2 2019, National Academy of Sciences, *Proceedings of the National Academy of Sciences*, https://www.pnas.org/content/116/1/233

[83] "One Health, Fermented Foods, and Gut Microbiota." Bell et al., Dec 2018, *Foods Magazine*, National Institutes of Health pubmed, https://www.ncbi.nlm.nih.gov/pmc/articles/PMC6306734/

A 2016 study[84] on zebrafish larvae showed that leptin levels increased after treatment with probiotics, thus suppressing appetites. Zebrafish are similar enough genetically to humans that this is thought to be a very significant finding.

> "In the present study we observed changes of zebrafish gut microbiota composition induced by [a bacteria found in probiotics]. The resultant microbiome decreased appetite and glucose by regulating the transcription of genes involved in the control of feed intake and glucose metabolism."

Specifically, they found that probiotics introduced into the digestive system increased leptin, decreased appetite, and increased glucose metabolism. A host of other studies I have already discussed have shown that an increase in leptin translates to a speeding up of the metabolic rate.

Obviously, it will be easier to kick the sugar habit and lose weight if your appetite is suppressed and your metabolism is sped up. Conversely, if sugar stays in the diet, and the good bacteria remain suppressed, and leptin remains lower, then your appetite for more sugar will remain strong. So be sure to add probiotics to your diet as you cut out the sugar.

Step 9. Think positively. In fact, use positive language to describe your decision to quit eating harmful sugars. "I've decided not to eat sugar", or "I am eating healthily these days" is a lot more empowering than "I can't eat sugar," "I had to stop eating sugar," or "I wish I could eat sugar." When you think and speak positively about your decision, you are much more likely to stay with it.

---

[84] "Probiotic treatment reduces appetite and glucose level in the zebrafish model." Silvia Falcinelli et al., January 5 2016, *Scientific Reports*, https://www.nature.com/articles/srep18061

Step 10. **Quit cold turkey.** Only take this step after you have already cut back substantially on your sugar consumption and you are thorough in your adherence to steps 1 through 9, and you are absolutely committed to sticking it out.

Clients have told me that the sugar cravings are the worst in the first two to three days, then almost completely subside in two or three weeks. Quitting your sugar addiction is absolutely doable. Take it seriously, and you will do fine.

Here are some tips for how to get through the cold turkey period:

- **Chew gum.** The act of chewing helps with resistance of cravings

- **Move.** Workout or walk around the block. Exercise curbs sugar cravings

- **Stay busy.** Do not allow your mind to be idle.

- **Drink water.** Dehydration can make you crave sugar.

- **Get seven to eight hours of sleep a night.** Being sleep deprived or staying up late at night spurs sugar cravings.

- **Cut back on caffeine intake if you have type 2 diabetes.** It can cause your blood sugar to swing, which increases sugar cravings.

- **Think ahead.** Decide in advance what sensations you may miss whenever you have cravings. If it is crunchiness, have crunchy Unlimiteds available like carrots or celery. If it is sweetness, have sweet Unlimiteds available to you. Try to avoid having foods with refined sugars available.

- **Accept that withdrawal symptoms will end.** You may experience headaches, fatigue, and irritability. These are just ways that sugar is calling to you. Don't answer! Remember, it will only be a few days before the symptoms will pass.

Quitting refined sugars is worth it!

Without refined sugars, you will think more clearly. Your emotions will be steadier. You'll have more usable energy every day. You'll be much healthier, probably live longer, and lose weight far more easily.

Poor health feels awful. So many people spiral down in their late years because of lack of exercise and poor habits with food. They are miserable and dependent on others. Have you known anyone like that?

I have clients committed to taking good care of their health. Their lives are rich, full, satisfying and filled with purpose. They are independent, self-sufficient, intelligent, active, and fun to talk to.

I choose to follow the latter path. How about you?

Takeaways for Chapter 11

- **Refined sugar negatively impacts health, happiness and energy.**

- **Refined sugar leads to obesity.**

- **Refined sugar is highly addictive.**

- **Quit sugar before you start a weight-loss diet.**

- **Follow the 10 steps above to kick the sugar habit!**

Chapter 12

Countables

Ideal Balance = Satiety, Health & Longevity

Give your body what it needs, and you won't be hungry. You'll also have greater health and longevity. Your body needs more than calories. It needs the micronutrients in Unlimiteds. In this chapter, we will learn that your body also needs certain amounts of low-GI carbohydrates, complex proteins and healthy fats.

What are Countables Ranges?

In the Eat As Much As You Want system, each person is given a target range for how many grams to consume in each meal of Countable Carbs, Countable Proteins, and Countable Fats. Foods and drinks in the Countables lists are higher in caloric density than Unlimiteds, and thus consumption of them should be limited.

What do the Countables Ranges do?

Countables ranges were created to optimize the balance of macronutrients in each meal in order to keep your appetite satisfied and give your body what it needs without taking in more calories than necessary. This, in combination with eating Must Haves and other Unlimiteds, facilitates weight loss or weight maintenance (depending on your goal) while keeping your metabolic rate as high as your genetics will allow.

Certain Countables lists are favored over others, and I will give you examples from each list below. Foods that are lower in caloric density, lower in Glycemic Index or Glycemic Load, and higher in nutrient-content are the most favored.

Balancing macronutrients

When you first go on a diet, cutting calories makes you lose weight, no matter how you do it. This has been established by quite a few short-range studies. But it doesn't keep working for long.

A balanced diet is necessary for good health and longevity; I think we all know that. You also need a balanced diet to avoid weight-loss plateaus and starvation mode.

Balance means getting the amount your body needs of each macronutrient: carbohydrates, proteins and fats. It also means getting all of the plant nutrients and other micronutrients you need.

If you eat the right mix of foods, your body will tell you when you have had enough to eat. When Countables are limited, and you eat as much as you want of Unlimiteds, your body is able to tell you when you have had enough to eat. My clients -- even the ones who believed their hormones have always been out of whack – have been able to avoid hunger and still lose weight. By keeping Countables in their ranges, you will get the right balance of carbohydrates, proteins and fats.

Let's talk some about what constitutes healthy balance and how this is reflected in the Eat As Much As You Want system.

Carbohydrates

As you will recall from Chapter 4, the best health and mortality outcomes were for people who consume between about 50 and 55 percent of calories from low-GI carbohydrates.[24] Total carbohydrates in any amount less than 40 percent or more than 70 percent has a significant negative impact on life expectancy.

The Eat As Much As You Want system uses the Countables ranges and Unlimiteds to target 50 to 55 percent of calories coming from carbohydrates without you even having to think about it. Most of the macronutrients from Unlimiteds are carbs. Thus, the amount of carbohydrates allowed in your Countable Carbs range is only a fraction of the total carbs you will get in a meal. Our experience is that when people are allowed to eat Unlimiteds ad libitum, and they stay in their Countables Ranges, they choose naturally to consume amounts that average out to the ideal balance... no thinking necessary!

I had my programmers analyze 1072 meals created by a number of different people in accordance with the rules of the Eat As Much As You Want system (Chapter 24). The average amount of total carbohydrates was 53% of total calories per meal, including those from Countable Carbs and Unlimiteds. This is as close to ideal as one could hope for.

How does it work?

Your body is an amazing machine with a tremendous capacity for engineering its own health and survival. If it had not been so severely impacted and damaged by the "American Diet" (which is full of refined sugars, processed foods, and chemical additives), it would probably work great to keep you relatively slender and healthy.

You have many innate mechanisms to tell you when you have eaten enough of all of the right kinds of nutrients. However, when you do not get enough to eat of certain foods, the American Diet has trained you to crave unhealthy foods. Before refined sugar, you would have hungered for carbs when your carbohydrate intake was too low. Now, you crave sugar. Before salty snacks such as salted nuts or potato chips, you would never have thought to eat endlessly.

The rules for the Eat As Much As You Want system are designed to help you create meals that will keep your hunger satisfied. They work with your natural mechanisms to bring your natural urges back into a healthy rhythm.

Your own appetite guides how much you eat. The rules bring balance to your meal even when you are deciding quantities of Unlimiteds based on how satisfied you are. By helping you to meet all of the actual nutritional needs of your body, we build a barrier against the unhealthy urges created by the American Diet. The Countables Ranges make sure you get the right amounts of complex proteins and low-GI carbohydrates to satisfy your appetite and keep you healthy.

I am amazed that so many people still try to lose weight by making themselves hungry. One highly marketed weight loss program advises that if you believe you will lose weight, then you will be successful doing so. Then they count your calories and praise you if you are below budget, no matter how hungry you may feel when you stopped eating out of sheer willpower. Wouldn't you rather lose weight by satisfying your appetite, being healthy, and lacking hunger?

In this chapter, I will go into some detail on the scientific studies that tell us what macronutrient balances our bodies need to be satisfied and healthy.

Is the Eat As Much As You Want system just a carb and protein gram counter?

No. The number of grams of actual carbohydrates is different from the number of Countable Carbs, because there are other carbohydrates in each meal. Unlimiteds and other non-Countables (see Rechargers below) almost always contain carbohydrates as their dominant macronutrient, and they can also add to the proteins and fats. The system does not dictate the quantity of Unlimiteds any one person may choose to consume. Nonetheless, among the 1072 meals people using the system created that we analyzed, 86% were within the range of 40 to 70% carbohydrates when calories from *all* carbohydrates are included.

The system works best when people allow their own bodies to tell them when they have eaten enough. You may recall that, out of all of the participants in the Minnesota Starvation Experiment, the ones who were allowed to eat ad libitum at the end of the experiment experienced the most rapid increases in their metabolic rates.

The High Protein Myth

For the past several decades, there have been millions of people who have followed the teachings of the now deceased Dr. Robert Atkins, the inventor of the low-carb Atkins Diet who first authored a book about a high protein diet in 1972.

Dr. Atkins died in 2003 nine days after falling and hitting his head on a sidewalk. He went into a coma and died due to complications from surgery to remove a blood clot in his brain. A year before that, he had a heart attack. After his death, it came out that he had cardiomyopathy, a heart muscle disease.

There has been much speculation about his heart muscle disease and whether his death related to it. I certainly do not know the answer, but I find it interesting that the muscles of his heart were malfunctioning after being on a high protein diet for 30 years or so. This brings to mind the 2019 study[25] by the South Australian Health & Medical Research Institute finding that high protein diets lead to errors in protein synthesis in the body, which in turn shortens lifespan.

Ketogenic diet experts argue that super high-protein, low-carbohydrate diets are safe. However, studies provided to support such claims are based on short-term results that do not reflect long-term effects. We have already seen strong evidence that long-term adherence to a ketogenic diet is bad for you[23,24,25] and that they shorten your life expectancy.[24,25] Scientists are also gathering an understanding of why the right balance of macronutrients is so important. The study of mice by Solon-Biet that we looked at in Chapter 4 showed us that the right balance is not super high-protein:

> *"There is… growing evidence from studies on a wide range of species that, rather than macronutrients acting singly, it is their interactive effects (i.e., their balance) that are more*

important for health and aging. In particular, it has emerged that the balance of protein to nonprotein energy in the diet is especially significant, influencing total energy intake, growth and development, body composition, reproduction, aging, gut microbial ecology, the susceptibility to obesity and metabolic disease, immune function, and resistance to infectious diseases (Blumfield et al., 2012, Gosby et al., 2011, Huang et al., 2013, Lee et al., 2008, Mayntz et al., 2009, Piper et al., 2011, Ponton et al., 2011, Simpson and Raubenheimer, 2009, Simpson and Raubenheimer, 2012).

"Median lifespan was greatest for animals whose intakes were low in protein and high in carbohydrate...

"Chronic exposure to high-protein, low-carbohydrate diets resulted in the lowest food intakes, but... with reduced lifespan."[61]

Dr. Atkins' cause of death was hotly debated in the media, especially by people who championed the cause of low-carb diets. The Wall Street Journal reported that he had a history of heart attack and congestive heart failure, but Dr. Stuart Trager disputed that. Dr. Trager was chairman of the Atkins Physicians Council, a group of physicians who work as consultants to the Atkins organization.

Still, Trager disclosed that Dr. Atkins had cardiomyopathy. Trager tried valiantly to support the idea that Dr. Atkins' diet had nothing to do with his death. However, according to the New York Times, Trager admitted "Old age was not particularly kind to him. This cardiomyopathy was a real bugger."[26]

Trager speculated the cardiomyopathy was from a past virus, but really did not know. Remember this was long before research established protein synthesis goes awry on a high protein diet. Protein synthesis is what should repair and replace defective muscle tissue in a normally functioning human body.

The Times also reported that hospital records indicate that the doctor gained 63 pounds from fluid retention in the nine days he was in a coma, going from 195 lbs the day after he entered the hospital to 258 lbs at the time of his death. Strange. Someone who knew Dr. Atkins disputed the fluid retention story, saying he was badly overweight when he entered the hospital, and that he was unable to stay on his own diet.[26]

Appropriate protein consumption

I think we can safely say Dr. Atkins consumed too much protein for good health. So what constitutes appropriate protein consumption? This has been a raging debate in our society for many years, and it is the subject of much research. In this section, I will give you some pieces of the protein puzzle. In the next section ("The assembled protein jigsaw puzzle"), I will put it all together into a clear picture.

Given that generally 50 to 55% of caloric intake will come from carbohydrates to optimize human longevity, this leaves about 45 to 50% available to come from protein and fat combined.

Daniel Pendick, Former Executive Editor of *Harvard Men's Health Watch,* argues as follows:

> *"The Protein Summit reports in [American Journal of Clinical Nutrition]… suggest that Americans may eat too little protein, not too much. The potential benefits of higher daily protein intake, these researchers argue, include preserving muscle strength despite aging and maintaining a lean, fat-burning physique. Some studies described in the summit reports suggest that protein is more effective if you space it*

out over the day's meals and snacks, rather than loading up at dinner like many Americans do..[85]

The Eat As Much As You Want system encourages frequent eating which includes some protein in every meal. This is right in line with what the studies cited by Pendick recommend.

Is Pendick right? For guidance on the protein-intake consensus among today's top nutrition scientists, let's look at the "Daily Nutritional Goals for Age-Sex Groups Based on Dietary Reference Intakes and Dietary Guidelines Recommendations" (DGR) issued by the Food and Nutrition Board of the Institute of Medicine of the National Academy of Sciences.[86] Their current recommendation is that a Female aged 19 and over needs at least 46 grams of protein every day and a male at least 56. Regardless of gender, they say that protein should be in the range of 10 to 35% of caloric intake.

Anyone trying to lose weight will typically consume fewer calories than most other people. If you are eating fewer calories than the average person, and your minimum protein requirement does not change, then the 46 or 56 grams requirement is a higher percentage for you than for someone with a greater caloric budget. There is a large body of research out there about why so much protein is needed.

Another governmental recommendation on protein is the Recommended Daily Allowance, or RDA. Pendick says the RDA "for

---

[85] "How much protein do you need every day?" Daniel Pendick, October 16 2015, Harvard Medical School, *Harvard Health Blog*, https://www.health.harvard.edu/blog/how-much-protein-do-you-need-every-day-201506188096

[86] "Daily Nutritional Goals for Age-Sex Groups Based on Dietary Reference Intakes and Dietary Guidelines Recommendations." Dietary Guidelines 2015-2020, https://health.gov/dietaryguidelines/2015/guidelines/appendix-7/#table-a7-1

protein is a modest 0.8 grams of protein per kilogram of body weight. The RDA is the amount of a nutrient you need to meet your basic nutritional requirements. In a sense, it's the minimum amount you need to keep from getting sick — not the specific amount you are supposed to eat every day."[85]

Studies that focus exclusively on the percentage of calories coming from protein do not take into account the absolute total caloric intake. It is well known, for example, that people and animals eat fewer calories in old age. To reach the daily protein goal specified by the RDA, a person who is eating fewer calories must consume a higher percentage of protein in their overall diet.

For example, a woman who weighs 200 pounds would have a protein RDA of 72 grams. That equates to 288 calories. To lose weight, she may be consuming less than 1100 calories a day, which means her minimum protein intake must be over 26% of her total calories consumed. This is a much higher percentage than would be needed for someone who is only maintaining current weight and thus eating more calories.

Another large group of people who tend to eat fewer calories is people over age 65. A 2014 study showed that excessive protein consumption is associated with higher mortality rates in people 65 and younger, but not in people over 65.[87] The RDA for older people is no different than for younger folks in terms of grams per pound of body weight, but that translates to greater protein requirements for older people as a percentage of caloric intake because of their lower overall food intakes.

For optimal long-term health, your protein intake should be selected following the example of Goldilocks: not too much, not too

---

[87] "Low protein intake is associated with a major reduction in IGF-1, cancer, and overall mortality in the 65 and younger but not older population." Levine et al., March 4 2014, Cell Metabolism, National Institutes of Health pubmed, https://www.ncbi.nlm.nih.gov/pubmed/24606898

little, but just right! The rules of the Eat As Much As You Want system (Chapter 24) lead you to creating meals that meet all of the protein requirements. Analyzed meals almost all met the quantity goals set by the DGR and the RDA and were within the optimal percentage ranges set by the DGR.

The assembled protein jigsaw puzzle

Now we have the pieces to the puzzle. Let's put them together into a clearer picture:

- Too much protein is bad for you and shortens your life.

- Not enough protein leads to muscle loss and metabolic slowing.

- Women need at least 46 grams of protein a day, and men need at least 56.

- Government recommendations call for at least 0.8 grams of protein to be consumed per day per kilogram of bodyweight.

- Government recommendations also call for 10% to 35% of caloric intake to come from protein.

- When considering the caloric budgets of people losing weight or trying to keep it off, the minimum government recommended grams requirements are very close to the maximum government recommended ranges of percentage of calories from protein.

Let's make this even simpler. If you weigh 200 pounds, that is 91.72 kilograms. 0.8 grams of protein per kilogram would be about 73 grams of per day minimum protein intake. Compare that to various protein sources. Chicken breast has eight grams per ounce. Milk has eight grams per cup. Tuna has seven grams per ounce. A large egg has six grams. It does not take a lot of protein-rich food to meet your governmentally recommended minimum protein or to exceed your maximum.

The Eat As Much As You Want system

- gives you the right amount of protein to meet all of the government recommendations,

- allows you to Eat As Much As You Want of Unlimiteds,

- guides your own innate urges to have you feel satisfied and stop eating when you are optimally nourished within your caloric budget.

Don't forget the research: Your body craves a certain amount of protein and a certain amount of low-GI carbs. Until you get these amounts, you will feel hunger. After you get these amounts, filling your stomach with low-caloric density, nutrient rich fruits and vegetables will satisfy your hunger without putting you over your weight loss caloric budget.

That is why you can eat as much as you want and still lose weight with no hunger when you follow the system.

Fat

The National Academy of Sciences set the DGR for fat at a higher level than the amount recommended in the Eat As Much As You Want system. However, the system fulfills the health objectives of the DGR.

Pendick points out that the conversation among scientists has moved more recently from percentages to quality of the protein sources, with an emphasis on lower fat content and higher nutrient content. Quality is a theme that characterizes the foods on the most favored Countables lists.

We have already talked a lot about quality. The 2018 study cited in the New York Times (see Chapter 5) indicated *"The research lends strong support to the notion that diet quality, not quantity, is what helps people lose and manage their weight most easily in the long run."*[27]

The 1998 study by Shick et al.[4] of participants who had successfully lost an average of 66 pounds and kept it off for an average of 5 1/2 years found as follows: *"Successful maintainers of weight loss reported continued consumption of a low-energy and low-fat diet."* In this context, low energy means low calorie.

The Eat As Much As You Want system is low energy and low fat even though the people who follow it feel like they have high energy. Just because you don't eat a lot of calories doesn't mean you need to be low on usable energy. It seem ironic that people who eat the most calories are the ones who are the most likely to feel lethargic.

The grams of protein that you need does not drop just because you are eating fewer calories, so the percentage of your calories that come from protein end up being at the high end of the recommended DGR at an average of about 32 percent. Carbohydrates, as we have seen, average 53%, again quite optimal. This leaves only about 15% for fats, which is in fact the average fat content of the 1072 analyzed Eat As Much As You Want system meals. 15% from fats is definitely in the low-fat category.

Why are Countable Fats Ranges lower than the DGR?

Optimal health and satiety requires certain amounts of low-GI carbohydrates and complex proteins, as we have discussed. This leaves little room in the diet for fats if weight loss is your goal.

Fat is much more calorically dense than protein. One gram of fat is nine calories, but one gram of either carbohydrates or protein is only four calories. Fats that are added to foods such as oil or butter are extremely calorically dense. Thus, fat intake must be tightly controlled to avoid pushing the fat-calorie percentages sky-high when planning a meal.

Nutrient value and fat content must play a big role in food selection. The DGR for fat is 20 to 35%. Yet, when we meet the optimal requirements for carbohydrates and protein, there is only room for 15% from fats. What went wrong with this math? Mainly the problem with the DGR is that it was not calculated for people either losing weight or attempting to maintain a loss.

The daily calorie intakes assessed by the National Academy of Sciences for the DGR ranged from 1600 to 2000 calories per day if female and 2200 to 3000 if male. Those caloric ranges are too high for the average currently or formerly overweight or obese person to maintain during weight loss. For example, the participants in Shick et al.[4] who successfully sustained substantial weight loss were consuming an average of 1306 calories a day if female and 1685 a day if male while in weight-maintenance mode. In the weight-loss mode, they would necessarily have had even lower caloric intakes than these. So the caloric budgets assessed for the DGR are substantially higher than those of anyone on a significant weight-loss journey.

"Healthy fats"

A fitness client of mine had decided to manage her own weight loss without input from me. She had read some articles and thought she knew what to do. But the weight wasn't coming off. Finally, one day while she was working out she blurted out "I'm not losing any weight! How can we change the workouts so I'll start losing?"

I paused before responding. She was certainly not working out as hard as she could. But I didn't think that was the answer.

"Let's start with what you're eating," I replied. "Can you tell me about that?"

"It has nothing to do with what I'm eating," she insisted. "I eat very clean."

"Indulge me," I replied. "It can't hurt to tell me what you're having."

"Well, first, I know that coconut oil is very good for you. I read that in an article. So I am using lots and lots of coconut oil in my cooking. But it seems like the more I use, the more weight I gain. It doesn't make sense!"

"Why do you think that using lots of coconut oil would make you lose weight?" I asked.

"Because it is so good for you. I read that in an article."

This was quite an eye opener for me. Americans have a wild notion that if a little of something is good, then a lot of it is great. At that time, coconut oil was thought by many people to be healthy. Since then, that has been brought into question. Regardless, healthy fats are only good for you in very small quantities.

"Large amounts of any fat, no matter how healthy it is, simply add calories," I told her. "Only use fats very sparingly. That's your first step. What else are you eating…"

That conversation got her back on the right track, and she started losing weight.

Quality fats

Given that there is not room in the caloric budget for 20% of calories to come from fat, make sure that whenever you have the choice in a meal, choose a healthy fat, and consume it sparingly.

An enormous amount of research has been done into the harmful effects of excessive fat consumption and of the consumption of saturated and trans fats. We know now that if we are to consume fats, we should lean toward polyunsaturated and monounsaturated fats.[88] It is also well known that omega-3 fatty acids from free range and grass fed animals and wild-caught fatty fish can be healthful while Omega 6 fatty acids from grain-fed farmed animals and fish can be problematic.

However, fat is an extremely calorically dense nutrient that quickly balloons our caloric intake. So limiting fat intake, even if it is so-called "healthy fat", is necessary to achieve weight loss. Nonetheless, some amount of fat in the diet is necessary. An absolutely fat free diet would not be healthy. Our bodies need some of the essential nutrients from fat.

"The minimum of 20% is to ensure adequate consumption of total energy, essential fatty acids, and fat-soluble vitamins

---

[88] "The truth about fats: the good, the bad, and the in-between." December 11 2019, Harvard Medical School, Harvard Health Publishing, https://www.health.harvard.edu/staying-healthy/the-truth-about-fats-bad-and-good

[12] and prevent… low… HDL-C… which occurs with low-fat, high carbohydrate diets and increases risk of coronary heart disease [13]. The maximum of 35% was based on limiting saturated fat and also the observation that individuals on higher fat diets consume more calories, resulting in weight gain [13]…

"The median intake of saturated fat currently is 9.7–11.1% depending on sex and race or ethnic subgroup, and approximately 42–65% of the adult population consumes greater than the recommended level of 10% of calories from saturated fat [22]."[89]

The just quoted meta-analysis of many different studies sheds considerable light on the question of how much fat is appropriate. Unpacking this statement by Liu et al., a few things jump out. First, when we are trying to lose weight and keep it off, our primary concern is not "to ensure adequate consumption of total energy". Rather, we strive to be satiated with as few calories as possible. Thus, that first reason given for the 20% minimum is not applicable.

Secondly, the 20% DGR assumes that a large percentage of the population is getting more than the maximum recommended 10% of calories from saturated fat. Much of the rest of this meta-analysis goes into great detail about the importance and great health benefits of cutting down substantially on saturated fat and replacing it with essential fatty acids found in monounsaturated fats and polyunsaturated fats.

In the Eat As Much As You Want system, this is actually why avocados, wild-caught fatty fishes, and various types of seafood are among the most favored Countables, the "Go For 'Ems", and their

---

[89] "A healthy approach to dietary fats: understanding the science and taking action to reduce consumer confusion." Liu et al., August 30 2017, *Nutrition Journal*, National Institutes of Health pubmed, https://www.ncbi.nlm.nih.gov/pmc/articles/PMC5577766/

macronutrients are not fully Countable. Canola oil and olive oil are among the "Oils and Fats" list, which is a list of more favored sources of fat. These foods have all been cited in the research highlighted in this meta-analysis as important sources of the essential fatty acids hoped for in crafting the DGR. Similarly, proteins that have very low saturated fat content are also on the Go For 'Ems list.

The Liu et al. meta-analysis[89] goes on to say the following:

"The new research suggests that rather than focusing on total carbohydrate, the guidance should be on specific foods: limiting foods rich in refined starch and sugars, while eating more of other carbohydrate-containing foods such as fruits, legumes, and fiber-rich whole grains. Likewise, the new research suggests that rather than focusing on total saturated fat, the guidance also could be on specific foods, as saturated fat from different major food sources is associated with higher risk, no risk, or even lower risk of CHD, depending on the food source [38, 39]."

That is precisely what the Eat As Much As You Want system does. We guide and encourage subscribers to consume from lists of specific healthy whole foods and away from "foods rich in refined starch and sugars".

Thus, even if the 15% average caloric content from fat is lower than the 20% DGR, it contains more mono- and polyunsaturated fats and omega-3 than the typical low fat diet at 20%. Thus, in effect, it satisfies the objectives outlined as the reason for the 20% minimum.

After being on the Eat As Much As You Want system for a while, many of my clients have told me their doctors were very pleased with their blood panels. Their serum cholesterol levels have consistently improved significantly. This is another very strong indication the Eat As Much As You Want system satisfies the objectives of the National Academy of Sciences for the DGR.

But... but... but... Fat is what satisfies!

"Just tell me what I can eat."

That is a phrase I have heard many times from new clients. Yet, as soon as they start to look at the lists of foods, some begin to raise objections based on what they have heard are healthy diet foods.

"What about almond butter? And granola? And hummus made with olive oil? Surely those should be in my diet."

"I like to eat spoonfuls of peanut butter as snacks. I only see fat free peanut powder on the list."

"I use lots of coconut oil and olive oil in my cooking. I can keep doing that, right?"

All of these comments and suggestions and downright insistences of what they ought to be able to eat in unlimited quantities boil down to one concern and misconception:

"Fat is what stops your hunger!"

This is a false concept that has been put forth in the popular culture. So let's talk about the truth. Fat tastes really good, but it does not satisfy hunger.

Fat versus satiety

Scientific research proves that satiety is most effectively achieved with carbohydrates and protein, but not with fat. In fact, fat makes you want to eat more:

> "Dietary fat has frequently been blamed for the increase in prevalence of obesity (Bray et al., 2004). Epidemiological studies have demonstrated a positive relationship between high-fat diets and excess energy intake due to their high energy density and palatability (Prentice and Poppitt, 1996)... [I]n a free-living environment, the presence of highly palatable foods, a characteristic of high-fat foods, could chronically activate the hedonic system which would promote higher appetite and more energy intake (Lowe and Levine, 2005). The hedonic system is regarded as pleasure associated with eating palatable foods. In an environment with unlimited availability of highly palatable foods, there is a concern of how much the homeostatic appetite regulatory mechanisms can override the hedonic components and hyper responsiveness to palatable foods (Blundell et al., 2005)."[90]

Once again, let's look at the ad-libitum fed mice in the 2014 study by Solon-Biet et al.[61] The researchers found that the mice ate just as much volume of food whether it was high in fat or not, so they consumed a lot more calories when it was high fat. Worst still, when the food had a lot of fat, but was low in either protein or carbohydrates, the mice overate to get their carbs or protein (whichever one was too low) regardless of how much fat was in the food. Conversely, when protein and carbohydrate was increased in the food, the mice ate less.

------

[90] "Chapter 15 Fats and Satiety." Rania Abou Samra, 2010, *Fat Detection: Taste, Texture, and Post Ingestive Effects*, National Institutes of Health pubmed, https://www.ncbi.nlm.nih.gov/books/NBK53550/

This is scientific evidence showing that fat consumed in our everyday lives has effectively zero satiation value, and it can lead us to excessive caloric consumption, but a diet rich in complex proteins and low-GI carbohydrates can satisfy without regard to how much fat is present. This matches the experience of my clients following my system. They have found that their appetites stay satisfied, and they experience little, if any, hunger.

Nonetheless, if you have a concern that you need more fat in your diet than is contained in the average Eat As Much As You Want meal, there is certainly room for creating meals that contain enough fat to put you over 20% on calories from fat. In fact, over 200 of the 1072 that were analyzed were over 20% calories from fat. If you so choose, you can add fats from the Oils and Fats list (the list of acceptable fats) to any meal to bring the fat content up to the Countables range maximum. Almost all meals that are at the Countables range maximum for fats will be in at or above the 20% DGR range minimum for calories from fat.

Long-term health

The Liu et al. meta-analysis[89] concurs with Solon-Biet[61] and also with the various studies I have already shared that show that the quality and balance of what you eat is far more important to your health than any arbitrary amount of fat:

> "We have presented evidence that the types of foods consumed and the overall dietary pattern followed are far more important for reducing [cardiovascular disease] risk than total fat. Also the types of fat and carbohydrates – and more relevantly, the types of foods supplying these nutrients – are more important than the total amounts of fats and carbohydrates in the diet. Healthful plant and seafood sources of monounsaturated and polyunsaturated fats have important health benefits in the context of a healthy dietary pattern."

If you have any concerns at all about your specific dietary needs, consult a physician or a Registered Dietician. Absent individualized guidance from a professional, no diet can address every person's specific needs. Keep in mind that the fats are low in order to keep calories down, optimize fat loss, and meet the carbohydrate and protein requirements that have been shown to be important for long-term health of the typical person.

If you do decide to add fats to all of the lowest fat meals, you will of course be adding calories and slowing down your weight loss. Nonetheless, your top priorities should be long-term health, longevity, and quality of life, so if your doctor or dietician tells you to do it, then go for it. Even with the additional fat, you should still be able to lose weight as long as you stay within your Countables ranges. Speed of weight loss should never be your top priority anyway.

Good versus bad fat

I have touched on the importance of including good fats and cutting down on bad fats, but let's go deeper on that subject:

The healthiest animal fats are Omega 3 fatty acids and certain fats contained primarily in fatty, wild caught fishes (such as salmon). Mia Syn, MS, RD of Life's DHA explained the need for these special fats very clearly:[91]

> *"Eicosapentaenoic acid (EPA) and Docosahexaenoic acid (DHA) are the forms of omega-3 fats particularly important for maintenance of normal brain function in adults. These fats build cell membranes and promote new brain cell formation…*

---

[91] "Why the Brain Needs Omega-3 Fatty Acids." Mia Syn, August 18 2017, *Life's DHA*, https://www.lifesdha.com/en_ZA/news/why-the-brain-needs-omega-3-fatty-acids.html

"Studies have revealed a link between an imbalance in omega-3s from diet and impaired brain performance and cognitive diseases.

"The brain contains more than 100 billion cells and omega-3 fatty acids are the building blocks of these cells. These fats bind to cell membranes increasing fluidity, which is important for the functioning of each brain cell. The benefit of membrane fluidity is that it helps the brain change and adapt to new information. Additionally, the omega-3s in cell membranes aid the function of neurotransmitter receptors, which helps facilitate how information is communicated in the brain. Neurotransmitters are brain chemicals that communicate information throughout the brain and body.

"Preliminary studies have shown that omega-3s may increase BDNF, the brain's growth hormone. In turn, this increases the production of brain messengers while decreasing their destruction."

The worst fats are saturated fats such as Omega 6 fatty acids contained in meats and eggs and fishes from grain-fed animals kept in feeding pens and deprived of grass or other more natural foods for the species. There has been a lot of scientific research to show a linkage between heart disease and high intake of saturated and trans fats. The *Harvard Health Letter* tells us that additional research is showing problems with brain health related to saturated fats:[92]

"A Brigham and Women's Hospital study published in Annals of Neurology offers evidence. Researchers found that one bad dietary fat in particular—saturated fat, found in

---

[92] "Protect your brain with 'good' fat." September 2012, Harvard Medical School, *Harvard Health Letter*, https://www.health.harvard.edu/mind-and-mood/protect-your-brain-with-good-fat

foods such as red meat and butter—may be especially harmful to your brain.

"Compared with those who consumed the least amount of saturated fat, 'women who had the highest consumption of saturated fat had the worst memory and cognition over time,' says Dr. Olivia Okereke, lead author of the study and assistant professor of psychiatry at Harvard Medical School.

"Researchers analyzed food surveys of over 6,000 older women and the results of their cognitive testing over time. Total fat intake didn't seem to affect women's brain function, but the type of fat did. Women with the most saturated fat in their diets performed worst; women with the most monounsaturated fat in their diets—from foods such as olive oil, nuts, or avocado—performed best. Trans fat and total polyunsaturated fat did not appear to have any effect on cognitive function."

If you choose to add oils to your otherwise lowest fat meals, you may want to consider adding DHA and EPA. You can purchase these online or at a health food store as fish oils.

Regardless of whether you have any concern about your minimum fat intake, it is a good idea to consume some foods that naturally contain DHA and EPA. Examples are grass fed beef, free ranges chickens and their eggs, and wild-caught fatty fish, such as salmon, mackerel, trout, sardines, and anchovies, or shellfish, such as mussels, oysters and crabs.

The Countables

There are thousands of Countable foods. For a complete list, you can use the free Eat As Much As You Want application at topfitpros.com, and easily search by list on the Nutrition tab to find any and all Countables as well as how much to count with each food.

However, I will describe each list in this chapter and give you a good number of examples of items on the most favored lists. The most highly recommended Countables are Go For 'Ems, Preferred Foods, Best Convenient Foods, and Jump Starters. Only the Jump Starters are high-GI.

Go For 'Ems

These are the highest quality Countables and are mostly made up of lean proteins and low-GI foods that have especially strong nutrient characteristics. They are all too calorically dense to qualify as Unlimiteds, but they are valuable foods that should play a major role in your meal plans. These are such high quality foods that the macronutrients are only partially countable. Examples are as follows:

Anchovy
Avocados
Canadian bacon
Chicken breast, meat only
Crab meat (not imitation)
Egg white
Fat free cheeses (certain ones)
Fish, many different varieties
Game meats, many varieties
Ground beef, super lean (3% fat)
Lobster
Lox
Oysters
Peanut powder, nonfat
Pears, raw
Poi
Pork loin, lean meat only

Tuna, canned in water
Turkey breast, meat only
Salmon, canned, cooked or raw
Shrimp
Tomato Juice
Vegan low fat imitation meats, many varieties
V8 Vegetable Juices, specific selections

Preferred Foods

This is a list of the healthiest low-fat, low-GI foods that are fully countable and either carbohydrate rich or protein rich. Examples are as follows:

Almond butter, powdered
Almond milk, unsweetened vanilla
Barley, pearled
Beef broth or bouillon, canned, ready to serve
Beef, certain lean cuts with the fat trimmed off
Beets, canned
Black beans
Black bean soup
Blackeyed peas (Crowder peas)
Buckwheat groats
Bulgur
Catsup
Cheddar or Colby cheese, low fat
Chestnuts, European, Japanese and Chinese
Chicken broth, canned
Chicken, canned with broth
Chicken, meat only
Chickpeas
Chunky vegetable soup
Clams
Cod
Cottage cheese, nonfat or 1%

Ginkgo nuts
Great northern beans
Greek yogurt, plain nonfat
Green peas
Ham, 96% fat free
Hummus, oil free
Kidney beans
Lentils
Lima beans
Mixed vegetables (corn, lima beans, peas, green beans, carrots)
Oat bran bread
Oat bran reduced calorie bread
Marinara sauce
Minestrone soup
Miso
Navy beans
Okara
Pastas, various types, use in very small quantities
Pickles
Pinto beans
Protein powder, soy
Protein powder, whey
Pumpernickel bread
Pumpernickel rolls
Quinoa
Refried beans, fat free
Roast beef, deli style
Rye bread, reduced calorie
Salad dressing, fat free, various varieties
Scallops
Shitake mushrooms
Sour cream, fat free
Split pea soup with ham
Soymilk, all flavors, nonfat or lowfat
Squid
Tamari soy sauce
Teriyaki sauce

Tofu, lite
Tomato bisque soup
Tomato soup, canned
Turkey breast
Turkey, fat free
Turkey ham, extra lean
Wheat bran
Wheat germ
Wheat germ cereal
White beans
Whole wheat tortilla
Wild rice
Yogurt, nonfat, various flavors made with low-calorie sweetener

Best Convenient Foods

These are like the Preferred Foods, but they are balanced between carbohydrates and protein. This makes them very convenient to eat. Here are some examples:

Greek yogurt, nonfat vanilla
Milk, nonfat
Scallops, imitation, made with surimi
Soymilk, original and vanilla, light, unsweetened
Yeast extract spread

Other permissible low-Glycemic Index foods

There are additional categories of low-GI foods that are permissible to include in meal plans, even while in the weight-loss mode. They are not as favored as the ones I have already listed. "Just-a-Littles" are good, healthy choices, but generally a little bit higher in fat content than the Preferred Foods. "Good Convenient Foods" are like the Just-A-Littles, but are balanced between Countable Carbs and Countable Proteins so that one food will give you all the Countables you need. "Quick Bites" are highly convenient foods that balance Countable Carbs and Countable Proteins for a quick meal on the go, but they tend to be higher in fat than your recommended Countables ranges would normally allow. We recommend that you include these in your meal plans only infrequently.

Jump Starters

Jump Starters are foods that are good for you, but they are hi-GI. If you are insulin resistant or have type 2 diabetes, you should not have these. They give your body a quick boost when your blood sugar is naturally lower. They also help your body to recover more quickly and effectively after a workout. One serving of any of these is good for anyone who has just completed a workout or has been 4 ½ hours or more without food (such as at breakfast). Here are examples:

Banana
Bagel
Baked beans
Brown rice
Cereals, many varieties
Coconut water
Corn
Cornbread
Corn tortilla
Couscous
Cracked wheat bread
Cream of Wheat
Farina
Figs
Frozen yogurts, various varieties
Fruit juices, various flavors
Grits
Japanese soba

Mashed potatoes
Oatmeal
Parsnips
Passion fruit
Pita, whole wheat
Plantains
Pomegranates
Potatoes
Rice bran bread
Rice cakes, brown rice
Rye bread
Soymilk, various flavors
Soups, many different varieties
Sweet potato
Succotash
Taro
Waffles, low fat or original
Wheat bran bread
Wheat bread, reduced calorie
Whole wheat bread

Rechargers: Limited but not Countable

Similar to Jump Starters, Rechargers are healthy fast carbs to help you rev up your body when your blood sugar is naturally lower. They get your day started out well, and they help your body to recover more quickly and effectively after a workout. You do not have to count any of the carbs, protein or fat in these foods. However, you should only have one serving per meal, and you should only have it first thing in the morning or immediately following a workout or if you have gone 4 ½ hours or more between meals. These are not appropriate for anyone with insulin resistance or type 2 diabetes. Examples follow:

Cantaloupe, raw
Casaba melon, raw

Figs, raw
Grapes, red, green, or muscadine
Honeydew, raw
Kiwi, raw
Kumquats, raw
Mango, raw
Papaya, raw
Pears, Asian, raw
Persimmons, raw
Pineapples, raw
Watermelon, raw

Fats and Oils

Use fats and oils in very small quantities. This list includes fats that are better for you than others. It also includes certain foods such as nuts and eggs with high-fat content that can be combined with other foods to make a healthy meal. Examples follow:

Almonds
Almond butter
Almond oil
Avocado oil
Beechnuts
Brazilnuts
Canola oil
Cashew butter
Cashew nuts
Chia seeds
Cocoa butter
Coconut meat
Cod liver oil
Flaxseed
Hazelnuts
Hickory nuts
Macadamia nuts

Menhaden fish oil
Olive oil
Peanuts
Peanut butter
Peanut oil
Pecans
Pilinuts
Pine nuts
Pistachio nuts
Pumpkin and squash seeds
Salad dressings, many varieties
Salmon oil
Sardine oil
Sesame butter
Sesame oil
Sesame seeds
Sunflower seeds
Sunflower seed butter
Tempeh
Walnuts
Walnut oil
Whole egg

Countables you should not eat when losing weight

There are thousands of foods that would hamper your ability to lose weight. "Caution Foods" are foods that tend to be fatty, sugary or too highly alcoholic. Caution Foods are not recommended, but may be included in your meal plans if your goal is weight maintenance.

"Weight Gain Foods" tend to be even higher in fat than Caution Foods, and may have more sugar. Both Caution Foods and Weight Gain Foods may be included in your plans if your goal is to gain weight.

"Fat Gain Foods" are foods or drinks that tend to contribute to weight gain that is disproportionately fat. These are foods everyone should try to avoid. They may be high in refined sugars and/or unhealthy fats, and/or they may be addictive in nature, and/or they may result in metabolic slowdown because they rob enzymes.

The lists and descriptions contained in this chapter are far from complete. They are intended to give you a reasonably good understanding of how any given food ought to be characterized. There are far too many foods in existence to list them all in a chapter of a book. For far more complete lists and selections, see the free Eat As Much As You Want System app.

Takeaways for Chapter 12

- **Health, longevity, satiety and sustainable weight loss require a balanced diet.**

- **Low-Glycemic Index carbohydrates and complex proteins are each necessary for satiety.**

- **Too much protein shortens your life expectancy.**

- **Insufficient protein leads to muscle loss and frailty.**

- **Fats make you want to eat more calories, not fewer.**

- **Use fats sparingly, and emphasize healthy fats.**

- **Ideal weight loss macronutrient intake: 50 to 55% of calories from low-GI carbs, 30 to 35% from complex proteins, and 15 to 20% from fats.**

- With the Eat As Much As You Want system, you don't need to know those percentages. It guides you to meet them automatically.

- Eating the right foods, if you stay in range on Countables and eat as much as you want of Unlimiteds, your average intake will stay in the optimal health, longevity and satiety ranges.

- There are many Countables and Unlimiteds to choose from.

- You can eat as much as you want and still lose weight with no hunger when you follow the system.

Chapter 13

Nature Can't Be Replaced

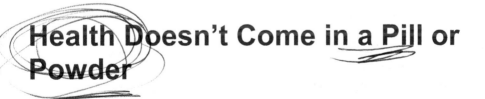

Health Doesn't Come in a Pill or Powder

Marketers have tried to convince me to sell my clients meal replacement powder, energy bars, and milk shakes, among other things. All of these supplements are touted to be better than real foods. Taking your food that way is no more effective for your body than it would be to stuff an apple or an orange into the gas tank of an old car. The car needs gasoline. The human body needs whole food.

The weight-loss dietary supplements market is huge and rapidly growing. Persistence Market Research says soft gel/pill sales alone are likely to surpass $18.5 billion by 2026.[93]

Sadly, much of this money is being spent in misguided ways. Always remember that supplements, by definition, are merely supplemental. They do not comprise complete or natural nutrition.

The National Institutes of Health (NIH) warns as follows:

> *"The proven ways to lose weight are eating healthful foods, cutting calories, and being physically active... But there's little scientific evidence that weight-loss supplements work. Many are expensive, some can interact or interfere with medications, and a few might be harmful."*[94]

---

[93] Global Market Study on Weight Loss Dietary Supplements: North America to Lean the Global Market in Terms of Revenue during 2017-2026." December 2017, Persistence Market Research, https://www.persistencemarketresearch.com/market-research/weight-loss-dietary-supplements-market.asp

[94] "Dietary Supplements for Weight Loss; Fact Sheet for Consumers." June 20 2019, National Institutes of Health Office of Dietatary Supplements, https://ods.od.nih.gov/factsheets/WeightLoss-Consumer/

Most weight loss supplements are sold with no research done to determine whether they are safe or effective. Research studies that have been done are usually very small studies with only a few participants. They may lack controls and other scientific methods generally accepted as basic requirements in determining safety and efficacy. They are generally paid for by the manufacturers and not peer-reviewed in the scientific community. This conflict of interest casts a shadow on the findings.

Studies done are typically short term, so they are not long enough to determine side effects that typically require longer periods of use to emerge. Research findings associated with various weight loss supplements tout health results that normally come from weight loss in any form, such as lower cholesterol and lower blood pressure, but it is often unclear whether the actual weight loss was the result of the supplements themselves or other factors such as dietary changes.

There is a long-term health cost to bypassing the many processes that a healthy human body must perform when you eat and digest real food. Maintaining or attaining long-term wellness requires healthy, balanced nutrition, which in turn means eating a balanced diet with plenty of natural foods.

Too many marketers of supplements focus on rapid weight loss without consideration of long-term consequences. They often call their plans or products "sustainable" even when independent scientific research may contradict such a claim. Before you decide to use a plan or a supplement, do some research to see if the claims are consistent with scientific facts other than those from small, short-term research studies paid for by the manufacturers.

The NIH further warns that

> "...dietary supplements don't require review or approval by the FDA before they are put on the market. Also, manufacturers don't have to provide evidence to the FDA

that their products are safe or effective before selling these products… Weight-loss supplements, like all dietary supplements, can have harmful side effects and might interact with prescription and over-the-counter medications. Many weight-loss supplements have ingredients that haven't been tested in combination with one another, and their combined effects are unknown.[94]

Health and Longevity are Not Accidental

All of our lives, we have been admonished that this is good for you and that is bad for you. It's easy to begin to ignore those warnings and pearls of wisdom in favor of living for the moment. Hey, I am definitely a fan of savoring every morsel of life. Each moment is precious.

But, really, are the pleasures of structuring your life around unhealthy behaviors worth the cost? For me, the answer is an emphatic no. In fact, I derive great pleasure from my healthy behaviors. Truly, ripe whole fruits, garden fresh veggies, and healthy meats and fishes prepared the right way are awesome.

Twenty-two years ago, a healthy, robust friend came to me excited.

"I'm supporting myself now selling supplements! You should try some."

"What are they?" I asked.

He pulled out some samples. They were all pills.

"Here's my spinach in a pill," he said, and he took one. "Here's my orange in a pill." He took another.

"Now I can eat whatever I want," he continued, "because I have all the nutrition I need."

"You don't like fruits and vegetables?" I asked.

"Never have," he replied. "Never will. And now I don't have to eat any... Tonight I'm having steak, potato and ice cream, but no veggies."

He was very pleased with himself.

"I like fruits and vegetables," I said. I didn't buy any of his pills.

Fast forward to today. He and his wife are both very frail and in poor health. I am if anything stronger and more fit than I was twenty-two years ago. I doubt all of the difference is the use of supplements, but the cumulative effect of unhealthy choices takes a huge toll over time.

To me, healthy or unhealthy choices are serious decisions. In my business, I have watched hundreds of people age. Some have maintained great health and have active, fun, enjoyable lives. Others such as my friend and his wife have experienced downward spirals that have led to pain, weakness, poor health and the accompanying limits to what they can do on any given day. I have seen people succumb to strokes, heart attacks, cancer and more.

When you are twenty, thirty or forty years old, substantial decline seems far off. I am now 63, and I feel great! I can do many things that most twenty year olds cannot do. But I have watched as those around me have chosen unhealthy habits, then have experienced the slow, steady parade of negative health consequences.

I want to live healthy and strong to a ripe old age, then die. I make choices consistent with that goal. Of course, I look for options that also allow me to have an enjoyable life now. That is very important, because life is a series of "nows".

I choose to make exercise and good nutrition a regular part of my life. I have learned to love exercise, and to love healthy foods.

Supplements are shortcuts, but they are generally shortcuts to the wrong destination.

Limits to the Benefits of Supplements

A supplement, by definition, cannot stand alone. The word supplement means "something that completes or enhances something else when added to it." In the context of healthy weight loss, supplements, pills and powders cannot replace excellent nutrition.

The use of supplements can be a good thing in certain circumstances, but NOT as a replacement for real food. All pills and supplements are limited in that they can only provide a relatively small list of nutrients. Natural foods have so many more potentially beneficial nutrients than any supplement can provide.

> "[N]utrients are most potent when they come from food. 'They are accompanied by many nonessential but beneficial nutrients, such as hundreds of carotenoids, flavonoids, minerals, and antioxidants that aren't in most supplements,' says Dr. [Clifford Lo, an associate professor of nutrition at the Harvard School of Public Health.]"[95]

The best way to achieve wellness is to have a balanced, healthy diet. The primary reason that supplements may be needed is

[95] "Should you get your nutrients from food or from supplements?" May 2015, Harvard Medical School, *Harvard Health Letter*, https://www.health.harvard.edu/staying-healthy/should-you-get-your-nutrients-from-food-or-from-supplements

because of dietary deficiency or an individual body's specific difficulty absorbing nutrients.

> "The typical American diet is heavy in nutrient-poor processed foods, refined grains, and added sugars—all linked to inflammation and chronic disease. Yet even if you eat a healthy, well-balanced diet, you may still fall short of needed nutrients. That's a consequence of aging. 'As we get older, our ability to absorb nutrients from food decreases. Also, our energy needs aren't the same, and we tend to eat less,' explains Dr. Howard Sesso, an epidemiologist at Harvard-affiliated Brigham and Women's Hospital."[95]

Diets may leave you vulnerable to nutrient deficiency if they emphasize dietary imbalance (such as a ketogenic diet) or nutrient-poor processed foods such as meal replacement shakes, frozen dinners, energy bars and the like. However, it would be better to switch off of such imbalanced diets than to try to use supplements to get what is missing, because natural foods contain so many more nutrients than any pill or powder.

Gut Microbiome

Back when my friend was offering me spinach and oranges in a pill, no one had any idea about all of the trillions of bacteria that live in our digestive tracts. So he did not offer me sauerkraut in a pill.

Supplement marketing has led any people to believe they need to take probiotic pills or powder to maintain good health. This is a tremendous distortion of the truth. The reality is that poor nutrition leads to poor gut health and proper nutrition from whole foods is the answer.

Much research is now ongoing on the topic of how our gut microbiome contributes to wellness. The gut microbiome is made up of trillions of microbes, or "microbiota". These are living organisms that are introduced into our bodies a variety of ways, but they are highly influenced by long-term diet. They are vital to our ability to avoid diseases, to maintain a strong metabolism, and to lose weight.

How many people do you know who are having troubles with their intestinal tracts? The number is probably a lot higher than you realize, because people usually don't talk about that. And most people don't even know it because their only symptom is that they are overweight or obese.

When we eat too much sugar and processed foods or have imbalanced diets, this can create an imbalance in our gut microbiomes, which contributes to the "progression toward a broad spectrum of diseases" and to "impair the normal functioning of gut microbiota" to maintain wellness. [96]

The gut microbiome can change over a period of years due to "diet, drugs, prebiotics or probiotics", and the degradation of the "microbiota from long-term consumption of a high-fat/high-sugar Western diet may need long-term dietary changes to restore their microbiota to a healthy state."[97]

Imbalances in the gut microbiome are brought about by long-term dietary nutritional imbalance such as extremes of plant or animal-based diets. This leaves a person vulnerable to disease.[97]

"Given the close symbiotic relationship existing between the gut microbiota and the host, it is not surprising to

[96] "The Human Gut Microbiome – A Potential Controller of Wellness and Disease." Kho and Lal, August 14 2018, *Frontiers in Microbiology*, National Institutes of Health, https://www.ncbi.nlm.nih.gov/pmc/articles/PMC6102370/
[97] "Introduction to the human gut microbiota." Thursby and Juge, May 16 2017, *Biochemical Journal*, National Institutes of Health, https://www.ncbi.nlm.nih.gov/pmc/articles/PMC5433529/

observe a divergence from the normal microbiota composition… in a plethora of disease states ranging from chronic GI diseases to neurodevelopmental disorders.

"Extreme 'animal-based' or 'plant-based' diets result in wide-ranging alterations of the gut microbiota in humans."

Certain microbiota are lost and others grow more plentiful, depending on which extreme of diet is maintained (high protein and fat or high carbohydrate).[98] This strongly implies that a balanced diet may yield a greater variety of microbiota, thus aiding in greater health. And it is clearly an argument against maintaining ketogenic diets or super high-starch diets for an extended period of time.

In the context of truly sustained weight loss, it is especially important to maintain a balanced natural diet that fosters an abundance of beneficial microbiota. *"Most gut microbes are harmless or beneficial to the host. The gut microbiota protects against"* bacteria that cause intestinal disease. It *"extracts nutrients and energy from our diets, and contributes to normal immune function… [O]bese persons harbor fewer types of microbes in their guts than lean persons, and lean and obese people differ significantly in abundances of specific"* species of microbes… *"[P]eople can be classified as lean or obese with 90% accuracy based solely on their gut microbiota."*[98]

Dietary changes must be long term to have significant changes to gut microbiota.[98] Specifically, a one-year change in how much protein versus carbohydrates are in your diet is thought to be significant enough to bring about significant microbiota change.[98] Conversely, studies of the introduction of regular consumption of

---

[98] "Diversity, stability and resilience of the human gut microbiota." Lozupone et al., September 13 2012, *Nature*, National Institutes of Health, https://www.ncbi.nlm.nih.gov/pmc/articles/PMC3577372/

probiotics over a duration of greater than 12 weeks showed reductions in Body Mass Index and body weight.[99]

Many gut microbiome studies in recent years have referenced probiotics as good for you. As we have already established, chronic consumption of refined sugar disrupts gut microbiome health, and the best solution for those specific missing bacteria is to stop eating sugar and to increase the consumption of probiotics. In most studies showing a beneficial relationship between good health and the use of probiotics, the probiotics are actual foods, NOT supplements.

> *"Probiotic use was associated with significant decreases in BMI, weight and fat mass. Studies of subjects consuming prebiotics demonstrated a significant reduction in body weight...*
>
> *"The gut microbiome has a crucial role in the functioning of the digestive tract and in harvesting energy from the diet . There is a large body of evidence demonstrating the link between the gut microbiome and obesity...*
>
> *"The ability to engineer a favorable metabolic environment by dietary modulation makes the gut microbiome an attractive target in the war against obesity... Probiotics are living microorganisms... which, when ingested, provide health benefits, either directly or through interactions with the host or other microorganisms."[99]*

Probiotics as supplements

---

[99] "Dietary Alteration of the Gut Microbiome and Its Impact on Weight and Fat Mass: A Systematic Review and Meta-Analysis." John et al., March 16 2018, *Genes*, National Institutes of Health pubmed, https://www.ncbi.nlm.nih.gov/pmc/articles/PMC5867888/

Today, supplement companies have done such a great marketing job, many people don't even realize taking probiotics in a pill or powder is not normal. If you suggested they take their "spinach in a pill" as my friend did, they would look at you like you had lost your mind. Yet, they don't see that taking fermented foods in a pill is essentially the same thing and is unlikely to be any more effective.

Inflammation in the body, as we have already seen, is caused by processed foods and refined sugars. It is ironic that some supplements are marketed by citing research on the health benefits of fermented foods, but the research on that subject relates to probiotics as living organisms that grow in the fermentation process in actual whole foods.

To be clear, true probiotics are organisms in foods that have been fermented with live cultures, including sauerkraut, kimchee, certain pickles and pickled vegetables, unpasteurized miso, certain yogurts and cheeses, and kefir. Check to be sure these are live cultured products when you buy them.

However, due to the distorted research claims by supplements manufacturers, people buy pills and freeze-dried powders to get their probiotics, and they have no idea that those ultra-processed food supplements are not the best sources of what they need. The Wildbrine company argues that supplements cannot retain the same potency as eating real fermented foods:

> "And don't forget the effectiveness of the microbes themselves when they gallop down your gullet along with fermented whole foods. Beneficial gut bacteria are already alive and working in [fermented foods]. With probiotic supplements, some bacteria are lost in the freeze-drying process, some die off during their stay on a store shelf, and some are lost when they wake up in the harsh environment

of stomach acid — all of which can lessen the product's effectiveness."[100]

Foods that you see, smell, taste, chew up and swallow are also more able to satiate than a powder or a pill. Chewing enhances satiety and stimulates the release of gut hormones related to satiety. In other words, a liquid or powder or pill theoretically containing the same nutrients will not satiate as well as whole natural foods that must be chewed before swallowing. And the reality is that whole foods carry many nutrients you will not get in the supplements.

Science Fiction vs. Satiation

Years ago, sci-fi writers imagined a future in which we could space travel and get our nutrition from pills instead of whole foods. Now we know nutrition is much more than vitamins, minerals and calories.

Think about it. How would you like to give up ever having a plateful of food again? No more chewing. No more delicious aroma of a home-cooked meal. No more fullness in your stomach.

Is that the future you want? It's not the one I want. That future would leave you hungry, constipated, malnourished and deprived of many of life's pleasures.

Seeing, tasting and smelling foods

Seeing, tasting and smelling foods can enhance satiety with a smaller amount of intake, according to a study by McCrickerd and Forde:[101]

---

[100] https://wildbrine.com/natural-probiotics-from-food-is-better/

"[T]he satiating effect of a particular food is highly dependent on the early experience of consumption. Cecil, French and Read demonstrated this nicely, showing that a previously satiating 425 g (400 kcal) portion of soup was experienced as progressively less satiating as parts of the eating experience were removed, such that the soup was most satiating when consumed orally with the belief that it was food, and least when infused into the stomach with no oro-sensory exposure and the belief that it was water."

In other words, scientists did an experiment in which some people simply ate the soup, and others had it infused directly into the stomach or small intestine. Some of those who had it infused were told it was water and some were told it was soup. Satisfaction of hunger happened when eating the soup, but there was zero satisfaction for those who had it infused into the small intestine. Slight satisfaction occurred for those who had it infused into the stomach, but not nearly the level of satisfaction as those who ate it. Those who were told it was soup experienced a small degree of satisfaction, and those who were told it was water experienced none.

McCrickerd and Forde went on to explain as follows:

"The initial experience of eating is important because animals (including humans) learn to eat in response to sensory cures, by forming associations between the early experience of a food's sensory characteristic and the post-ingestive effects of nutrient delivery. Sensory characteristics that consistently cue nutrient delivery acquire meaning and can be used to predict the consequences of consumption. This learned integration of pre-ingestive and post-ingestive

---

[101] "Sensory influences on food intake control: moving beyond palatability." McCrickerd and Forde, December 11 2015, *Obesity Review,* Wiley Online Library, https://onlinelibrary.wiley.com/doi/full/10.1111/obr.12340

signals can be expressed as increased liking for nutrient-rich foods and explicit beliefs about a food's potential satiating power, which in turn modify food selection and intake."

Life has taught you that certain foods will satisfy your appetite. Imagine that someone tells you about the foods you are going to eat, or you recognize them, then you see and smell them, then you chew and taste them, then you swallow them and feel the fullness in your stomach. This is all part of the integrated network of signals or triggers that satisfy your hunger. Conversely, if you have unhealthy food associations such as a sugar addiction, perhaps from childhood or even from adult trauma, these associations can undermine your ability to satisfy your appetite with healthy foods. In such a situation, it becomes especially important to get in the habit of keeping hunger satisfied by healthy foods before the primitive part of your brain has the chance to prompt a yearning for the unhealthy choices.

Whole, natural, nutrient-rich foods are associated with high potential satiating power. They can keep you satisfied as a pre-emptive strike against potential urges to eat food you should not. Supplements do not offer this multifaceted support for natural prompting of satiety.

A full stomach

Similarly, a full stomach stimulates the release of leptin, an appetite suppressant hormone, and the reduction of ghrelin, an appetite enhancement hormone, as covered in Chapter 6. Liquid, powder, and pill form supplements do not fill the stomach like whole natural fruits, vegetables and fermented foods do.

Remember also that leptin is highly associated with increasing metabolic rates, and a reduction in leptin levels causes a metabolic slowdown, fat accumulation, obesity, and lethargy.[102]

"Magic diet pill"

Do you remember that my friend was excited that he would be having steak, potatoes and ice cream for dinner twenty-five years ago? That is the false allure of supplements, that you can eat whatever you want, because you have all of your nutritional needs covered.

As a result, people who take supplements often choose to eat high-GI and high Glycemic Load foods such as ice cream, pastries, muffins, potatoes, and white bread. They may consume lots of saturated fats (i.e.: steak), and salty high-GI snacks such as chips.

We are led to believe by marketers that we can eat whatever we want when we buy their products. The NIH warns us against this:

> "Be very cautious when you see weight-loss supplements with tempting claims, such as 'magic diet pill,' 'melt away fat,' and 'lose weight without diet or exercise.' If the claim sounds too good to be true, it probably is. These products might not help you lose weight—and they could be dangerous."[94]

Unfortunately, the nutrients in the supplements cannot control the way the body handles the onslaught of inflammatory foods, blood sugar spikes, and salt driven hypertension. All of these lead longer term to excess weight and poor health.

---

[102] "Adiponectin, Leptin, and Fatty Acids in the Maintenance of Metabolic Homeostasis Through Adipose Tissue Crosstalk." Stem et al., May 10 2016, *Cell Metabolism*, National Institutes of Health pubmed, https://www.ncbi.nlm.nih.gov/pmc/articles/PMC4864949/

Low-Glycemic Load

Energy levels throughout the day are modulated according to the rise and fall of blood sugar. Fiber and low-GI carbohydrates contained in whole natural foods, when eaten frequently, help to smooth out potential blood sugar fluctuations to extend the periods of satiety each day. Frequent eating of meals using whole foods keeps you satisfied for longer periods of time with less intake of food, and you will naturally choose to eat fewer calories. This happens, not because of willpower, but because you'll be satisfied with the amounts you have eaten.

As a reminder, the Glycemic Load (GL) is a measure of how much glucose enters your blood over a short period of time after consuming 100 grams of a food. High-caloric density high-GI foods typically have high-GL.

Weight-loss supplements themselves may or may not be low-GL, but the person taking the supplements often will use the supplements for convenience once or twice a day, but will likely not adequately change other eating habits. Other meals may continue to be imbalanced, may contain a lot of processed foods, and are likely to be high-GL. This haphazard approach to dieting is quite common with dietary supplement user. It typifies the average Western Diet, and it leads to inflammation and, potentially, a slowing metabolism.

Reversing the bad habits of the Western Diet and moving more toward a varied and nutritious intake focused primarily on low-GI and low-GL whole foods is a more effective solution for enhancing satiety than taking supplements without a reduction in GL by modifying the rest of the diet. [103]

---

[103] "LOW GLYCEMIC LOAD EXPERIMENTAL DIET MORE SATIATING THAN HIGH GLYCEMIC LOAD DIET" Chang et al., May 7 2012, *Nutrition and Cancer*, National Institutes of Health pubmed, https://www.ncbi.nlm.nih.gov/pmc/articles/PMC3762696/

Supplements are not as bulky as whole foods, so they do not fill you up as well, and they do not contain the broad variety of more easily digestible nutrients as whole foods. Thus supplements are not as effective in satisfying your appetite, keeping your metabolism strong, and keeping you healthy.

Takeaways for Chapter 13

- Supplements will never replace whole foods.

- Exercise and a balanced diet of whole foods that reduces your caloric intake is the only proven path to sustained weight loss.

- The American Diet compromises your gut microbiome.

- A compromised gut microbiome makes you vulnerable to obesity, disease and poor health

- Probiotics are best delivered in whole foods.

- Only take supplements in addition to eating a balanced, nutritious diet.

- Supplements are often untested, unproven, and potentially harmful.

Chapter 14

Good Habits

Habits Produce Results

Good habits are necessary to lose weight and to keep it off. Success at weight management is almost always due to a deliberate, ongoing process. So be sure to select habits that you can live with for the long-term.

You do not control your weight or your health. You DO control your habits, and your habits will ultimately drive whether you are healthy and slender or unhealthy and overweight. Many people argue that their health is completely out of their control, and that their body fat is determined by genetics, but the science does not support that.

Certainly, accidents happen and diseases happen, and some people have genetically slower metabolisms than others. However, healthy eating, hunger avoidance, and regular exercise substantially diminish the likelihood of accidents, diseases, and excess fat. Put another way, unhealthy eating, chronic hunger, and a sedentary lifestyle virtually guarantee a compromised immune system, a slowed metabolism, and obesity. Your adoption of good habits puts you on the path to a much better life!

Consistent with the goal of having a better life, it should feel good to be alive. I do not recommend that you adopt habits that you believe will make you miserable. That is not sustainable. Instead, you should look at the habits discussed here, and pick the ones that will actually improve your life... right now. Really, I want your life improved immediately, not after some far off time when you have reached all of your weight loss goals. Adopting habits that actually make you feel better about your life will make your journey sustainable.

Temporary willpower yields temporary results

Don't kid yourself. None of us can just use willpower to lose weight, then go back to our old ways and expect it to stay off. Weight gain is the natural result of our genetics and behaviors. Fortunately, we control how we choose to live, what habits we will adopt as our own, and what habits we will reject. The sooner we recognize that we are in charge of our own bodies, the sooner we can move toward success.

Choose the right habits

Choosing your habits is a major strategic decision. You do not need to adopt every one of the good habits that are associated with sustained weight loss, but you probably should adopt most of them. Try hard to see how to make each of them into an immediate positive in your enjoyment of life.

Each habit is an incremental step in the direction of burning more calories than you consume. Only if you adopt a majority of these habits are you likely to lose the weight you want to and keep it off. Studies have shown that each of these habits is shared by the majority of people who have been successful at losing substantial amounts of weight and keeping it off. The more good habits you adopt – and stick with – the greater the likelihood that you will be successful.

Over 10,000 people participated in a series of major research studies conducted by the National Weight Control Registry (NWCR). Every one of these people lost at least 30 pounds and has kept it off for at least a year. The average loss is 66 pounds for 5 ½ years. What they have in common is a set of habits that work.

People who have been successful at sustained weight loss generally focus at least as much on their good habits as they do on the actual end results they are looking for. The habits lead to the results.

Take Control of Your Life

Are you really serious about losing weight and keeping it off? Then take control of your situation. According to the International

Food Information Council 2015 survey[104],

> "Americans are trying to take control of many aspects of their lives, including their diet and physical activity. Over half try to take some control over the healthfulness of their diet (55%), their weight (57%), or their level of physical activity (55%). Only a quarter (24%) take a great deal of control over the healthfulness of their diet. In comparison, 41% try to take a great deal of control over their happiness…

> "So why the gap between thinking about healthfulness and taking action? For many, it is the lack of willpower (37%). Others cite lack of time (31%) or money (26%) as being barriers to meeting their weight management goals."

You already know that you can avoid severe tests to your willpower by avoiding hunger and plateaus. With five-minute meals and good planning, eating right does not have to take time, although exercise does require some time. Decide now whether your good health and happiness are priorities. Preparing your own meals can be less costly than the alternatives. If you want to take control of healthfulness, there is no better time than now.

"You can do anything if you set your mind to it"

My mother used to say that to me when I was a boy, and I came to believe it. This attitude allowed me to win a state championship in wrestling when my own best friend had told me it was an unrealistic goal. It allowed me to pay my way through Harvard. It allowed me to do quite a few things that others said were unrealistic.

---

[104] "2015 Food and Health Survey: Executive Summary."
International Food Information Council Foundation,
https://foodinsight.org/wp-content/uploads/2015/05/2015-Food-And-Health-Survey-Executive-Summary-Final.pdf

I have known many other people who have accomplished surprising things that would not have been possible if they did not believe they could do it. I am sure you do too. In fact, I bet you have done things that others were amazed about, because you believed in yourself.

When you have a proven approach like the Eat As Much As You Want system that is purely based on science and thoroughly tested so you already know it works, that assurance gives you the confidence to stick it out and do what is necessary to get to your goal and stay there. The system plus the following habits are what is necessary:

The Main Good Habits

Here is a list of a dozen habits that are so important, I have devoted at least a major part of a chapter to each of them:

1. Avoid hunger.
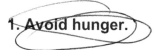

Not being hungry is great! What's not to like about that? It may take some getting used to though. Some people say they feel guilty eating before they get hungry. Don't feel that way. There is nothing to feel guilty about. When you are not hungry, your judgment about food improves, and your metabolism burns faster.

2. Log the following: meals, weight, measurements, exercise, sleep, activity.

Track your progress by looking back at your logs from time to time. When your weight or measurements improve over time, it will feel good to see it. If you stall, you can look at your logs and see that, then adjust accordingly. Keeping close track will usually help you to figure out what went wrong, so you can change course effectively.

3. Weigh yourself frequently, preferably every day.

Frequent weighing keeps us honest with ourselves and keeps us from straying too far. It always feels better to have some control in our lives.

4. Seize control of the trajectory of your life by focusing on the formation and maintenance of good habits.

The right habits make your life better. Feeling some power over your life's direction also feels good. Choose to implement habits that you believe strongly will make your life better. Have a clear understanding of what will be better about your life as a result of each of them. Write down your reasoning, and put that record with your life mission statement.

5. Plan your meals, and eat frequently.

Frequent, planned meals keep us moving toward our goals efficiently without hunger. The key on this is to find some really quick and easy meals that you like. Use those for the times when you have no extra time to deal with food. Eating this way gives you much more usable energy, keeps you more alert, and makes you more productive.

6. Eat low-fat, low-caloric density, nutrient-rich, mostly low-Glycemic Load, nutritionally balanced meals.

The Unlimiteds lists are quite long, so you should have no trouble finding foods you like. These foods fill you up and satisfy. The Countables lists are even longer. It feels good to eat foods you like, and know they are taking you to your goals without the suffering that goes with hunger.

7. Exercise regularly. Make appointments with yourself to exercise, and keep them.

When you identify activities that you enjoy, exercise will truly enrich your life's experience. It will help your social life, and it will make you feel better throughout each day. Start easy, and build from there.

As you progress through life, especially from age 40 onward, the less time you have been sitting each day (or curled up on your side) the less likely it is that you will suffer from chronic back pain. Don't underestimate the value of living without pain!

Once you have established a habit of exercising, doing it the right way accelerates your progress, and it makes you stronger. I have had so many clients tell me stories about how they would have been injured in some situation in their daily lives if they had not been doing the kinds of exercises recommended in Chapter 18. It is a huge plus in quality of life to be able to get through life with few if any injuries.

8. Keep your friends and loved ones informed about what you are doing with weight management.

Having the support of people you care about and who care about you will help you to get over many trials. Being able to talk about your experience is good for your soul. And having someone you are accountable to will help you to stay motivated.

9. Have no more than one alcoholic beverage a day. Minimize the carbohydrate content of your drink.

A little alcohol boosts the metabolism, but too much causes a world of hurt. Most people find that drinking a little alcohol is pleasurable.

10. Stay away from refined sugars.

Refined sugar is bad stuff. Once you fully understand the damage it causes you, you will begin to appreciate how much better life is without it. The immediate benefit of sugar avoidance is steadier energy throughout the day and less sleepiness or lethargy. Once you get past the addiction, your ability to taste the natural flavors of whole foods will improve, and healthy food will begin to taste much better to you.

11. Maintain a strategy targeting seven to eight hours of sleep a night.

Getting too much or too little sleep causes obesity, depression, cognitive dysfunction and a whole host of other problems you are better off without. Feeling rested is a huge plus in quality of life.

12. Create and maintain tools for self-motivation.

Living life with a purpose is huge. If you want a satisfying life, this is a must.

If you establish these 12 habits, you are well on your way to a successful weight loss and weight maintenance journey.

Nine Additional Secrets to Success

Are you all in? Do you want to know all the secrets to success in weight loss and maintenance? Scientists have done countless studies of how to be effective in losing weight and keeping it off. Here are nine additional good habits that scientists have found to be keys to that success.

Every one of these habits is adhered to by a significant percentage of people who have been successful in losing substantial amounts of weight and keeping it off for many years. Most such successful weight losers adhere to the majority of these habits:

1. Take personal responsibility.

When you accept and acknowledge that you alone are responsible for the behaviors that lead to being either trim or overweight, then you will be well started on a successful sustained weight-loss journey. The degree to which we believe that we control are destinies with respect to weight loss and weight loss management is highly correlated with success in doing it. [105]

It is easy to put the blame on our genes or on our partners or on society, but ultimately we are responsible for the choices we make. Seizing your personal power takes guts sometimes, but doing it is vital. Don't allow others to control what you do with your body. Your body is yours and yours alone. Take control of your own body and your own life.

This may mean proactively removing food temptations from your home. It may mean making healthy choices when you go out. You

---

[105] "Weight loss maintenance in relation to locus of control: The MedWeight study." Anastasiou et al., August 2015, *Behaviour Research and Therapy,* National Institutes of Health pubmed, *https://www.ncbi.nlm.nih.gov/pubmed/26057439*

may have to resist peer pressure at times. Do not allow people around you to undermine your self-determination.

2. Find physical activities you enjoy.

We all have difficulty adhering to unpleasant requirements, so try to build a life filled with things you enjoy. That includes how you get your exercise. The following quote from a 2016 study[106] discussed dancing, but if dance does not resonate with you, find an activity that does. If you find a group to do it with, so much the better!

> "In order to increase motivation and adherence, individuals experiencing problems during weight loss maintenance may be addressed to pleasant programs of leisure-time physical activity. Among leisure-time activities, dancing has a remarkable place; dance stimulates positive emotions, social interaction, and relationships in the community, while the acoustic stimulation and the music might strengthen the beneficial effects of aerobic exercise on cognitive functions. In a pilot nonrandomized trial, a 6-month dance course was associated with similar weight changes but with lower dropout rates compared with self-selected physical activity programs. This underlines the importance of social support and pleasant activities to increasing adherence to lifestyle intervention programs and to maintaining long-term weight loss in motivated patients."

3. Build confidence in your ability to exercise.

During my career in fitness, I have occasionally seen people start new workout programs determined to show on the first day that they

---

[106] "Long-term weight loss maintenance for obesity: a multidisciplinary approach." Montesi et al., February 26 2016, *Diabetes, Metabolic Syndrome, and Obesity: Targets and Therapy*, National Institutes of Health pubmed, https://www.ncbi.nlm.nih.gov/pmc/articles/PMC4777230/

could workout as hard as anyone else. A 2012 study showed that this is not a good approach:

> *"Individuals who build greater confidence in their ability to exercise, even in the face of barriers, may be more likely to exercise and therefore lose more weight..."*[107]

I recommend that you ease into increasing the amount of exercise that you do. Do not push yourself so hard at the beginning that you hate it or are overly sore or hurt yourself. None of those are good outcomes. The people who have put in amazing workouts the first day after a long period of sedentary living typically quit because they are so sore they cannot get out of bed the next day.

It is not how hard you work out that is most important. It is the fact that you DO workout that matters, no matter how lightly at first. The key is to make exercise a habit, then you will be able to build from there. You can do it!

4. Eat consistently throughout each week.

A major 2004 study disproves the popular idea that cheat days are good. People who cheat on the weekends are far more likely to gain weight than those who do not.[108]

---

[107] "Predictors of Weight Loss Success: Exercise vs. Dietary Self-Efficacy and Treatment Attendance." Byrne et al., April 2012, *Appetite*, National Institutes of Health pubmed, https://www.ncbi.nlm.nih.gov/pmc/articles/PMC3726181/

[108] "Promoting long-term weight control: does dieting consistency matter?" Gorin et al., February 2004, *International Journal of Obesity and Related Metabolic Disorders: Journal for the International Association for the Study of Obesity*, National Institutes of Health pubmed, https://www.ncbi.nlm.nih.gov/pubmed/14647183?dopt=Abstract

5. Eat consistently year around, including during the holidays.

178 successful weight losers (SWL) who lost an average of 77 pounds and kept off at least 30 pounds of it for an average of 5.9 years were asked about their "weight control strategies during the winter holidays." This was compared to the responses of 101 normal weight individuals (NW) with no history of obesity. Here is what the scientists learned:

> *"More SWL than NW reported plans to be extremely strict in maintaining their usual dietary routine (27.3% vs. 0%) and exercise routine (59.1% vs. 14.3%) over the holidays... SWL maintained greater exercise, greater attention to weight and eating, greater stimulus control, and greater dietary restraint, both before and during the holidays."[109]*

6. Sit to watch 10 hours or less a week of TV.

The average successful weight loser averages less than 10 hours of TV a week. Period. However, as long as you are up and moving, I do not believe that TV watching has to be a problem for you. This is why I say that if you feel the need to watch more than 10 hours of TV in a week, just make sure you are up and moving for all but 10 hours.

Here is what was revealed in a survey of the participants in the National Weight Control Registry:

---

[109] "Holiday weight management by successful weight losers and normal weight individuals." Phelan et al., June 2008, *Journal of Consulting and Clinical Psychology*, National Institutes of Health pubmed,
https://www.ncbi.nlm.nih.gov/pubmed/18540737?ordinalpos=2&itool=EntrezSystem2.PEntrez.Pubmed.Pubmed_ResultsPanel.Pubmed_RVDocSum

"A relatively high proportion (62.3%) of participants reported watching 10 or fewer hours of TV per week on entry in the NWCR. More than one third of the sample (36.1%) reported watching <5 h/wk, whereas only 12.4% watched > or =21 h/wk, which contrasts markedly from the national average of 28 hours of TV viewing per week reported by American adults. Both baseline TV viewing and increases in TV viewing over the follow-up were significant predictors of 1-year weight regain, independent of physical activity and dietary behaviors."[110]

7. Drink plenty of low calorie beverages.

What you drink can be sweetened or unsweetened. Generally speaking, you should get at least 96 ounces of water a day if you are female and 120 ounces if you are male. Water in all foods and beverages count. What you should not do is drink a lot of calories. Save the calories for the things you can chew, so they will satiate you and fill your stomach.

Drinking water immediately increases your metabolic rate, according to a study by Boschmann et al. in 2003.[65]

"Drinking 500 ml of water increased metabolic rate by 30%. The increase occurred within 10 min and reached a maximum after 30-40 min."

Water or herbal tea counts as an unsweetened beverage. There is no rule that says your beverages must be sweetened, and I do not recommend that you artificially sweeten, but it is permissible to do so. 53% of NWCR participants drink low- to no-calorie sweetened beverages:

[110] "Television viewing and long-term weight maintenance: results from the National Weight Control Registry." Raynor et al., October 2006, *Obesity*, National Institutes of Health pubmed, https://www.ncbi.nlm.nih.gov/pubmed/17062812

"Regular consumption of [low/no-calorie sweetened beverages] is common in successful weight loss maintainers for various reasons including helping individuals to limit total energy intake. Changing beverage consumption patterns was felt to be very important for weight loss and maintenance by a substantial percentage of successful weight loss maintainers in the NWCR."[66]

8. Pat yourself on the back regularly.

Congratulate yourself for any good habit(s) that you have maintained. Each new good habit puts you closer to attaining your goals. Adopting numerous (even if not all) good habits puts you in that small minority of overweight and obese people who are most likely headed for success in weight management. Merely forming and keeping the new good habits is a significant accomplishment. Acknowledging that fact to yourself is important in maintaining a positive attitude about yourself and your progress.

Scientists have found that self-esteem is important to maintain, not just for its own sake, but also for the sake of being able to stick with a program that will lead you to your weight and health goals. For example, people with positive feelings about themselves are much more likely to plan and log meals, which in turn increases the likelihood of successful weight loss:

"Self-esteem was related to attrition [that occurs in obesity treatment studies] such that the odds of attrition were significantly higher for those who reported negative feelings about themselves than those with positive feelings...

Early adherence (i.e., completion of food records) and weight loss predicted weight loss success at 1 year. Each additional day of food recording during the first three weeks of treatment was associated with a 7% increase in the odds of attaining at least a 5% weight loss at 1 year."[111]

If you establish the habits, then the weight loss and weight control will automatically follow. So your focus should be on the process, and the results will come. Elevate your own self-esteem by recognizing your own success in establishing a good habit even before the weight losses have happened.

9. Continue the good habits after reaching your goal.

Quitting the good habits means the weight will not stay off. This is why any habits you establish – even from the start – should be ones you are comfortable with and are confident you can maintain for the rest of your life. Choose only the habits that pass that test.

"A substantial proportion of people do not adhere to weight loss interventions… Adhering to healthy weight loss behaviors is required for weight loss initially and in the long term. If participants are unable to adhere to weight loss strategies, they will not lose weight."[112]

Scientists have found that -- after substantial weight losses – the people who kept the weight off maintained their good habits. The people who gained the weight back had largely given up on the good habits that enabled them to achieve the losses.

---

[111] "Predictors of Attrition and Weight Loss Success: Results from a Randomized Controlled Trial." Fabricatore et al., August 2009, ScienceDirect, *Behavioral Research and Therapy*, https://www.sciencedirect.com/science/article/abs/pii/S00057967090 01259?via%3Dihub
[112] "Weight loss intervention adherence and factors promoting adherence: a meta-analysis." Lemstra et al., August 12 2016, *Patient Preference and Adherence*, National Institutes of Health pubmed, https://www.ncbi.nlm.nih.gov/pmc/articles/PMC4990387/

"[G]ainers reported greater decreases in energy expenditure and greater increases in percentage of calories from fat. Gainers also reported greater decreases in restraint and increases in hunger, dietary disinhibition, and binge eating. This study suggests that several years of successful weight maintenance increase the probability of future weight maintenance and that weight regain is due at least in part to failure to maintain behavior changes."[113]

This study on weight regain underscores the importance of choosing hunger avoidance, enjoyable activities, and other habits that can truly be maintained for a lifetime.

Takeaways for Chapter 14

- **You control whether you will be successful at losing weight and keeping it off.**

- **Knowing the right way to eat, all you need to do is establish good habits to go along with eating right.**

- **The 12 habits and nine additional secrets to success described in this chapter will get you to your goal and keep you there:**

[113] "What predicts weight regain in a group of successful weight losers?" McGuire et al., April 1999, *Journal of Consulting and Clinical Psychology*, National Institutes of Health pubmed, https://www.ncbi.nlm.nih.gov/pubmed/10224727?dopt=Abstract

Habits:

1. Avoid hunger.

2. Log meals, weight, measurements, exercise, sleep, and activity.

3. Weigh yourself frequently, preferably every day.

4. Seize control of the trajectory of your life by focusing on the formation and maintenance of good habits.

5. Plan your meals and eat frequently.

6. Eat low-fat, low-caloric density, nutrient-rich, mostly low-Glycemic Load, nutritionally balanced meals.

7. Exercise regularly. Make appointments with yourself to exercise, and keep them.

8. Keep your friends and loved ones informed about what you are doing with weight management.

9. Have no more than one alcoholic beverage a day. Minimize the carbohydrate content of your drink.

10. Stay away from refined sugars.

11. Maintain a strategy targeting seven to eight hours of sleep a night.

12. Create and maintain tools for self-motivation.

Additional Secrets to Success:

1. Take personal responsibility.

2. Find physical activities you enjoy.

3. Build confidence in your ability to exercise.

4. Eat consistently throughout each week.

5. Eat consistently year around, including during the holidays.

6. Sit to watch 10 hours or less a week of TV.

7. Drink plenty of low calorie beverages.

8. Pat yourself on the back regularly.

9. Continue the good habits after reaching your goal.

Chapter 15

A Little Alcohol

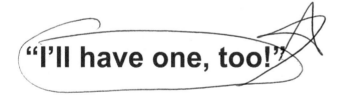

"I'll have one, too!"

Great news! You can have that drink or glass of wine or beer. It's okay! In fact, it's good. But you need to stop at one.

All of our lives, alcohol has been little understood. Recently, science has brought clarity to key questions about whether or not alcohol causes weight gain and whether or not alcohol shortens your life.

I remember decades ago when I was quite young. I saw Johnny Carson, the late night talk show host, joking about alcohol. He said a study had just come out that life insurance actuaries thought having one drink a day added a year to your life, but two drinks a day took 2 years away. I never forgot it. Now, all these decades later, it turns out that he was not far off from the truth.

Binge drinking is bad for you

Now, we know for sure that heavy drinking is associated with poor health. A 2005 study[114] showed that men who engaged in "episodic heavy drinking" were 28% more likely than the average person to have poor health, and women were 86% more likely.

A 2012 study in Korea associated binge drinking with abdominal obesity and metabolic syndrome. [115] Binge drinking was defined as seven or more drinks for men and three or more for women per typical occasion" at least once a week.

The damage done by clustering heavy drinking into one day a week cannot be undone by having an overall low alcohol

---

[114] "Poor health is associated with episodic heavy alcohol use: evidence from a National Survey." Okosun et al., June 2005, Science Direct, *Public Health*, https://www.sciencedirect.com/science/article/abs/pii/S00333506040 02288

[115] "Gender-specific relationships between alcohol drinking patterns and metabolic syndrome: the Korea National Health and Nutrition Examination Survey 2008." K. Lee, October 2012, *Public Health Nutrition*, National Institutes of Health pubmed, https://www.ncbi.nlm.nih.gov/pubmed/22321717

consumption average. It is clearly unhealthy to have a lot of alcohol on any given day or night.

Daily low level drinking is good for you

However, most people who average seven or fewer drinks a week actually spread their consumption out over the course of the week. This is clearly a far healthier approach.

You didn't really think you could drink seven drinks in one night, then make up for it by skipping the next six nights and call it healthy, did you?

A major 2018 study[116] seems to generally support what Johnny Carson said all those years ago. It looked at individual-participant data from 599,912 current drinkers without previous cardiovascular disease, and it found that the magic number for best life expectancy was at or below 100 grams of alcohol per week. That equates to no more per day than 12 ounces of 5% alcohol beer, or 5 ounces of 12.5% alcohol wine, or one 80 proof shot (1.5 ounces).

If you average more than one drink a day, though, your life expectancy will begin to drop:

> *"In comparison to those who reported drinking >0–≤100 g per week, those who reported drinking >100–≤200 g per week, >200–≤350 g per week, or >350 g per week had lower life expectancy at age 40 years of approximately 6 months, 1–2 years, or 4–5 years, respectively..."*[116]

---

[116] "Risk thresholds for alcohol consumption: combined analysis of individual-participant data for 599 912 current drinkers in 83 prospective studies." Wood et al., April 14 2018, *The Lancet*, https://www.thelancet.com/journals/lancet/article/PIIS0140-6736(18)30134-X/fulltext

Alcohol and insulin sensitivity

Why would a little bit of alcohol each day be good for you? One benefit is that it improves insulin sensitivity.

Type 2 diabetes is when your lean tissues have become resistant to insulin. This creates a cascade of health problems that can lead to metabolic syndrome, which is a combination of some of the following: excessive amounts of abdominal fat, high blood pressure, high LDL cholesterol, low HDL cholesterol, high serum triglycerides, and high blood sugar. This combination often leads to cardiovascular disease. If your brain becomes insulin resistant, that can lead to dementia. So enhancing insulin sensitivity is good:

"Low to moderate amounts of alcohol, when taken on a regular basis, improve insulin sensitivity. Insulin is a potential intermediate component in the association between alcohol consumption and vascular risk factors (metabolic syndrome)."[117]

Brown Fat

Until recently, nearly everyone believed that even a little bit of alcohol would cause weight gain. However, a 2017 study proved that assumption to be false.[118] To understand why the answer is no, let's talk about brown fat.

---

[117] "Insulin sensitivity and regular alcohol consumption: large, prospective, cross sectional population study (Bruneck study)." Kiechl et al., 1996, *The BMJ*, https://www.bmj.com/content/313/7064/1040.short

[118] "Moderate alcohol intake induces thermogenic brown/beige adipocyte formation via elevating retinoic acid signaling." Wang et al., October 2017, *The FASEB Journal*, https://www.fasebj.org/doi/pdf/10.1096/fj.201700396R

We have more than one kind of fat. The kind that we are constantly struggling with is white fat. That is the unhealthy kind of fat that can make us overweight or obese.

However, when we were babies, we also had brown fat, which increased our metabolic rates and helped us to burn the white fat. We tend to lose brown fat as we get older. Scientists formerly thought that all of our brown fat was gone by the time we became adults, but now it is known that many adults still have it.[119] The more brown fat we have at any point in time, the more slender we are likely to be and vice versa. The formation of brown fat is a great help in the fight to lose weight and keep it off.

In 2017, Wang et al. discovered that one drink or less of alcohol per day aids in the formation of new brown fat.[118] It also *"improves human health with protection against metabolic syndromes, including type 2 diabetes."*

Wang et al. found that one drink per day or less (but greater than zero) provides protection against *"obesity, diabetes, and fatty liver disease"*, and it *"increased caloric intake but reduced body weight by increasing energy expenditure"* and speeding the metabolism... *"which explains the beneficial effects of alcohol intake on glucose and lipid clearance, and improving insulin sensitivity..."*[118]

---

[119] "Overlooked 'Brown Fat' Tied to Obesity", Harrison Wein, Ph.D, April 20 2009, National Institutes of Health, *NIH Research Matters*, https://www.nih.gov/news-events/nih-research-matters/overlooked-brown-fat-tied-obesity

Technical Explanation

Wang et al. gave a technical explanation of how alcohol speeds the metabolism, so you automatically burn extra calories totaling more than the amount of the alcohol you consume:

Moderate alcohol consumption elevates levels of a chemical called retinoic acid (RA) by converting some of your vitamin A to RA. This increases signaling of RA, which boosts the metabolism, including oxidation of lipids and glucose. Elevated RA levels cause the formation of new brown fat and raises the body temperature, which implies that the metabolism has sped up. In mice, it reduces obesity and metabolic dysfunction. Vitamin A itself is also associated with a faster metabolism.

What could be better?

Awesome, right? You drink alcohol, then you burn more calories and it helps you to lose weight! Wow!! Who'd have thought?

Hold on, though. Don't get too excited. There's a catch.

Wang et al. say that more than one drink of alcohol a day can lead to vitamin A deficiency and liver disease, so the entire process breaks down. One drink spurs vitamin A to speed the metabolism, but having more than one interferes with liver function, ultimately causing vitamin A deficiency. Ouch!

With heavy drinking, RA signaling is not able to function and brown fat is not able to form, so all of those extra calories go to fat, and weight gain happens.

Prior to the Wang et al. study in 2017[118] and the Wood et al. study in 2018[116], there was lots of confusion about whether or not alcohol caused weight gain. We did get a glimpse from the Bendsen study in 2013 which found that it was only people who were drinking over a pint of beer a day were gaining belly fat:[120]

"Data from a subset of studies indicated that beer intake > 500 mL/day may be positively associated with abdominal obesity."

Bendsen et al. was trying to decipher many different studies that mixed up all levels of drinking and were simply looking at whether alcohol causes weight gain. Now, in light of Wang and Wood, we know that the ideal number to shoot for is one drink or less per day, because a little alcohol helps us to avoid excess weight, but anymore than a little leads to weight gain, poorer health, and shortened life expectancy. In other words, that second drink turns the first one from a good thing to a bad thing.

In short, consume anywhere from zero alcohol to one drink on any given day. Avoid any extra calories in your drinks though such as sugary mixers or sweet dessert wines. Keep the carbohydrate levels of your alcoholic beverages to an absolute minimum.

One caution

Having said that, I feel obliged to warn you about the "apéritif effect". It is well established that alcohol consumption spurs appetite.[121] The apéritif effect does not affect everyone. Just in case

---

[120] "Is beer consumption related to measures of abdominal and general obesity? A systematic review and meta-analysis." Bendsen et al., February 2013, *Nutrition Reviews*, National Institutes of Health pubmed, https://www.ncbi.nlm.nih.gov/pubmed/23356635
[121] "The apéritif effect: alcohol's effects on the brain's response to food aromas in women." Eiler et al., July 2015, *Obesity*, National Institutes of Health pubmed, https://www.ncbi.nlm.nih.gov/pmc/articles/PMC4493764/

though, be sure to have some Unlimiteds handy to quench your appetite anytime you have a drink.

Takeaways for Chapter 15

- **Limit your alcohol per day to no more than 12 ounces of 5% alcohol beer, or five ounces of 12.5% alcohol wine, or one 80 proof shot (1.5 ounces).**

- **One drink or less per day speeds the metabolism enough to make up for the calories in the drink.**

- **More than one drink on any given day converts the calories to weight gain.**

- **You cannot average out a day of excess by abstaining on other days.**

Chapter 16

Motivation

Weight Loss is Not Your Purpose

What motivates you? I mean, really motivates you. And I don't just mean about weight loss. We all have things we know we ought to do, but we can't seem to bring ourselves to do them. Why are these different from the things we actually get done?

Each person has many goals and one purpose. Weight loss may be one of many goals you have. Find your purpose, and connect the dots from your purpose to your goals. If your goals seriously support your purpose in life, then this process will help you to tap into unshakable motivation. Finding your deepest, most effective motivation will help you to achieve a meaningful, fulfilling life, live longer, be healthier, and reach your dearest long-desired goals.

When starting a new weight-loss program, most people believe they are highly motivated. There are many obvious reasons why weight loss is appealing. However, after spending a few weeks making sacrifices, establishing new habits, and encountering challenges, those reasons may seem less compelling.

Yo-yo weight loss is a prime example of the cycle of failed motivation. We start out determined, maybe even excited, to achieve our weight-loss goals and keep the weight off. But if we hit some roadblocks, then motivation may weaken.

Motivation Maintenance

While you still feel motivated, establish a strategy to keep your motivation high.

Prepare for roadblocks on the way to your goal. These may include peer pressure, social challenges, a slowing metabolism, a plateau, or chronic hunger pangs. Be sure you have a good strategy for eliminating or getting past these obstacles.

Know why you are doing it. Before you start, document specifically how your goal relates to your life's purpose. Do not jump ahead into a weight-loss program without clearly enunciating why you are doing it. Explore the deep reasons why it is imperative that you lose weight. Knowing and documenting this truth in advance is the best way to build a box of tools to use whenever your feelings of motivation falter. When superficial reasons for weight loss are not

278

enough anymore, it is vital that you be able to draw from a deeper well.

Find a strategy that works. Believing you can do it is not enough. To be successful at anything, you need to have a "How" and a "Why". The How is the step-by-step strategic plan that will take you there. We should always do sufficient research to have faith in the How before we charge ahead with it. Once we are convinced that the plan will work, we can stay committed if we have a sufficient "Why".

The Eat As Much As You Want system is the "How" that gets you to your goal without hunger or plateaus. It provides a healthy, guided path to your goal and onward to the rest of your life in maintenance mode. This enables you to take the weight-loss journey with as few tests as possible to your willpower. However, it still takes a lot of motivation and determination to change habits that you have built up over a lifetime, to stay consistent, and to be committed even in the face of many temptations.

The fact that you are reading this book tells me you are probably open to making positive changes in your life. And you are motivated. However, if you have experienced the yo-yo in the past, then you know motivation can break down.

Your motivation is the "Why." Arm yourself with motivation that is too strong to break. With a "How" that surely works and a "Why" that will not break, you will be successful at attaining your goal of sustained weight loss.

The Importance of Having a Purpose

With a clear life purpose, you are more likely to avoid yo-yo weight loss and to live a long life. A major 2019 study[122] concluded the following: "[A] stronger purpose in life was associated with lower all-cause mortality." Put another way, "This study's results indicated that stronger purpose in life was associated with decreased mortality." Those participants with a purpose had much better survival rates than those without.

Not only are you likely to live longer if you have clear purpose, but your health, quality of life, social support and resilience are likely to be greater, according to a major peer-reviewed study in 2018:[123]

> "[Purpose in life] has been associated with positive health outcomes among older adults, including fewer chronic conditions, less disability, and reduced mortality... The strongest characteristics of medium and high [purpose in life] from the separate regression models were high social support followed by high resilience... In numerous prospective research studies, higher [purpose in life] has been associated with better self-rated health, fewer chronic diseases (eg, stroke, myocardial infarctions), reduced pain, less disability, less dementia and Alzheimer's disease, and reduced mortality. In addition, those with higher [purpose in

[122] "Association Between Life Purpose and Mortality Among US Adults Older Than 50 Years." Aliya Alimujiang et al., *Journal of the American Medical Association*, May 24 2019, https://jamanetwork.com/journals/jamanetworkopen/fullarticle/27340 64

[123] Source: "Purpose in Life and Positive Health Outcomes Among Older Adults." Musich et al., *Popular Health Management*, April 1 2018, National Institutes of Health, https://www.ncbi.nlm.nih.gov/pmc/articles/PMC5906725/

life] are more compliant with preventive services, are more likely to be physically active, engaged in meaningful activities, and have fewer sleep problems. Those with medium and high [purpose in life] had significantly lower health care utilization and expenditures... and higher [quality of life]... [Purpose in life] is strongly associated with better physical and mental health outcomes among older adults."

A 2017 study conducted by Turner et al. found that people with a strong sense of purpose in life sleep better. [124] This study looked at 800 people and found a high correlation between purpose in life and current and ongoing sleep quality.

"Furthermore, these findings are consistent with anecdotal observations that people who have meaning and purpose in their waking activities appear to sleep well at night. It appears that for both African American and White American older adults, the more meaning and purpose one has in daytime activities, the better one tends to sleep at night. Collectively, the emerging data indicates the benefits of positive psychology on sleep health.

"We found that higher levels of purpose in life were generally protective against the occurrence of sleep apnea and RLS [(Restless Leg Syndrome)] as well as the onset of sleep apnea and RLS over the following 1 to 2 years. One interpretation of our findings is that individuals with a high purpose in life tend to have better overall mental and physical health. The premise of positive psychological well-being includes the notion that improved well-being will be

---

[124] "Is purpose in life associated with less sleep disturbance in older adults?" Turner et al., July 10, 2017, *BMC, Sleep Science and Practice*, https://sleep.biomedcentral.com/articles/10.1186/s41606-017-0015-6

accompanied by the optimal functioning of the persons' physiological systems (Phelan et al. *2010*; Ryff et al. *2004*)."

Finding the "Why"

Having a clear life purpose, or life mission, transforms our lives for the better. It allows us to focus our energies on what is important, and to disregard the things that might be wasting our time. It helps us to prioritize and organize. When we recognize and internalize the relationship between achieving our specific goals and our life purpose, our motivation – the "Why" -- becomes unshakable.

Motivation and purpose are inextricably linked. The "Why" is answered by knowing your purpose in life. If you know your purpose, and you understand clearly how it relates to your goals, then you are far more likely to follow through on achieving the goals. Thus, creating a life mission statement is a critical part of laying a foundation for achieving your goal of sustained weight loss.

Each of us is faced with a choice of whether or not to drift through life without ever looking seriously at why we are here. If we choose not to look carefully at that question, then we likely have no coherent understanding of what our life mission is. There is a big price to pay for not knowing this.

Goals vs. Purpose

We all have goals. Losing weight may be a very important one. Other goals could be things like getting a promotion, earning a lot of money, becoming good at our work, putting our kids through college, remembering people's birthdays, winning an election, achieving certain community or church-related objectives, or doing bucket-list items such as hiking the Appalachian Trail, surfing, or running a race.

These are all worthy goals. You will reach some of them, but, if you are like most people, there may be some on your list that you miss achieving. A goal is not your life mission, because it is usually achievable in a finite period of time.

Your life purpose lasts a lifetime. It gives meaning to your existence--past, present and future. It is bigger than any one goal. The goals that best support your purpose are the ones you are most likely to achieve. The goals that do nothing to help you to live out your mission are the ones you may give up on.

If you struggle with obesity, I would wager that sustained weight loss is central to optimally serving out your purpose. Clients of mine who have been successful at substantial sustained weight loss have been able to tell me how that goal relates to their life aspirations. Anyone who loses a lot of weight and keeps it off has abiding reasons for doing so.

Meaningfulness

As you think about what the overarching purpose is for your life, keep in mind that sustained weight loss is a goal, not a purpose. It probably supports your purpose, but it is not your overall reason for being. For now, set aside weight loss and think of why your life has meaning. Usually, the most fulfilling purposes are ones that focus on meaningfulness.

At the end of this exercise, you will look at how your goals line up with your life's purpose, but please do not do that right now. For now, let's look at what is most important to you, so you can see what you want the theme to be of the remainder of your life.

It is often said "I just want to be happy." However, research has shown that happiness is primarily a short-term feeling. You may feel happy, for example, if you win a prize or your workweek ends or you achieve a goal or your child makes an A. Such happiness does not last, because there is always something around the corner to make you unhappy, such as a defect in the prize, the start of a new workweek, a setback in your efforts toward another goal, or your child being defiant.

Fortunately, all of the benefits of having purpose in life relate to meaningfulness, not to happiness. When you focus on the meaning in your life, the ups and downs of happiness become much easier to manage. Meaningfulness provides perspective. Perhaps the prize you received was recognition for personal work, and it is not the prize itself that matters so much as the sense of satisfaction you got from your work. Perhaps your work relates to your passions and personal interests, in which case the end of the week may be great because of personal activities you are looking forward to, but the start of a new workweek gets you back to the work you love.

If your goals are part of an overall tapestry of tasks that relate to your life purpose, then you may be able to consider the journey, as Steve Jobs said, to be the reward. Then, each setback can be put into your mental framework as another step in the path to success. For example, when you weigh the aggravations of child rearing against your unconditional love for your children, short-term unhappiness or disappointment may be outweighed by the abiding joy of knowing that your presence in their lives has made an overwhelmingly positive difference.

Happiness and meaningfulness often go together, but the former fluctuates far more than the latter. At any given point in time, we can experience great unhappiness within the context of a highly meaningful existence. Purpose is your intentional life driver that takes you in the direction of creating the meaning you have decided your life will have.

"The quest for meaning is a key part of what makes us human," Stanford researchers concluded in a study on "the key differences between lives of happiness and meaningfulness."[125]

> *"Happiness without meaning is characterized by a relatively shallow and often self-oriented life, in which things go well, needs and desires are easily satisfied, and difficult or taxing entanglements are avoided, the report noted.*
>
> *"And so, the meaningful life guides actions from the past through the present to the future, giving one a sense of direction. It offers ways to value good and bad alike, and gives us justifications for our aspirations. From achieving our goals to regarding ourselves in a positive light, a life of meaningfulness is considerably different than mere happiness."*

That does not mean that you must abandon happiness in order to live with purpose. Quite the opposite is true:

> "'You don't become happy by pursuing happiness. You become happy by living a life that means something,' says Harold Kushner…
>
> "'Many persons have a wrong idea of what constitutes true happiness. It is not attained through self-gratification but through fidelity to a worthy purpose.' — *Helen Keller*"[126]

---

[125] "Stanford research: The meaningful life is a road worth traveling." January 1 2014, Stanford University, *Stanford Research*, https://news.stanford.edu/news/2014/january/meaningful-happy-life-010114.html

[126] "Your Life Will be Incredibly Better if You Pursue Meaning Instead of Happiness." Thomas Oppong, January 16 2018, *Thrive Global*, https://medium.com/thrive-global/this-year-pursue-meaning-instead-of-happiness-71e1bb3a3d8f

Meaningfulness takes us beyond our selves. It is the distillation of how our lives touch other people's lives and make a difference. Positive meaningfulness is driven by a purpose that guides us to aspire to help others to have better lives. In the pursuit of positive meaning, we are incidentally led to greater health, longevity, satisfaction and long-term happiness.

Creating a Life Mission Statement

Step 1: Think about key events in your childhood that influenced your thinking. Write about them. Two or three events may be enough. You do not need to write yourself a long story. Write enough to be reminded of what happened and how your values, beliefs and desires were influenced by each event.

Step 2: Think about key events in your adulthood that influenced your thinking. Write about them. Again, two or three may be enough.

Step 3: Considering Steps 1 and 2, make a list of what you are passionate about.

When doing step 3, do not place limits on yourself. Almost anything could be on that list. It is all about you and your passions only. Maybe it is your desire for your children or grandchildren to have a better life, or your concern for the environment, social justice, societal norms, medical issues, or people in need. It could have to do with your faith, or helping the sick or downtrodden, or entertaining people, or teaching children. The possibilities are endless.

Step 4: Looking at your list of passions, ask yourself the following: "Which of these can I do something about?"

Is there a way for you to make a difference, either small or large? Would making a difference require certain skills that you already have or could acquire?

Step 5: Focus on the passions that you can do something about, whether by pursuing new skills or by some other means such as community involvement or outreach, or a career change, or the adoption of new habits. Think about things you did in the past that gave you a sense of satisfaction.

Step 6: Narrow the list from Step 5 to passions and pursuits that are in line with your talents and interests. Would pursuing them feel rewarding to you? I do not mean financially rewarding, although there is nothing wrong with getting financial rewards when helping others. What I mean is, would they make you feel good?

Step 7: Write your life mission statement. It should be no more than one sentence. It may specifically reflect your talents, interests, passions, and abilities. It should be meaningful in that it will direct you to have a positive impact on the lives of others. And it should be broad enough to be meaningful throughout the balance of your life.

Save your mission statement to an easily accessible file. Put it where you can retrieve it whenever you are trying to focus your life in positive and personally rewarding ways.

Examples

My life's purpose is to gather and use knowledge to help others to have better lives. My area of interest has been the workings of the human body, so this is where I have focused much of my attention over the years. This has given me the courage to lose 40 pounds and keep it off for the past 12 years. It has also driven me to become a weight-loss and fitness coach, to found topfitpros.com, and to create the Eat As Much As You Want system. I derive great satisfaction from helping my clients to change their own health trajectories. In the process, I have also become a Licensed

Massage and Bodywork Therapist (NC #14700) certified in medical massage. Knowing my purpose guides me and motivates me, even when there are challenges.

This same purpose supports my goal of having a positive impact on my kids. I love them dearly, so of course I am passionate about this goal. They are all grown now, and each of them is very independent, but I know this goal will never end for me. Ironically, part of the knowledge I have gathered is that, as valuable as my input may be, my kids now make their own decisions and find their own ways in life. As they become ready to hear, only then can I effectively share what I have learned.

In much the same way, those of you who are reading this book must decide for yourselves whether or not you will be open to – and put into practice – the knowledge that is available here. That is your decision to make. My purpose is the same, regardless, and it provides substantial meaningfulness to me.

One of my clients, Nancy G, says that her purpose is to be a positive force in the lives of her daughters, so she set goals to maintain health and vitality so as not to be a burden to them. Her own mother spent the last five years of her life bedridden and attached to a catheter, and this was a very difficult experience for Nancy. This motivated her to determine in March of 2015, at age 65, to lose weight and get into shape. She lost 27 pounds following the Eat As Much As You Want system and has kept it off ever since.

As a result, she is able to travel frequently to visit her daughters in San Antonio, Texas and New York City. They exercise together, go hiking together, and she is able to keep up with them while walking the streets of New York City and climbing the many flights of stairs in their apartment buildings. Rather than being a burden to her children, she is able to help them in a variety of ways, including working in one daughter's thriving business and helping another daughter recently with wedding planning. This brings a great deal of joy to her life, and she is confident that her daughters do not need to worry about her suffering the same fate as her mother.

Implementation

Once you have your mission statement, consider how your life should change to enable you to live out your stated purpose. Perhaps you should be going back to school to develop certain skills, or you may need to change jobs. You may need to change certain habits.

Or maybe you don't need to make major changes, because you are already on the right track. Perhaps all you need to do is to focus your energy more on specific areas of your life that support your purpose. Looking at your life through the lens of purpose gives you solid guidance as to how to prioritize your actions and your goals.

Examine each of your goals in light of your purpose. Keep in mind that some of the goals may be important supports to your purpose even though the support may be indirect. List out all of the ways that each goal does or does not support your purpose. Elevate the goals to high priority if they support your purpose, and discard goals or demote them to low priority if they do not.

Goal: Sustained Weight Loss

Look at your goal of losing weight and keeping it off. Does it support your life purpose? If it does, great! List out the many reasons why.

If you do not believe that it supports your life purpose, it is unlikely you will be successful at losing the weight and keeping it off. But I have great confidence that it does support your life purpose, because I have guided many clients to weight loss, and all of them identified numerous ways that sustained weight loss supported their life purposes.

Here are some of the reasons my clients have given as to why sustained weight loss supports their life purposes:

- More energy throughout each day

- Better health supports greater ability to accomplish things

- Greater mobility allows them to do more
- Higher self confidence

- Improved self esteem

- Enhanced public image

- Ability to keep up with children and grandchildren

- Self sufficiency and independence

- Social benefits

- Greater mental acuity

- Greater longevity

The list could go on and on. Perhaps you can think of a lot of reasons not on the list that apply to you. Be specific. For example, less fat is associated with lower blood pressure, lower cholesterol, more consistent blood sugar, and less incidence of dementia. If excess weight is making you vulnerable to major negative health events, this limits the options of what goals you will ultimately be able to achieve, but good health opens up all kinds of possibilities.

Are there any specific health-oriented reasons why excess weight could ultimately block you from living out your purpose? If so, list them all, and then store them with your life mission statement. Having this list will be a powerful tool if you ever question your motivation to lose weight and keep it off.

Go through a similar exercise for any other goals that you have placed as a high priority.

Perseverance

When you fully understand the importance of healthy weight loss (or any other goal) in the quest to fulfill your life's purpose, this sure knowledge will get you through the tough times. Setbacks and challenges often derail people from reaching goals unless they are determined. When you know absolutely that a goal must be reached because it offers such support to your life's purpose, then you will find a way to reach it.

Takeaways for Chapter 16

- **Your life's purpose is broad and lasts for the rest of your life.**

- **For it to truly add meaning to your life, a life's purpose should enable you to have a positive impact on the lives of others.**

- **Having a strong sense of purpose makes you healthier, sleep better, live longer, and feel better about your life.**

- **Goals should support your life's purpose.**

- **Developing an understanding of how a goal supports your life purpose will greatly improve your long-term motivation to achieve it.**

- **This detailed understanding will help you to persevere and overcome obstacles and challenges in your path without wavering.**

- **Healthy weight loss is a goal, not a purpose.**

- **Healthy weight loss strongly supports most people's life purpose.**

Chapter 17

Devise Sleep Strategies

Shortness of Sleep Makes Us Fat and Unhealthy

Poor sleep is associated with excess weight and obesity as well as shortened lifespan and many

health disorders:[127]

> *"It is estimated that 50 to 70 million Americans chronically suffer from a disorder of sleep and wakefulness, hindering daily functioning and adversely affecting health and longevity. The cumulative long-term effects of sleep deprivation and sleep disorders have been associated with a wide range of deleterious health consequences including an increased risk of hypertension, diabetes, obesity, depression, heart attack, and stroke."*

Yikes!! That is awful! We are taking on fat and emotional stress and illness because we are not sleeping well. Obviously, diet and exercise are not enough. We also need good sleep strategies.

Not convinced yet?

You would be amazed at how many studies prove that poor sleep habits, obesity and poor health all go hand in hand. Here are excerpts from a few:

> *"Laboratory studies in healthy young volunteers have shown that experimental sleep restriction is associated with… increased hunger and with alterations in parameters of glucose tolerance suggestive of an increased risk of diabetes. Epidemiologic findings in both children and adults are consistent with the laboratory data."*[128]

---

[127] "Sleep Disorders and Sleep Deprivation: An Unmet Public Health Problem." Colten et al., 2006, The National Academies Collection: *Reports Funded by the National Institutes of Health*, National Institutes of Health pubmed, https://www.ncbi.nlm.nih.gov/pubmed/20669438

[128] "Impact of sleep and sleep loss on neuroendocrine and metabolic function." Cauter et al., 2007, *Hormone Research*, National

And

"Accumulating evidence from both epidemiologic studies and well-controlled laboratory studies indicates that chronic partial sleep loss may increase the risk of obesity and weight gain. The present chapter reviews epidemiologic studies in adults and children and laboratory studies in young adults indicating that sleep restriction results in metabolic and endocrine alterations, including decreased glucose tolerance, decreased insulin sensitivity, increased evening concentrations of cortisol, increased levels of ghrelin, decreased levels of leptin and increased hunger and appetite. Altogether, the evidence points to a possible role of decreased sleep duration in the current epidemic of obesity."[129]

And

"Individuals with [short sleep duration] are heavier and gain more weight over time than normal-duration sleepers. This sleep-obesity relationship may have consequences for obesity treatments, as it appears that short sleepers have reduced ability to lose weight… [C]ompared to normal sleep duration, sleep restriction increases food intake beyond the energetic costs of increased time spent awake."[130]

Institutes of Health pubmed,
https://www.ncbi.nlm.nih.gov/pubmed/17308390
[129] "Role of sleep and sleep loss in hormonal release and metabolism." Leproult et al., 2010, *Endocrine Development*, National Institutes of Health pubmed,
https://www.ncbi.nlm.nih.gov/pubmed/19955752
[130] "Sleep disturbances, body fat distribution, food intake and/or energy expenditure: pathophysiological aspects." St-Onge and Shechter, January 2014, *Hormone Molecular Biology and Clinical Investigation*, National Institutes of Health pubmed,
https://www.ncbi.nlm.nih.gov/pubmed/25372728

Impact on brain health

If the research I have shown you already is not enough to make you want to change your sleep-related habits, let's look at what inadequate sleep does to your brain:

> "[P]oor sleep in middle-age is linked to neurodegeneration-related biomarkers (e.g., amyloid deposition) and subsequent cognitive decline... Acute sleep deprivation and chronic sleep restriction have diverse effects... including increases in blood pressure, evening cortisol levels, insulin, proinflammatory cytokines, and sympathetic tone... , all which are hypothesized to accelerate cognitive aging... Furthermore, sleep deprivation/restriction in young animals can cause protein misfolding... and increased amyloid deposition... , which impair memory consolidation... and underpin Alzheimer's disease..."[131]

And look what it does to your ability to think:

> "Recent findings with clinically oriented neuropsychological tests suggest that one night without sleep causes particular impairment to tasks requiring flexible thinking and the updating of plans in the light of new information."[132]

And to your mood:

---

[131] "Sleep, Cognition, and Normal Aging: Integrating a Half-Century of Multidisciplinary Research", Scullin and Bliwise, January 2015, *Perspectives on Psychological Science*, https://www.ncbi.nlm.nih.gov/pmc/articles/PMC4302758/

[132] "One night of sleep loss impairs innovative thinking and flexible decision making", Harrison and Horne, May 1999, *Organizational Behavior and Human Decision Processes*, https://www.ncbi.nlm.nih.gov/pubmed/10329298

"[O]verall sleep deprivation strongly impairs human functioning. Moreover, we found that mood is more affected by sleep deprivation than either cognitive or motor performance and that partial sleep deprivation has a more profound effect on functioning than either long-term or short-term sleep deprivation."[133]

And to your ability to react appropriately:

Rapid eye movement sleep deprivation *"causes widespread abnormalities in coping and defensive responses in threatening situations; these deficits are not reversed and, in some cases, may be exacerbated by amphetamine."[134]*

How Much Sleep Do You Need?

I think we all know we need sleep, but how much? Bob K is a good friend who never sleeps more than six hours. If I did that, I would be constantly tired. Yet Bob is always high energy, productive and sharp.

"How can you survive on so little sleep?" I once asked him.

"I get asked that all the time," he answered. "I feel rested when I get up, and I just can't sleep any more than that. My doctor assures me that I am getting the right amount for me."

---

[133] "Effects of sleep deprivation on performance: a meta-analysis", Pilcher and Huffcutt, May 1996, *Sleep*,
https://www.ncbi.nlm.nih.gov/pubmed/8776790
[134] "REM sleep deprivation induces changes in coping responses that are not reversed by amphetamine", Martinez-Gonzalez et al., June 15 2004, *Sleep*,
https://www.ncbi.nlm.nih.gov/pubmed/15282995

Sleep

Bob convinced me before I began my own independent research that, for him, six hours is enough. I don't know anyone else like Bob though, and I couldn't enjoy life if that was all the sleep I was getting.

This is a personal decision. How much sleep do you need? Let's see what the experts say.

Dr. Daniela Marschall-Kehrel, a medical researcher Frankfurt, Germany says:

> *"Adequate sleep is a basic requirement for good health. Adults generally require 7 to 8 hours of sleep per night. Sleep deprivation is associated with a decreased ability to perform tasks controlled by the frontal lobe, such as planning, concentration, motor performance, and high-level intellectual skills. Constant poor-quality sleep can also cause excessive daytime sleepiness, depression, and immune function compromise. In addition, continued sleep disruption has been associated with an increased risk for mortality."*[135]

All the experts seem to agree with Marschall-Kehrel about what sleep deprivation causes, but not everyone agrees about the precise amount of sleep each of us needs. Here is what virtually all of the experts agree about:

We all need sleep. If we do not sleep well, our health and longevity are at risk. Many studies have found that inadequate sleep or poor-quality sleep leads to weight gain and obesity. So if you want to lose weight or maintain at your weight goal, it is vital that you have strategies to attain healthy sleep.

---

[135] "Update on nocturia: the best of rest is sleep." Marschall-Kehrel, December 2004, *Urology*, National Institutes of Health pubmed, https://www.ncbi.nlm.nih.gov/pubmed/15621224

Many experts say that most of us need seven to eight hours of sleep. However, a meta-analysis done jointly in 2017[136] by major universities in the U.S. and China found that the risk of death from all causes is lowest at seven hours of average sleep per night. Below seven hours, the risk goes up by 6% per hour. Above seven hours, the risk goes up by 13% per hour. This was true of both men and women.

The meta-analysis implies that seven hours is the magic number, and that eight may be too much.

However, some experts will tell you that the amount of sleep needed each night is very individual. The real question is "Do you feel rested?" They say that if all of the following is true, you are probably getting enough sleep:

- You don't have daytime impairments,

- You feel rested during each day,

- You are sleeping the same amount you have slept most of your adult life, and

- You couldn't sleep anymore even if you stayed in bed longer.

If all four of those conditions are true, as they are for Bob, and you are only sleeping six hours a night, then six hours a night may be the right amount for you even though it is less than seven. Conversely, if it is not all true, then you may need more sleep. To make all of those true, I generally need somewhere between seven

---

[136] "Relationship of Sleep Duration With All-Cause Mortality and Cardiovascular Events: A Systematic Review and Dose-Response Meta-Analysis of Prospective Cohort Studies." Yin et al., September 9 2017, *Journal of the American Heart Association*, National Institutes of Health pubmed, https://www.ncbi.nlm.nih.gov/pubmed/28889101

and eight hours. I can make do with seven, but I feel better with about seven and a half.

If you are in bed nine hours or more a night, and you feel sluggish during the day, you probably should shorten your amount of time in bed. Remember what the 2017 meta-analysis said: "Above 7 hours, the risk [of all cause mortality] goes up by 13% per hour." [136]

In light of these facts, what is your ideal number of hours of sleep? For most of us, it is probably about seven hours like the meta-analysis said. You decide. You can always adjust your number later. Whatever your ideal number is, set a goal to get that much each night.

I realize that your life may be very busy and demanding. Still, sleep must be a priority if you want to be able to optimally function physically, mentally and emotionally, and to stay healthy and lose weight. Being overly tired at work is counterproductive, and it can be a major source of accidents. See if there is a way to adjust your work and social schedules as needed so there is time for enough sleep.

Suggested Strategies for Better Sleep

This chapter is full of suggestions for how to start sleeping better. Every suggestion is backed by scientific research.

Suggestion #1: Be consistent.

Before you start setting up your ideal bedtimes and wake up times, let's talk about consistency. A lot of us like to vary our sleep throughout the week. I know I have been guilty of that throughout most of my adult life. I work hard during the week, but then on the weekends, especially Saturday nights when I can sleep in on Sunday, I like to stay up a little later.

Until recently, I saw nothing wrong with that. A 2019 study[137] now has shown that this kind of variability in your weekly bedtime and wake-up schedule can contribute to obesity, among other things:

> "[N]ot sticking to a regular bedtime and wakeup schedule—and getting different amounts of sleep each night—can put a person at higher risk for obesity, high cholesterol, hypertension, high blood sugar and other metabolic disorders. In fact, for every hour of variability in time to bed and time asleep, a person may have up to a 27% greater chance of experiencing a metabolic abnormality... [T]he variations in sleep duration and bedtimes preceded the development of metabolic dysfunction. According to the authors [of the study], this provides some evidence supporting a causal link between irregular sleep and metabolic dysfunction. "

Consistency is very important, both for good health and quality of sleep. Why? Our bodies have circadian rhythms. A healthy circadian rhythm allows you to get up at a certain time, then enables your body and mind to function well during the day. At some point your alertness begins to fade, then your body begins to release melatonin

---

[137] "Study links irregular sleep patterns to metabolic disorders", June 2019, *National Institutes of Health, National Heart, Lung, and Blood Institute News*, https://www.nhlbi.nih.gov/news/2019/study-links-irregular-sleep-patterns-metabolic-disorders

and you become sleepy at bedtime. That is the way it is supposed to work.

Constantly varying your sleep schedule confuses your body about when it is supposed to prepare you for sleep. This may make you feel tired all day long and then wide-awake at bedtime resulting in dysfunction during the day and lost or poor-quality sleep most nights. Try to be consistent, so your body clock can set itself appropriately.

Suggestion #2: Experience bright light after you get up

Your circadian rhythm is like an alarm clock. Your habits will actually set your clock if you are intentional about it.

Make sure you set your circadian rhythm appropriately to fit your lifestyle. Whatever is your normal wake-up time, embrace the early part of the day by being in bright light during the first few hours. Sunlight is ideal, but normal electric lights in your house or your office are also very effective. The main requirement is the lights should include the blue light portion of the light spectrum (Suggestion #3), which almost all lights do. If you are trying to adjust to a new wake-up time, it may take a few days to make the adjustment, because only by establishing a routine will the body begin to release melatonin at the appropriate time to make you sleepy when it is time to go to bed.

People who are night owls tend to take longer to settle down to sleepiness after the lights dim than do morning people. Why? This is partly genetic. However, in large part, it is because they stay in the dark (with closed shades or a night mask) for some or all of the morning hours.[138]

---

[138] "Phase Angle of Entrainment in Morning- and Evening-Types Under Naturalistic Conditions." Emens et al., April 2009,

For sleep scientists, being a night owl is called "eveningness," and they say it can be unhealthy. For teenagers,

> "[e]veningness was associated with later bedtime and wake-up time, especially on weekends, shorter time in bed during the week, longer weekend time in bed, irregular sleep-wake schedule, subjective poor sleep. Moreover, evening types used to nap more frequently during school days, complained of daytime sleepiness, referred more attention problems, poor school achievement, more injuries and were more emotionally upset than the other chronotype. They referred also greater caffeine-containing beverages and substances to promote sleep consumption."[139]

According to a 2010 study[140] of mice, eveningness is associated with weight gain as compared with the same activity levels and same caloric intake as morning types, and the night owl mice eat more too, so they really put on the pounds. This weight gain with eveningness is all tied to exposure to light throughout each night as opposed to being in a normal light and dark cycle.

> *"These results suggest that low levels of light at night disrupt the timing of food intake and other metabolic signals, leading to excess weight gain. These data are relevant to*

Chronobiology International, National Institutes of Health, https://www.ncbi.nlm.nih.gov/pmc/articles/PMC2699216/
[139] "Circadian preference, sleep and daytime behaviour in adolescence." Giannotti et al., September 2002, Journal of Sleep Research, National Institutes of Health pubmed, https://www.ncbi.nlm.nih.gov/pubmed/12220314
[140] "Light at night increases body mass by shifting the time of food intake." Fonken et al., October 26 2010, *Proceedings of the National Academy of Sciences of the United States of America*, National Institutes of Health pubmed, https://www.ncbi.nlm.nih.gov/pubmed/20937863

the coincidence between increasing use of light at night and obesity in humans."

You can make yourself into more of a morning person by being intentional about the cycle of lights you are exposed to during each 24-hour period. Get up early, then allow yourself to be exposed to bright light during the first few hours of your day.

However, if your lifestyle, job or career requires you to be up late at night, then find a way to make your circadian rhythm work within those constraints. Get up at the same time each day, and subject yourself to continuous bright light during the first few hours of your day. Conversely, wear a sleep mask to block the light before it hits you in the morning. That way, your body can experience a quasi-normal light/dark schedule that will allow you to experience darkness during your sleeping hours, but brightness when it is appropriate given your personal 24-hour cycle. The light cycle is the key to establishing your circadian rhythm.

Being exposed to bright light early in the morning makes you sleep MUCH better that night:[141]

> *Morning "[e]xposure to bright light resulted in substantial changes in sleep quality. Waking time within sleep was reduced by an hour, and sleep efficiency improved from 77.5% to 90%, without altering time spent in bed. Increased sleep time was in the form of Stage 2 sleep, REM sleep, and slow wave sleep. The effects were remarkably consistent across subjects."*

Here's another study with a similar outcome:

---

[141] "Alleviation of sleep maintenance insomnia with timed exposure to bright light." Campbell et al., August 1993, *Journal of the American Geriatrics Society*, National Institutes of Health pubmed, https://www.ncbi.nlm.nih.gov/pubmed/8340561

"Sleep-wake patterns during the 24-h day were evaluated by nursing staff ratings and wrist-worn motor activity devices (actigraphs). Sleep improved substantially with bright light exposure [from 8am to 11am]. Waking time within nocturnal sleep was reduced by nearly two h, and sleep efficiency improved from 73% to 86%."[142]

Clearly, you can become more of a morning person if you choose to and your working life allows. The science is clear: Unless you master your personal light/dark cycle, you will not sleep as well as you could.

If you decide to transition to morningness, you must not waver in your decision to reset your body clock even though you may feel exhausted for a few days. If you sleep in to make up for feeling tired, then you will miss the bright morning sunshine that is the very thing that resets your body clock.

I have seen friends and loved ones time and again make that decision to sleep in, stay under the covers, and/or take long naps during the day to make up for the exhaustion of either jet lag or eveningness. Every single time, they were unable to make the transition either to the new time zone or to morningness *until* they began to get out of bed every day at the correct time. Within a few days of starting to enter into the light and to get up in the earlier morning, they began to be able to go to sleep earlier and to sleep better. Remember, it is the early hours of exposure to the bright light of daytime that resets your body clock. If you miss those hours, then it will not reset.

---

[142] "Bright light treatment improves sleep in institutionalised elderly--an open trial." Fetveit et al., June 2003, *International Journal of Geriatric Psychiatry*, National Institutes of Health pubmed, https://www.ncbi.nlm.nih.gov/pubmed/12789673

Suggestion #3: Lower the lights as bedtime approaches, and block the blue

The same lights that start your circadian rhythm early in the day will prolong wakefulness if continued into the night. A 2011 study[143] showed that simply being exposed to bright light later in the day substantially delays sleepiness:

> "Compared with dim light, exposure to room light [for 8 hours] before bedtime suppressed melatonin, resulting in a later melatonin onset in 99.0% of individuals and shortening melatonin duration by about 90 min. Also, exposure to room light during the usual hours of sleep suppressed melatonin by greater than 50% in most (85%) trials."

For that reason, as you approach bedtime, lights should become less bright.

> "[R]oom light exerts a profound suppressive effect on melatonin levels and shortens the body's internal representation of night duration. Hence, chronically exposing oneself to electrical lighting in the late evening disrupts melatonin signaling and could therefore potentially impact sleep, thermoregulation, blood pressure, and glucose homeostasis… [E]lectrical light between dusk and bedtime strongly suppresses melatonin levels, leading to an artificially shortened melatonin duration and disruption of the body's biological signal of night."[144]

---

[143] "Exposure to Room Light before Bedtime Suppresses Melatonin Onset and Shortens Melatonin Duration in Humans." Gooley et al., March 2011, *Journal of Clinical Endocrinology and Metabolism*, National Institutes of Health, https://www.ncbi.nlm.nih.gov/pmc/articles/PMC3047226/
[144] "Exposure to Room Light before Bedtime Suppresses Melatonin Onset and Shortens Melatonin Duration in Humans." Gooly et al., March 2011, *Journal of Clinical Endocrinology and Metabolism*,

Any light will suppress melatonin, but it is specifically blue (short wavelength) light that most triggers the suppression. In a 2011 study[145] of computer monitor use at night, it was found that wearing glasses that block blue light caused the melatonin levels to not be significantly suppressed in college students.

Since that time, blue light blocking glasses have become popular. Some studies indicate that lesser quality blue light blockers do little good, but more recent studies of higher quality blue blockers indicate that they can be effective in improving sleep and the body's ability to produce melatonin.

> "The use of short wavelength blocking glasses at night increased subjectively measured sleep quality and objectively measured melatonin levels and sleep duration... Results suggest that minimizing short wavelength light following sunset may help in regulating sleep patterns."[146]

If you use blue blocking glasses, try to start at least three hours – but not more than five -- before bedtime. You need the bright light prior to that, including the blue part of the spectrum, to enhance your circadian rhythm. (See Suggestion #2.)

There are also numerous blue light blocking apps for computers, and they automatically block the blue only in the evening. If you need to use your computer after dark, it would be a good idea to

National Institutes of Health,
https://www.ncbi.nlm.nih.gov/pmc/articles/PMC3047226/
[145] "The impact of light from computer monitors on melatonin levels in college students." Figueiro et al., 2011, Neuro Endocrinology Letters, National Institutes of Health pubmed,
https://www.ncbi.nlm.nih.gov/pubmed/21552190
[146] "Attenuation of short wavelengths alters sleep and the ipRGC pupil response." Ostrin et al., June 27 2017, *Ophthalmic and Physiological Optics*, Wiley Online Library,
https://onlinelibrary.wiley.com/doi/abs/10.1111/opo.12385

download one of these apps. Additionally, wear blue light blocking glasses after dark, and keep lights in your home as dim as is practical the closer you get to bedtime.

Suggestion #4: Limit any naps to less than 30 minutes

Short naps can be a good thing, but long naps can undermine you in a variety of ways. First, as we saw in Suggestion #2, a long nap may mean significantly reduced exposure to bright light during the day, which may push back your perceived bedtime and transition you back to being a night owl. Second, it may make you groggy for 30 minutes afterward:[147]

> *"[A]fter a night of restricted sleep (6 hrs)... Working memory... and subjective workload were assessed approximately 5 and 25 minutes after 90-minute morning and afternoon nap opportunities...After afternoon naps, participants performed less well on more executive-function intensive working memory tasks..., but waking and napping participants performed equally well on simpler tasks. After some 30 minutes of cognitive activity, there were no longer performance differences between the waking and napping groups."*

Third, frequent naps will make you sleepy during the day even on days you do not nap:

> *"[F]requent napping appears to be associated with lighter daytime sleep and increased sleepiness during the day."*[148]

---

[147] "Effects of sleep inertia after daytime naps vary with executive load and time of day." Groeger et al., April 2011, *Behavioral Neuroscience*, National Institutes of Health pubmed, https://www.ncbi.nlm.nih.gov/pubmed/21463024

[148] "The effect of nap frequency on daytime sleep architecture." McDevitt et al, August 20 2012, *Physiology & Behavior*, National

However, short naps that last less than 30 minutes can actually refresh you and improve performance:[149]

"A nap during the afternoon restores wakefulness and promotes performance and learning. Several investigators have shown that napping for as short as 10 min improves performance. Naps of less than 30 min duration confer several benefits, whereas longer naps are associated with a loss of productivity and sleep inertia… In contrast, the habit of taking frequent and long naps may be associated with higher morbidity and mortality, especially among the elderly."

Naps less than 20 minutes long are common among healthy adults, and they do not affect nighttime sleep.[150]

Suggestion #5: Eat a small, balanced meal close to bedtime

Many studies have examined the timing and types of evening meals. The findings have been that the size and caloric content of the meals is critical in determining the impact on weight and sleep. The impact can be good or bad.

The older studies were focused on the impact on sleep of bingeing late at night. Not surprisingly, bingeing disturbed sleep patterns, disrupted nocturnal metabolic hormone secretion and

Institutes of Health pubmed,
https://www.ncbi.nlm.nih.gov/pubmed/22659474
[149] "Good sleep, bad sleep! The role of daytime naps in healthy adults." Dhand and Sohal, November 2006, *Current Opinion in Pulmonary Medicine*, National Institutes of Health pubmed,
https://www.ncbi.nlm.nih.gov/pubmed/17053484
[150] "The prevalence of daytime napping and its relationship to nighttime sleep." Pilcher et al., Summer 2001, *Behavioral Medicine*, National Institutes of Health pubmed,
https://www.ncbi.nlm.nih.gov/pubmed/11763827

caused weight gain. Newer studies have shown that a nutrient-rich small meal just before bedtime is beneficial for sleep, heart, muscle and metabolic health. [151]

Suggestion #6: Relax your mind

A little before time to go to sleep, engage in mental relaxation activities such as listening to music, meditating[152][153], or reading. If you have stressful subjects on your mind such as your job or relationship struggles or financial concerns, make a note to focus on those during the daytime only.

When you are in bed under the covers with the lights out, close your eyes and visualize something soothing such as a beautiful scene or a flowing stream. The human mind is always thinking, so choose to fill your mind with pleasant imagery, prayer or some kind of positive fantasy that relaxes you.

Discipline yourself not to dwell on your difficulty sleeping or on the negative things that can happen if you do not get enough sleep.

---

[151] "The health impact of nighttime eating: old and new perspectives." Kinsey and Ormsbee, April 2015, *Nutrients*, National Institutes of Health pubmed, https://www.ncbi.nlm.nih.gov/pubmed/25859885

[152] "Mindfulness Meditation and Improvement in Sleep Quality and Daytime Impairment Among Older Adults With Sleep Disturbances: A Randomized Clinical Trial." Black et al., 2015, *JAMA Internal Medicine*, https://jamanetwork.com/journals/jamainternalmedicine/article-abstract/2110998

[153] "The effect of mindfulness meditation on sleep quality: a systemati review and meta-analysis of randomized controlled trials." Rusch et al., December 2018, *The Annals of the New York Academy of Sciences*, Wiley Online Library, https://nyaspubs.onlinelibrary.wiley.com/doi/abs/10.1111/nyas.13996

That train of thought will only keep you awake. Set a goal to relax and rest. Sleep may come on its own if you relax, but do not try to force it. Positive meditation or visualization is restful and healthy, and engaging in it can take your mind away from the challenge of going to sleep. As long as you are lying down comfortably and engaging in restful mental activity, you are moving in the right direction.

Suggestion #7: Seek either quiet or soothing sound at bedtime

Noise causes poor sleep quality, less sleep duration and increased cortisol.[154]

For that reason, it is best to sleep in a very quiet place. However, if that is not feasible, relaxing music has been found to be effective in improving sleep:

> "[M]usic statistically significantly improved sleep quality [in young participants with poor sleep]… Relaxing classical music is an effective intervention in reducing sleeping problems."[155]

If you are in a place where there is a lot of noise, such a parties or traffic, masking the noise with whatever sound is soothing to you is a better alternative than simply enduring the noise:

> "Environmental noise, especially that caused by transportation means, is viewed as a significant cause of

[154] "Effects of nighttime low frequency noise on the cortisol response to awakening and subjective sleep quality." Waye et al., January 10 2003, *Life Sciences*, National Institutes of Health pubmed, https://www.ncbi.nlm.nih.gov/pubmed/12493567

[155] "Music improves sleep quality in students." Harmat et al., May 2008, *Journal of Advanced Nursing*, National Institutes of Health pubmed, https://www.ncbi.nlm.nih.gov/pubmed/18426457/

sleep disturbances. Poor sleep causes endocrine and metabolic measurable perturbations and is associated with a number of cardiometabolic, psychiatric and social negative outcomes both in adults and children."[156]

If the familiarity of having a TV on soothes you, it may be what you use to go to sleep. Be aware, however, that there are drawbacks to sleeping with a TV on, and there may be other alternatives for background sound that will work better for you. The glowing blue light that the TV emits before and during sleep can impact sleep quality, shorten sleep duration, and potentially put you into a state of depression. (See Suggestion #3.) The sounds of the TV are not consistent, and there is no way to know what messages are penetrating to your subconscious mind from the TV while you are sleeping. A more rhythmic sound such as relaxing instrumental music or waves crashing is usually a better choice, but try to play those sounds without having a screen turned on.

Suggestion #8: Avoid caffeine for at least eight hours before bedtime

"[A] moderate dose of caffeine at bedtime, 3 hours prior to bedtime, or 6 hours prior to bedtime each have significant effects on sleep disturbance."[157]

Caffeine is thought to have many benefits, but try to get it early in the day and stop immediately following lunch. If you feel you need a pick-me-up in the afternoon six hours or less from bedtime, then you

---

[156] "Environmental noise and sleep disturbances: A threat to health?" Halperin, December 2014, *Sleep Science*, National Institutes of Health pubmed, https://www.ncbi.nlm.nih.gov/pubmed/26483931
[157] "Caffeine effects on sleep taken 0, 3, or 6 hours before going to bed." Drake et al., November 15 2013, *Journal of Clinical Sleep Medicine*, National Institutes of Health pubmed, https://www.ncbi.nlm.nih.gov/pubmed/24235903

are probably eating too much high-GI food at lunch, which has caused a blood sugar spike and subsequent crash.

Eat according to the Eat As Much As You Want system or snack on Unlimiteds so the pick-me-up won't be necessary. That will even out your blood sugar much more effectively, and allow you to get through the afternoon without the customary energy crash. Standing up for three minutes every 30 also helps with energy levels.

Suggestion #9: Have no more than one drink of alcohol at least three hours before bedtime.

There have been many studies on sleep disturbance caused by excessive alcohol consumption. It is definitely a bad idea to have two or more drinks within three hours of bedtime. One study found that having roughly two drinks or more after 7:00 p.m. inhibited melatonin production significantly for the first half of the night.[158]

One drink for healthy women had no impact on melatonin or estrogen, but two or more did:

> *"Consumption of alcoholic beverages may suppress circulating melatonin levels at night, possibly resulting in an increase in circulating estrogen. An increased estrogen burden could increase the risk of breast cancer. This study was designed to investigate whether alcohol consumption is associated with a decrease in nighttime melatonin levels in a group of healthy women… A categorical analysis revealed no effect of one drink, but a 9% reduction with two drinks, a 15% reduction with three drinks, and a 17% reduction with*

---

[158] "Ethanol inhibits melatonin secretion in healthy volunteers in a dose-dependent randomized double blind cross-over study." Ekman et al., September 1993, *Journal of Clinical Endocrinology and Metabolism*, National Institutes of Health pubmed, https://www.ncbi.nlm.nih.gov/pubmed/8370699

four or more drinks. It remains unknown whether such a change could affect estrogen levels or breast cancer risk."[159]

Thus, it is best to consume no more than one drink of alcohol, to have it well before bedtime, and to avoid excessive drinking entirely.

Additional studies have been done with regard to sleep apnea. A 1982 study found that people already diagnosed with apnea had it worse when they excessively consumed alcohol.[160] Another found that excessive drinking caused sleep apnea in otherwise healthy men.[161]

Two drinks or more disrupts nocturnal emission of growth hormone and TSH (thyroid stimulating hormone). These are hormones which are vital for maintaining your metabolic rate and for lean tissue repair, growth, and long-term health.[162]

---

[159] "Alcohol consumption and urinary concentration of 6-sulfatoxymelatonin in healthy women." Stevens et al., November 2000, *Epidemiology*, National Institutes of Health pubmed, https://www.ncbi.nlm.nih.gov/pubmed/11055626

[160] "Alcohol, snoring and sleep apnea." Issa and Sullivan, April 1982, *Journal of neurology, neurosurgery, and psychiatry*, National Institutes of Health pubmed, https://www.ncbi.nlm.nih.gov/pubmed/7077345

[161] "Alcohol increases sleep apnea and oxygen desaturation in asymptomatic men." Taasan et al., August 1981, *Journal of American Medicine*, National Institutes of Health pubmed, https://www.ncbi.nlm.nih.gov/pubmed/7258218

[162] "Ethanol decreases nocturnal plasma levels of thyrotropin and growth hormone but not those of thyroid hormones or prolactin in man." Ekman et al., July 1996, *The Journal of Clinical Endocrinology and Metabolism*, National Institutes of Health pubmed, https://www.ncbi.nlm.nih.gov/pubmed/8675588

In short, if your bedtime is 10 or 11pm, two drinks or more after 7:00 p.m. will have a significantly negative impact on the quality and restorative value of your sleep.

Suggestion #10: Set the bedroom temperature to what feels comfortable

Sleep is of poorer quality when the room feels hot. For a better night's sleep, find a temperature that is cool enough and feels comfortable to you.

> *"[B]oth objective and subjective measures of sleep were more disturbed by heat than by noise."*[163]

Suggestion #11: Take a hot bath or shower before bed.

Numerous studies have shown that a hot bath, shower or footbath facilitates and enhances sleep and fights insomnia, especially among the elderly. [164, 165] *"A hot footbath is especially*

---

[163] "Relative and combined effects of heat and noise exposure on sleep in humans." Libert et al., February 1991, *Sleep*, National Institutes of Health pubmed, https://www.ncbi.nlm.nih.gov/pubmed/1811316

[164] "Bathing before sleep in the young and in the elderly." Kanda et al., July 1999, *European Journal of Applied Physiology and Occupational Physiology*, National Institutes of Health pubmed, https://www.ncbi.nlm.nih.gov/pubmed/10408315

[165] "Effects of passive body heating on body temperature and sleep regulation in the elderly: a systematic review." Liao, November 2002, *International Journal of Nursing Studies*, National Institutes of Health pubmed, https://www.ncbi.nlm.nih.gov/pubmed/12379298

recommendable for the handicapped, elderly, and disabled, who are unable to enjoy regular baths easily and safely."[166]

Suggestion #12: Make sure your bed is comfortable.

There is no question that pain and discomfort in bed disrupt sleep. (See Suggestion #17.) If the pain is being caused or exacerbated by the bed, you should consider getting a new one. [167],[168]

Suggestion #13: Exercise (preferably not just before going to bed)

Exercise improves sleep. There has been a huge amount of research on this, and the results are quite conclusive.

> *"Older adults with moderate sleep complaints can improve self-rated sleep quality by initiating a regular moderate-intensity exercise program."[169]*

---

[166] "Effects of bathing and hot footbath on sleep in winter." Sung and Tochihara, January 2000, *Journal of Physiological Anthropology and Applied Human Science*, National Institutes of Health pubmed, https://www.ncbi.nlm.nih.gov/pubmed/10979246

[167] "Effect of prescribed sleep surfaces on back pain and sleep quality in patients diagnosed with low back and shoulder pain." Jacobson et al., December 2010, *Applied Ergonomics*, National Institutes of Health pubmed, https://www.ncbi.nlm.nih.gov/pubmed/20579971

[168] "Grouped comparisons of sleep quality for new and personal bedding systems." Jaconson et al. March 2008, *Applied Ergonomics*, National Institutes of Health pubmed, https://www.ncbi.nlm.nih.gov/pubmed/17597575

[169] "Moderate-intensity exercise and self-rated quality of sleep in older adults. A randomized controlled trial." King et al., January 1 1997, *Journal of the American Medical Association*, National

And

"*Acute moderate-intensity aerobic exercise appears to reduce pre-sleep anxiety and improve sleep in patients with chronic primary insomnia.*"[170]

Exercise at anytime is a major net positive, so if the only time you can do it is just before bed, go for it. It is a great stress reducer, which is good for sleep, and it is vitally important for good health. However, if you have a choice on timing it is best to do it earlier in the day, or at least a couple of hours before bedtime. It can be invigorating, so it is likely to make you more alert for a couple of hours after your workout. Because of the alertness boost, I have some very successful clients who like to workout in the afternoon, then go back to work recharged.

Suggestion #14: Limit your late evening liquid consumption

Hydration is extremely important for good health, and especially important when trying to lose weight. You should consume water and other liquids throughout the day and into the early evening. However, be thoughtful about how much liquid you take in as you get closer to your bedtime and during the night. The more you drink late, the more likely you are to need to go to the bathroom during the night. This is true of many people.

Then, there are extreme cases. Nocturnal Polyuria Syndrome (NPS) happens in about 3% of the elderly population. NPS is excessive urination at night that disturbs sleep.

Institutes of Health pubmed, https://www.ncbi.nlm.nih.gov/pubmed/8980207
[170] "Effect of acute physical exercise on patients with chronic primary insomnia." Passos et al., June 15 2010, *Journal of Clinical Sleep Medicine*, https://www.ncbi.nlm.nih.gov/pubmed/20572421

"The treatment of NPS may include avoidance of excessive fluid intake, use of diuretics medication in the afternoon rather than the morning, and desmopressin orally at bedtime."[171]

Suggestion #15: Consult your doctor or a sleep specialist.

If you are concerned that you may have a chronic sleep disorder that will not be resolved by implementing the suggestions in this chapter, then by all means you should consult a physician or sleep specialist. You can look for a specialist at the American Academy of Sleep Medicine (http://www.aasmnet.org/bsmspecialists.aspx).

Common sleep disorders include sleep apnea, restless leg syndrome, acute insomnia, chronic pain (see also Suggestions #12 and #17), hormone imbalance, and many others. Workers who have late night shifts or who must work different shifts on different days often struggle with establishing circadian rhythms (see also Suggestions #2 and #3). Maybe you do not even know why, but your sleep has been of poor quality for a very long time. In any of those cases, reach out for some help.

Suggestion #16: See a therapist.

If you cannot relax at night because you are plagued by angst related to large issues of your life, the best answer may be to seek the help of a Licensed Professional Counselor. I highly recommend therapy for everyone, even people who believe they've got it all together. Sleep difficulty is often related to deeper issues you may be struggling with that come up in your mind at night when all is

---

[171] "Nocturia, nocturnal polyuria, and sleep quality in the elderly." Asplund, May 2004, *Journal of Psychosomatic Research*, National Institutes of Health pubmed, https://www.ncbi.nlm.nih.gov/pubmed/15172208

quiet. Health and quality of life can be much better if you speak with a professional who can help you to sort out any negative emotions you may be feeling. It is far easier to sleep when you are at peace within yourself.

Lots of very healthy people use therapists. I do, and it has been beneficial. It is important to sort out your emotions, but not when you are lying in bed preparing to sleep. That is the time for peaceful relaxation. (See Suggestion #6.)

Suggestion #17: Get a periodic massage.

Massage therapy can help your body to stay more relaxed, which in turn can allow you to relax more effectively at night. I recommend either medical massage for specific work to resolve seriously tight muscles or joint pain, or relaxation massage for general physical tension.

As I mentioned before, pain and discomfort can keep you awake at night. Painkillers may mask the symptoms, but they do not solve the underlying problem. Remember, pain is your body's alarm system that something is damaging your body and should be resolved.

Medical massage can make a huge difference for many chronic pains such as back, hip, knee, foot, shoulder, elbow, wrist, thumb, neck and jaw pain. Also, tight muscles in the upper back, neck and jaw are common causes of chronic headaches and migraines. Any one of these pains can and do interfere with sleep. I have helped numerous clients to get back to sleeping through the night.

You can address many of these issues with a process called Self Myofascial Release (a form of self-administered massage therapy). You might look online for how-to videos if you prefer not to see a massage therapist. You may be surprised at how many pains can be resolved with the right kind of massage. However, if a massage therapist cannot help you with your pains, you should definitely see a doctor.

Suggestion #18: Log your sleep

Write down what time you go to bed and how much sleep you get each night, or log it with an online application. Some devices even track the quality of your sleep. Any of these tools can help you to keep track of whether you are progressing toward getting the correct amount of sleep. If you look back on the history of your sleep, and you are making good progress, great! If not, review the suggestions above to see if there are any other changes you can still make to your sleep-related habits.

Takeaways for Chapter 17

- **Sleep deprivation, either from poor-quality sleep or too little sleep, causes health issues, shortened lifespan, cognitive decline, and weight gain.**

- **For most people, seven hours of sleep is ideal. More or less than that shortens life expectancy.**

- **Everyone's sleep needs are slightly different.**

- **It is vital to have a regular sleep schedule. You can help your body to establish a healthy circadian rhythm by using bright light when you get up, and low light or blue blocking in the evening.**

- **Comfort improves sleep quality.**

- **Comfort can be achieved with noise masking or quiet, darkness, a good bed, and the right room temperature.**

- **Prepare your mind for sleep with relaxing thought, music and therapy.**

- **Prepare your body for sleep with exercise earlier in the day, massage, a hot bath, shower or footbath, and a small nutrient-dense meal.**

- **Avoid caffeine after noon and alcohol three hours before going to bed.**

- **Limit water consumption just before bedtime.**

- **Log your sleep.**

Chapter 18

Optimize Exercise Results

Look Good. Feel Good. Have Fun. Live Long.

This chapter is about getting the most you can out of exercise. This is a scientific approach to taking your fitness to the next

level. I will teach you how to become stronger, increase stamina and retain all of your musculature as you lose fat.

Most people following diets lose about a third of a pound of muscle for every two thirds of a pound of fat they lose. Such muscle loss can add up very quickly, and it is hard to get it back. My goal for you, if you choose to accept it, is to lose only fat and no muscle. That is what my clients typically do.

Like everything else that I recommend, this is not done with pills or shots or surgery. You will use all of your muscles and all of your muscle fibers in all planes of motion. In this chapter, I will explain fitness science, and I will introduce you to multiplanar high intensity interval training. More detail on this kind of training is found in the Exercise Appendix at the back of the book.

"Multiplanar" exercises are movements in all planes of motion. These could be straight ahead, side to side, or twisting motions. These use and strengthen large and small muscles all over your body that traditional exercise does not address.

The phrase "high intensity" can be intimidating, so let me explain. High intensity is very individual, and the intensity level must be appropriate for you. I always advise my clients to start out easy, and only do the exercises at a pace that will allow them to avoid excessive soreness. I want you to pick an appropriate pace at the outset that will allow you to enjoy it even if you feel like you are hardly pushing yourself at all. Once you have worked out a few times, you can start to push yourself a little harder.

Over a long period of time, you can work up to exercising at a high level of intensity. It may take you weeks or months or a year or two to get there, and that is perfectly okay.

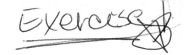

A major key to longevity and greater health is to make exercise a habit. As your fitness improves, you will begin to feel the increases in strength and stamina, and you will realize that tasks and exercises that used to overwhelm you no longer even make you breathe hard. That is when you'll be hooked. At that point, you won't mind pushing yourself, because you'll feel a sense of accomplishment and inner peace when you put in a hard workout. Stick with it, and that day will come.

If you have not done so already, begin by laying a foundation of movement in accordance with Chapter 7, and establish a habit of exercise and regular physical activity. The rewards for making a serious commitment to your health and wellness are immense.

We have already spoken about the importance of making at least some portion of your exercise fun. When you enjoy it, it becomes a positive in your life that you can look forward to doing. Again, find what you like, whether it is tennis, pickleball, basketball, walking around a shopping mall, gardening, hiking, biking, running, volleyball, yard work, cleaning, handyman tasks, walking around the neighborhood, throwing a Frisbee, or any other exercise. Your goal should be to find something that keeps you moving that you will continue to do because you like it.

Now let's talk about how to optimize your fitness results:

The Science of Fitness

When you exercise, your body reacts and improves. When you do not exercise, your body reacts and deteriorates. As you gain a better understanding of this process, my hope is that you will recognize the tremendous control you have over how good or bad you will feel in the future.

Adaptation

The basic foundation of fitness is a principle called SAID, which stands for "specific adaptation to imposed demands". Your body is constantly adapting to its environment. Adaptation can be either positive or negative. First, let's talk about the positive kind.

When you workout really hard, you use some muscles extensively and they may become sore. The soreness is your body adapting. Lactic acid, which is a by-product of the energy used in your muscles, seeps out into the local area of the muscle and irritates it, because your body is not used to working that area so hard.

As you get used to the exercises, your body will grow more blood vessels around those muscle cells, and it will begin to carry lactic acid away more efficiently. Then you will not become sore so easily. That is positive adaptation.

Along with the growth of vascularity, your muscles will be fed better, so you will gain stamina. That is also positive adaptation.

The initial straining that you did to complete the exercises may have broken down some of the muscle tissues. During recovery between workouts, your body repairs those tissues and grows more, making you stronger. Again… positive adaptation.

Motor nerve synapses that have not been used much in a long time will be put to the test during your workout, and they will have to fire to recruit all of the muscle fibers that you need to complete the exercises. At first, those synapses will not work very well, and you will feel weak. However, over the first couple of weeks, those synapses will wake up, and sleepy muscles tissues will respond better to motor nerve impulses. You will likely experience significant strength gains as the nerve signal pathways from the brain to the muscles begin to carry the signals more efficiently. Basically, your electrical wiring gets upgraded. Yet again… positive adaptation.

Atrophy and sarcopenia

Adaptation, unfortunately, cuts both ways. Slowly, but continuously, during any period in the past that you have been sedentary, your muscles and capillaries and nerves have been adapting in the other direction. When tissues are not used, the body interprets that as meaning you do not need them. So the body breaks them down and carries them away for energy usage.

That is called atrophy, and it is negative adaptation. As anyone gets older, atrophy accelerates due to the declining circulating levels of various hormones. The more sedentary a person becomes, the more atrophy occurs, and the weaker the body becomes. This continuous destruction and dissolution of muscle tissue with aging is called sarcopenia. Again, this is negative adaptation.

This acceleration of the process of atrophy is why older adults cannot afford to go as long without exercise as younger adults. Sadly, the older we are, the longer it takes and the harder we have to work to get back any muscle tissue we lose. So regular exercise is increasingly important the older we get.

When we restrict our caloric intake, and we start to lose weight, the body looks around for fuel to burn, i.e, any tissues not needed. If they are not being used, the body will determine they are not needed. That again is negative adaptation, and it is why the typical weight-loss program results in so much loss of muscle. It is really difficult to get lost muscle back, and it becomes increasingly so as we age.

Muscle Weight

Your job, then, while you are losing weight and beyond, is to tell your body that it needs that muscle tissue much more than it needs the fat. The way you communicate this is simple: You use the muscle tissues vigorously. When you do this, your body will quickly recognize that your muscle tissues are needed, and it will look elsewhere for fuel.

Meanwhile, your muscular capabilities will be developing. That does not necessarily mean your muscles will be getting bigger. Most women, for example, rarely increase muscle size even when they work out very hard. Women have small amounts of testosterone, but normally not enough to naturally develop big muscles.

You will probably gain muscle weight during the first two weeks of vigorous exercise, because the muscles are fed needed nutrients at a ratio of about three parts water per one part nutrients. Thus, the water swells the muscle cells to feed them, and this usually translates to a couple of initial pounds of muscle weight gain. After roughly two weeks, that water-weight gain in the muscles will level off. In the meantime, if you are eating appropriately, fat will be burning off.

Inches before pounds

Because your initial two weeks is characterized by increases in muscle weight as fat is burned off, you may see no change in the scale, but your clothes may become a little looser. That is because muscles are denser and heavier than fat, so if you gain two pounds of muscle weight and lose two pounds of fat, your measurements may go down.

That is a good thing. That means your efforts are bearing fruit. In weight loss social media groups, this is an NSV, or "non-scale victory". That means you are losing fat and keeping your muscle. That is exactly what we want to have happen.

Why? We want you to keep the muscles so you will be healthy, strong and capable. People who lose muscle and fat together become weaker and see their metabolisms slow down along with the loss of muscle. We do not want that for you. And people who lose muscle and fat end up looking gaunt and emaciated after they lose weight. We don't want that for you either.

Look good. Feel good.

We want you to look good, feel good and be strong and healthy, also with a stoked metabolism. We want you to be able to meet the challenges of your daily existence more easily than you have in the past because your body is simply more capable than it has been. So we must impose demands on the body that will spur the specific adaptations that we want to have happen.

This chapter will teach you how to obtain the adaptations you want for your body. That way, instead of atrophy and sarcopenia, you will earn muscle retention and growth, nerve and capillary development, enhanced cardiorespiratory capability, better health and a faster metabolism.

As long as you have all of those things happening, and you are eating according to the Eat As Much As You Want system, your body will have no choice but to burn fat to fuel the caloric deficits your nutrition and exercise are creating. But you must exercise all of your muscles to get these results. You will not have the luxury of simply using your legs to walk or run, for example, while leaving your upper body vulnerable to atrophy and disintegration. You will not have the luxury of only using your bigger muscles for straight-ahead exercises such as crunches or push ups, leaving undefended the little ones that stabilize and rotate your back and shoulders. You must use them all to retain and develop them equally with the goal of keeping your body stable and injury free.

Remember, Specific Adaptation to Imposed Demands, or SAID, is the key to making your body as good as it can be.

Use It or Lose It

The SAID principle has taught us that we must use our muscles or the body will discard them. But it is not enough to use a certain muscle, because you may be using some of the muscle fibers and not others. The ones you do not use will be discarded.

I would like for you to take a long view of your life. If you are saving money for retirement now, then you should also want to save your body for retirement. When you get to retirement age, you will surely want to be able to do what you enjoy and to have choices about what activities you can participate in.

Whether you are 20, 40, or 60 years old, the exercises you do now, if they become habit, will give you compounded returns every decade. Health, strength, and vitality a decade from now may be extraordinarily better for you than for other people your age, and that contrast will only increase decade after decade.

I know this is true, because I live it every day, and so do my clients.

Muscle Fiber Types I and II

Most people think of a muscle as either contracting or not contracting, but that is not the way it works. When any muscle contracts, only some of the fibers do the work. Developing an understanding of different fibers and how they react to exercise will prepare you to more effectively guide your body to greater health and fitness for a lifetime.

For very easy tasks, Type I fibers do it all. These "red slow twitch" fibers are highly vascular, meaning they have ample blood flow to replenish any energy used in each contraction. For this reason, they have tremendous endurance. You can effectively use these fibers all day long for easy tasks such as working on the computer, walking or eating.

If you want to improve your endurance, then you do steady state exercises such as aerobics, distance running or bicycling, that push the Type I fibers to a capacity for a higher workload. To be clear, steady state exercises are ones that elevate your heart rate to a moderate level of exertion (possibly 110 or 120 beats per minute) and keep it there throughout the workout.

As tasks become more immediately challenging, such as heavier weights or bursts of speed, then fibers with less and less vascularity are recruited to help. This recruitment is achieved by increasingly strong motor nerve-firing impulses. In other words, your brain sends a signal to the muscle saying "This is going to be hard, so I need more fibers to help."

Type IIA ("red fast twitch") muscle fibers are next in line to be recruited. They have less blood flow than Type I, but enough to be used in sustained bursts of activity. If you have activities that require stamina for both strength and speed in bursts over a period of time, then you will use Type IIA fibers in addition to the Type I. Examples of this need are basketball, soccer, tennis, or even carrying luggage for a long trip or moving all of your belongings from one house to another. It is important to build Type IIA for stamina.

The only real difference between Type I and Type IIA muscle fibers is how much blood flow there is. Over time, with enough exercise, some of the Type IIA fibers will develop more vascularity, thus becoming Type I.

After Type IIA is Type IIX, or "white fast twitch", which is all of the remaining muscle fibers. (It is pronounced "type two ex".) In the past, we referred to this as Type IIB, but now we know there are many variations in the vascularity of this final category, so the "X" is a variable meaning the fibers could be IIB, C, D, E, etc. The less the vascularity, the further out the fiber type is in the alphabet.

Similar to Type I and IIA, if you regularly use any of these Type IIX fibers, they can increase their vascularity and move up. For example, some IIE fibers may become IID, and some IID may become IIC, and so on. That increase in vascularity means that more blood will be flowing to each of these muscle fiber types, which in turn means that the size of your muscles may increase. (But not always. See Gender and Genetics below.)

Type IIX is the strongest group of muscle fibers, because there are so many of them packed into a small space. However, the reason they are so tightly packed is that they have very little blood flow. Thus, they tire out quickly and take much longer to recover. These are only recruited when you are either lifting extremely heavy objects or moving explosively. You need your Type IIX fibers if you want to be very strong or very fast, or if you want to be able to jump high.

Aging

Unfortunately, most people are constantly losing Type IIX muscle fibers starting somewhere around age 30 or 35. I have made it a mission not to let that happen to me, and I regularly encourage my clients to follow my lead on loss prevention.

I mentioned atrophy and sarcopenia already. After about age 35, it becomes increasingly important to exercise regularly and to either lift relatively heavy weights or do explosive movements. The body is constantly adapting to stressors or to the absence of stressors. Exercises that stress muscles make the body adapt in a variety of ways. For example, vascularity will improve to bring more blood flow to the stressed muscle fibers. More fibers may grow. Motor nerve connectivity will improve.

Conversely, any muscle fibers that are not used for a long time are dissolved by the body and used for energy (atrophy). As we get older, it takes less and less time for the body to dissolve unused tissues (sarcopenia), so the older we get, the less time we can afford to not use something.

Not only does the loss of unused muscle fibers accelerate with age, but getting the lost muscle fiber back becomes anywhere from increasingly difficult to potentially impossible. You definitely do not want to lose muscle fibers if you can avoid it.

At any age, we can gain strength and increase muscle weight with resistance training. However, growing new muscle fibers requires an abundance of training and plenty of growth hormones and testosterone, both of which naturally diminish as we get older. It is much, much easier to keep what we've got than to grow it back.

The muscle fibers that are most vulnerable to sarcopenia and atrophy are the ones we use the least. These are the fibers that are furthest out on the alphabet (Type IIA, IIB, IIC, etc.) because they have so little blood flow. You may wonder why we would care about muscle fibers we use so seldom, but we care because we need these fibers if we hope to maintain our strength. They are vital to strength, and they are only used in situations when we need strength.

If we lift heavy, or if we do explosive movements like jumping, hard throwing, and sprints, then we recruit the furthest out Type IIX muscle fibers, and we signal to the body they are needed. That helps to keep us from becoming feeble in our old age. Find a way to regularly use all of your muscles and all of your muscle fibers if you want a strong, healthy, vital body as you get older. Every time you lose a group of muscle fibers, then the next least used becomes a target of sarcopenia.

Lots of people over the years have joked about how dedicated I am to staying fit. Some have jokingly proclaimed they believed in the benefits of rest, TV and "12 ounce curls". Others have said they would love to be able to find the time to exercise, but they are always too busy with work and family and/or church obligations. I have sadly watched these friends and family lose their vitality and grow old before their time.

At 63 years old, I am fairly muscular, about as strong as I ever have been, able to jump repeatedly onto a 36-inch-high box, trail run up and down mountains, and lead several workouts a day with clients. I tell you this not to brag, but because I want you to understand there is a great cost when you do not make time for exercise. I have made exercise a high priority, and it has paid me amazing dividends. Many people I have known who have not made it a priority have either died or are suffering with poor health, back or joint pain, obesity, dementia, depression, impotence, or any number of other ailments.

This choice to exercise or not is one of the most important choices you make *every day*. Old age can be wonderful, or it can be a nightmare. I strongly urge you to find a way to make time to exercise.

Gender and Genetics

Our genes dictate our natural mix of Type I, Type IIA and Type IIX muscle fibers. Some people have much more Type I fibers, but not a lot of Type II. They make great distance runners and have lots of endurance for any number of tasks. If that is your genetic make up, you will probably never have huge muscles, because it is by further developing the size and number and vascularity of the Type IIX muscle fibers that we make our muscles bigger.

Females on average have far fewer Type IIX muscle fibers than males.[172] That, coupled with hormonal differences, makes it difficult

---

[172] "Sex-Based Differences in Skeletal Muscle Kinetics and Fiber-Type Composition." Haizlip et al., January 2015, *Physiology*,

to impossible for most women to develop very large muscles, especially when they lose fat and get down to "normal" body weight based on the Body Mass Index (BMI).

A very small minority of women experience increased biceps size initially during the start of a new exercise program. This is almost always due to the fact that they hold a disproportionate amount of fat around and between muscle fibers. This is called interstitial fat. This fat will burn off with weight loss and regular exercise, and the upper arms will begin to look toned but not nearly as large.

Interstitial fat is often the quickest fat to burn off when losing weight. It is usually much healthier to carry our fat between muscle fibers than in our bellies, and it is often hardest to lose the belly fat. I have had female clients concerned that they did not want their arms to get bigger because of weight training. However, almost all have found that no matter how hard they workout, if they lose fat, then their arms get smaller.

Over the years, I have had two different female clients whose biceps got noticeably bigger after working out for several weeks. Both of them had stocky builds to begin with. One of them loved the increase, and the other did not. In both cases, they were not making dietary changes to lose weight, so none of the interstitial fat had burned off.

Certain males are born with an abundance of Type IIX fibers, which makes them really strong or really fast, but they may not have much endurance. The same is true among females in comparison to other females, but the ones with the most Type IIX fibers have far fewer than the strongest males. People with lots of Type IIX fibers are handy to know if you need heavy objects moved around, and they make great sprinters and football players. If you are in this

National Institutes of Health,
https://www.ncbi.nlm.nih.gov/pmc/articles/PMC4285578/

category, then you could choose to be competitive as a bodybuilder or powerlifter.

General Fitness

Most people just want to generally get in shape, enhance their health and vitality, boost their metabolic rates, become stronger and slimmer, and enjoy greater stamina and stability. In the fitness world, this is called general fitness.

If you are seeking general fitness, you will not typically workout for more than one hour three to five times a week. I am speaking in the ideal, now, because according to the US Department of Health and Human Services,

> *"More than 80% of adults do not meet the guidelines for both aerobic and muscle-strengthening activities."*[173]

The CDC guidelines are not terribly strenuous. For ages 18 to 64, they are as follows:

> *"At least **150 minutes a week** of moderate intensity activity such as **brisk walking.***
>
> *"At least **2 days a week** of activities that **strengthen muscles.***[174]

---

[173] "Facts and Statistics; Physical Activity." January 26 2017, *US Department of Health and Human Services,* https://www.hhs.gov/fitness/resource-center/facts-and-statistics/index.html

[174] "Physical Activity Recommendations for Different Age Groups." July 30 2020, *Centers for Disease Control and Prevention,* https://www.cdc.gov/physicalactivity/basics/age-chart.html

For ages 65 and over, they are the same, but the balance exercise such as standing on one foot.

If you desire to be in the upper 1% of fitness for your age, eventually work your way up to the following workouts over the course of each week: (i) three one hour multiplanar "high intensity interval training" (or "HIIT") workouts, (ii) one hour of traditional weight lifting with dumbbells and barbells, and (iii) two hours of brisk walking.

You can certainly reach great goals of health and vitality without such a major commitment to exercise, but I wanted to make you aware of the ideal so you know what it is. To start with, it would be great to set a goal to follow the CDC minimum exercise guidelines, and that step alone will put you ahead of 80% of the US population on fitness. Once you establish such habits and become more fit, you may choose to reach higher. As you know, exercise is an integral part of how to optimally lose weight, keep it off, and establish a very healthy outcome for your body in which you are fit, trim, and able to retain your musculature into the future.

For more detail on the types of workouts I am recommending, see the Exercise Appendix. To be clear, the one hour multiplanar HIIT workouts that I recommend generally include five minutes of warm-up at a lower intensity, then 45 minutes of HIIT (including a short water break in the middle), then 10 minutes of stretching at the end. Workouts that include all planes of motion stressing both the upper body and lower body musculature are great for muscle retention as well as strength and stamina development.

I believe strongly in the ideal that I am recommending. My personal goal is general fitness, because I am all about keeping what I've got in all different categories of fitness and health. So I do multiplanar HIIT a few times a week (plus leading classes), and I lift heavy for an hour a week, and I trail run up and down mountains on Sundays for about 60 to 75 minutes. I feel great!!

ormones

Testosterone and growth hormones play a big role in workout recovery and muscle development. And yes, women have testosterone too, just not as much as men. It is unhealthy, ill-advised and unnecessary to artificially supplement hormones unless there is a specified medical need.

Hormones can be enhanced in ways that are both healthy and natural. Proper nutrition and good sleep are big parts of this. We have already talked extensively about the need to resolve inflammation in order to enhance your sensitivity to various metabolic hormones such as leptin and insulin. Unlimiteds and fermented foods help with improving sensitivity by resolving inflammation.

Sleep is vital, because growth hormones are primarily released in your body during deep sleep. If your sleep is disturbed or is of poor quality, you will have less growth hormone in your system, and your recovery between workouts will not be as effective. A balanced diet with plenty of plant nutrients, in addition to adequate carbs and protein, will help your body to carry out all its natural functions including hormone synthesis and muscle repair and growth.

Workouts that engage a greater amount of muscle fibers also spur more testosterone release. Anyone who wants to healthily build or retain all of their muscle fiber should lift heavy at least once a week and use all body parts in all planes of motion over the course of the week.

When I say "lift heavy", please understand that the amount of weight is only what makes sense for you. Most of the people who have come to my heavy lifting classes are women. Heavy is a relative term, which just refers to a weight that is a challenge for the individual to lift. The amount that may be an appropriate challenge for you may be more or less than what is a challenge for me. Some of the people starting out in my classes lift no more than a 5-foot barbell with no weight plates on it. The point is to challenge yourself safely in such a way that you can preserve what you have.

Make appointments to exercise

Put your workouts on your calendar, and treat the workouts as noncancellable appointments. There will always be a pressing need -- work, personal or social -- that will offer you a perfect excuse not to exercise. But your body does not take excuses. It will put on weight, atrophy, and grow weaker no matter how good your reasons are for not exercising.

By making appointments with yourself and letting people know that those are inviolable times when you will not be available to do other things, you can evolve to have your calendar work for all the different parts of your life. Remember that you will be more alert, more energetic and more productive in the rest of your life if you are getting regular exercise.

Here is an old story, maybe even a folk tale (no one seems to know its source) that I have heard many times in many different forms:

A woman found a treasure of gemstones, including big rocks, little rocks, pebbles, and sand. Each of these items had value for her, and the only way she could carry them was in a large jar she had. The bigger the rocks were, the more value they had, so she put the biggest ones in first. They barely fit into the jar, yet there was room around them. So, she added the little rocks. Again, there was room around them, so she added the pebbles, then the sand. She happily left for her village with the entire treasure.

Another woman from the village heard of this great find, and she set out with a large jar hoping to find a similar treasure. Indeed, she found what she was looking for, and greedily began filling her jar with the sand, pebbles and small rocks. They filled the jar more than halfway. Then, when she got to the big rocks, there wasn't room. Sadly, she returned to the village leaving behind the most valuable part of her treasure. After emptying her jar, she hurried back to get the big rocks. By the time she arrived, they were gone.

In life, there are certain things that must be your big rocks. Exercise is one of them. Set your priorities, and put the big rocks in your calendar first.

No end point

Vary your exercise. Don't do all of it at home or at a gym, or with your small group. Continue to do whatever activities you identified in Chapter 7 that you love to do. Exercise must be a habit, and the easiest healthy habits to maintain are the ones you enjoy.

Find activities you can do for a lifetime that naturally fit with your life. Regular ongoing exercise is key, so there should be no artificial end point. In other words, a weekend workshop, a 6-week class, or a 3-month program may not be ideal unless you can take what you learned and apply it to another class or program. You should never be done with exercising if you want to be healthy and fit for a lifetime.

Practice will increase your confidence that you are competent when you work out. Gravitate away from short-term programs with a steep learning curve followed by an endpoint. Instead, do something that you can become increasingly good at over time, so the longer you are involved with it, the better you will feel about it.

Not one path

How you get your exercise can be different from other people, depending on your needs. The large majority of my clients come for multiplanar fitness training because they are primarily interested in general fitness. Older clients typically come for balance, stability and core classes. Some come for traditional weightlifting. Some come for more than one type of exercise class. It is also popular to alternate between different intensity levels, such as doing a HIIT class one day, then joining a moderate intensity interval training class as a recovery workout on another day. Many begin with low or moderate intensity workouts, then graduate to HIIT.

As you are structuring your own program, or joining trainer led classes, keep in mind that the top priorities are to get varied exercise, to workout in all planes of motion, and to make exercise a habit.

Avoid injuries!

The biggest obstacle for realizing a goal of general fitness is injury. Anytime you get hurt, your fitness journey is disrupted. The most common muscle injuries are pulls, strains and tears. These typically happen because of tight muscles and poor form. Prevention is the best cure, so learn how to use good biomechanics, and loosen up your muscles.

To loosen, try self-myofascial release and stretching. The best tools for this are a foam roller, a Theracane, a massage star, and a baseball (ideally a T-ball, which is a baseball for little kids designed to hit off of a T). You can look up how-to videos on the internet for this.

Be sure to stretch well after each workout, so the muscles will be loose enough for healthy use the next time. The best time to stretch is always when your body is fully warmed up or you have just had some myofascial releases. Stretching cold before you exercise is not nearly as effective and may leave you vulnerable to exercise.

If you do get injured, you can generally tell the difference between that and plain old muscle soreness, because injuries tend to happen suddenly, and you usually feel it in one specific place.

DOMS, or "delayed onset muscle soreness", will be distributed to various body parts, is likely to be relatively symmetrical on the body, and generally becomes especially noticeable 24 to 48 hours after your workout.

To prevent DOMS, rub the muscles thoroughly to purge lactic acid before going to bed on the same day as your workout. Post-workout stretches and brisk walking after a workout help a lot to minimize the development of DOMS. Hot tubs are great, too. Try hard to avoid sitting down immediately following the workout, because that can trap lactic acid in the local tissues and make you very sore a day or two later.

Treat an acute injury with rest, ice, compression and elevation, and see a doctor if it is serious. A medical massage therapist can do release work on the tissues to loosen the pressures on the injured area and help accelerate recovery. Get back to using the muscle as soon as you safely can without reinjuring it. In the meantime, modify your workouts to use other muscles more and do less with the injured one.

Takeaways for Chapter 18

- **Find physical activities that you enjoy.**

- **Exercise in all planes of motion challenging all of your muscles.**

- **Exercise at an intensity that you can sustain and enjoy.**

- **Include fast movements or heavy lifting that challenge all of the fibers in your muscles, so you will not lose any through weight loss or the aging process.**

- **Vary your exercise.**

- Start out easy, and work your way over time toward greater challenge.

- Build confidence by learning proper biomechanics, then repeating and practicing.

- Exercise is a habit to be continued for a lifetime.

- Enhance your hormones naturally by resolving inflammation, challenging all muscles in each workout, and sleeping better.

- Put your workouts on your calendar, and keep the appointments.

- Avoid injury and reduce muscle soreness by using proper biomechanics and by stretching after exercise.

Chapter 19

Get Social Support

Your Commitment Will Be Tested

While you are losing weight, and even more so after you reach your goal, people you consider to be friends will test your commitment to your goal. That is certain. No one loses weight and escapes the peer pressure to break down and go off plan.

Will you be prepared? It's far more likely that you will be if you are not keeping your weight-loss efforts a secret! Social support is critical. People who succeed at losing the weight and keeping it off almost uniformly say support of others has been a key part of their success. Share your goals and mission with others, or they will not know how to help you. Even one person holding you accountable can make a huge difference in your ability to withstand temptations as they occur.

Your People

Talk to people in your household, and tell them what you are doing. Make sure they are on board with your efforts. Otherwise, they are likely to put temptations in your path without realizing they are doing anything harmful.

Similarly, talk to people in your workplace, and express to them how important this is to you. Enlisting allies in your efforts can help, and it may well help them also. Remember, more than 70% of American adults are obese or overweight, so it is likely that someone you work with is also working on weight management.

Numerous studies have shown that social support is highly correlated with success in sustaining weight loss. In 2014, Catherine J. Metzgar, a graduate research assistant in food science and human nutrition at the University of Illinois studied women for 18 months after they had completed a weight-loss program. Their success at keeping the weight off after substantial weight loss was inconsistent.

"The women who maintained their weight loss indicated that a high level of social support from many sectors was critical in their success.

"'Our women didn't find that accountability to themselves was so important, but having support from others was - just having that social support from someone who was going through the same experience,' said Metzgar... 'What this study shows is that if you can find that one friend who has the same goals or can just hold you accountable, it is really helpful.'"[175]

The women had been attending program meetings during the weight loss period, but there was no such support group provided when they finished. This proved to be their undoing for many of them, and they resumed the bad habits they had abandoned to lose the weight.

"Renewing their self-motivation day after day and staying focused on their goals without others' support were significant struggles for these women.
"Likewise, a major obstacle for some of these dieters was a lack of social support from significant people in their lives. Rather than encouraging the dieter's efforts to get healthier, some friends and family members responded negatively, intentionally or unintentionally sabotaging her progress by making unhelpful comments or tempting her with high-calorie foods."

It is extremely common for people to get involved with support groups during weight loss, then disengage from them when they reach their goals. This makes them vulnerable to the yo-yo effect. Make sure that you find or build a social support network for yourself that will not go away or undermine you once you go from weight loss to weight maintenance.

---

[175] "Social support critical to women's weight loss efforts, study says." Sharita Forrest, November 5 2014, Illinois News Bureau, https://news.illinois.edu/view/6367/204477

Online Social Media Group

Find someone to be accountable to. It is especially helpful to find other people with similar goals. Being able to share your successes, failures, struggles and tips can help you to navigate the challenges successfully.

"Internet health communities offer new opportunities to share social support via discussion forums, chat rooms, and blogs. Potential advantages of online support include access to many peers with the same health concerns, convenient communication spanning geographic distances, and anonymity (if desired) for discussion of sensitive issues... Members of a large Internet weight loss community exchange social support in the form of encouragement and motivation, information, and shared experiences. The support is similar to face-to-face social support, but also offers the unique aspects of convenience, anonymity, and non-judgmental interactions... Internet weight loss community plays a prominent role in participants' weight loss efforts—roles which might not be adequately filled by clinicians or offline family and friends... Participants report that the support from... Internet community helps them lose weight as well as cope with being overweight."[176]

In various studies, social support has been highly correlated with sustained weight-loss success:

"Social support may be associated with increased weight loss after bariatric surgery... 10 [studies] reported on social support and weight loss outcomes... All studies found a

---

[176] "Social support in an Internet weight loss community." Hwang et al., November 27 2009, *International Journal of Medical Informatics*, National Institutes of Health, https://www.ncbi.nlm.nih.gov/pmc/articles/PMC3060773/

positive association between post operative support groups and weight loss."[177]

One study in 2011 demonstrated that even people participating in online social media weight-loss groups who merely passively read the comments of other dieters were helped:

"The results of this study highlight how a social network can provide informational and emotional support to its members, even though users may differ in how they provide this support to other members (if indeed they do). Thus, while some members of a social network may take an active role in providing as well as receiving social support, the results of this study suggest that many members also accrue informational and emotional benefits by taking the role of a passive recipient. Indeed, the benefits enjoyed by being a member of a social network can still be obtained by those users who choose to act as passive observers of the social exchanges of others."[178]

Go ahead. Join a group now. There is no time like the present to get support on your weight-loss and weight-maintenance journey.

---

[177] "Is social support associated with greater weight loss after bariatric surgery?: a systematic review." Livhits et al., January 24 2011, *Obesity Reviews*, World Obesity, Wiley Online Library, https://onlinelibrary.wiley.com/doi/abs/10.1111/j.1467-789X.2010.00720.x

[178] "Help me, I'm fat! Social support in online weight loss networks." Ballantine and Stephenson, 2011, *Journal of Consumer Behaviour*, https://ils.unc.edu/bmh/courses/706/Ballantine2011-SocialSupportWeightLoss_review.pdf

Learn the Lingo

As you prepare to make the jump into an online weight-loss support group, learn the language:

NSV means non-scale victory, and it can refer to any progress made in health and fitness other than actually losing weight (such as ending type 2 diabetes, lowering blood pressure, or lowering cholesterol). The Holy Grail of dieting is to lose fat while gaining muscle, because most diets lead to the loss of three pounds of muscle for every 10 pounds of total loss. It is a major NSV to lose more inches than pounds, because this implies fat loss and muscle gain.

SV is scale victory, which implies the shedding of actual pounds.

SW is start weight. This is the weight you were when you started to intentionally lose weight. This is an important landmark that is important to record. When you compare it to CW, you will see how far you have come on your weight-loss journey.

CW is current weight, or how much you weigh today. I encourage clients to weigh themselves every day, because studies have shown that the more frequently we weigh ourselves, the more likely we are to reach our weight goals and sustain the losses. Weighing yourself is a form of self-monitoring, and it keeps you in tune with whether your weight is fluctuating in the right or wrong direction. Weigh yourself at the same time each day and under similar conditions, such as first thing in the morning after you have gone to the bathroom and before you have had anything to eat or drink. Our weights can fluctuate by a few pounds throughout the day based on what we have consumed.

HW is the highest amount you have ever weighed. When we gain a lot of weight, our fat cells can multiply, which gives us a propensity to put on weight more easily in the future. Knowing this amount gives us an understanding of what we could easily return to if we fall off the wagon again.

GW is goal weight, which can mean either a short-term goal or a long-term one. The most common target dieters set for themselves is the weight they were when they were most slender as adults. For example, it's common for dieters to talk about how much they weighed in high school or in their early 20s.

UGW is under goal weight. If you are the one reporting this, it means you got to your goal and surpassed it. This can obviously be a good thing, especially if you had set a modest goal that still left you overweight. However, a person can lose too much weight, which is unhealthy, so it is important to be prepared to stop losing once you get to a weight that is objectively light enough. One way to calculate that bottom limit is to look at your lightest weight when you were in high school or your twenties. If you truly felt that you were overweight then, by how much did you think you were overweight? Subtract that overweight amount from your slenderest weight back when you were younger and still overweight. This should be your most aggressive goal. Do *not* allow yourself to go below that goal weight. We often lose objectivity when we get to a healthy weight and cannot accept that this is the best weight for us. If you reach your aggressive goal, and you still feel flabby, or you don't like your "love handles", work on putting on muscle, not on losing more pounds. Any weigh-in below that amount could indicate you have lost too much. Remember to always stay healthy even if you think you could lose more.

BMI is Body Mass Index, which is a popular system of determining if you are underweight, normal weight, overweight, or obese. Most people's natural genetic set points are in the normal range, although inflammation and endocrine system dysfunction may create de facto set points at far higher weights, even in the obese or morbidly-obese ranges.

Takeaways for Chapter 19

- **Social support is vital both during and AFTER weight loss.**

- **Tell key people in your life what you are doing.**

- **Join an online or in-person support group that will not end when you reach your goal.**

- **Learn online weight control lingo.**

Chapter 20

Anti-Inflammation

Shorten or Lengthen Your Life Expectancy

Each of us has the power to choose to lengthen our life expectancy. That means avoiding inflammation. Resolving inflammation is vital to health and sustained weight loss. This chapter gets very specific about what we should consume because it is anti-inflammatory, and what we should avoid because it causes inflammation.

Our bodies fight for our health 24 hours a day, seven days a week. They do it by carrying out many vital internal processes and battling foreign bodies that are bad for us. Inflammation is part of our immune system response to injuries, germs and harmful cells that get into our bodies.

Our immune systems get triggered in ways that may surprise you. Our bodies need a broad array of nutrients to function optimally. If we do not get the right nutrients, or if we consume processed foods with refined sugars, low quality fats and chemical additives that our bodies are poorly equipped to handle, this can trigger inflammation that is harmful to our health. This kind of inflammation short-circuits our endocrine systems because inflammation undermines sensitivity to many healthy hormones. This can lead to joint pain and serious chronic diseases.

There are over 25,000 phytonutrients (nutrients from plants), and the body needs a broad variety of them to function and stay healthy. Eating anti-inflammatory foods helps the body fight disease, avoid harmful inflammation, and sustain weight loss.

"I'm a weed!"

Decades ago, I had a girlfriend who said she never got sick.

"I'm a weed!", she declared.

She likened herself to weeds in a garden that grew strong and healthy while other plants struggled against pestilence and disease.

At first, I thought it was an odd thing to sa~ was true. She ate a balanced diet of whole get sick despite the abundance of colds population.

[handwritten marginalia: "Statement", "Little colon, cance, mo, ki"]

Now, I too am a weed. Despite working closely with p~ day in my profession, I do not get sick. Of course I reali~ sickness is always possible, but while others frequently mis~ workouts or workdays due to the flu or a cold or some other malady, I have remained healthy and strong. Once or twice a year, I might feel poorly in the evening, but when that has happened I have gone to bed early and felt healthy again in the morning. I don't recall feeling poorly like that even once in the past year or two.

In my earlier years this was not the case. I attribute this to healthy nutrition and plenty of exercise. Like me, I'm sure you know many people who get sick frequently despite their best efforts to avoid germs. The vast majority of people I have known who get sick frequently have poor eating habits. I feel extremely fortunate to have such great health.

In contrast, many clients have told me over the years they beat cancer or otherwise overcame chronic illnesses by increasing exercise and eating nutritious and balanced diets including anti-inflammatory foods. These personal stories have been a powerful reinforcement to my belief in the Eat As Much As You Want system.

When you think about your ideal for living a high quality of life, how much value do you place on good health? I personally put that very high on my list of priorities. I want to live a long, healthy life with a clear sharp mind. When I die, I would like for my time to come without a long health struggle.

People who struggle with chronic health problems usually don't connect my intentional lifestyle choices to my good fortune:

"You're lucky to have such good genes," they say.

do they know how many members of my family have died of stomach, and lung cancer. My first cousin died of brain er in her early fifties. My mother died of colon cancer. My her's father died of stomach cancer. My father's father died of ney failure long before I was born. My father's mother died from he long, slow march of dementia. My father's brother died of stomach and colon cancer. Siblings struggle with life-threatening maladies. I do not delude myself that good health will come to me without effort and intention.

Avoiding chronic inflammation is a vital part of staying healthy. Your body constantly strives to maintain homeostasis, a steady equilibrium of all of the interdependent processes that keep your body healthy and strong.

When inflammation causes any of the normal functions of your body to fail, this compromises your entire immune system, and it opens you up not only to predictable syndromes such as diabetes, obesity and mental decline, but also to unpredictable diseases such as cancers, colds, flus and coronavirus disease. I invite you to join me in the quest for homeostasis and optimal health by living an anti-inflammatory lifestyle.

Unlimiteds

These Unlimiteds are highly nutritious, low-caloric density, low-Glycemic Index, anti-inflammatory foods. You can eat as much as you want of these without gaining weight. In addition to their great phytonutrient values, they fill you up and satisfy you.

1. Darkly pigmented berries such as blueberries, strawberries, raspberries, and blackberries contain anthocyanins, a type of antioxidants that fight inflammation. Antioxidants counter free radicals, which are inflammatory molecules that can cause damage to healthy cells. Free radicals, left unchecked, can lead to heart disease, cancer and other serious diseases. These berries are also low-Glycemic Index and fiber rich, so they will help in more than one way with the battle against obesity.

2. Stone fruits such as cherries, peaches, plums and nectarines are also low-Glycemic Index, fiber rich, and contain potent antioxidants such as anthocyanins, procyanidins, flavanols and hydroxycinnamic acids. All of these stone fruits are sweet and delicious, but cherries have the lowest Glycemic Index values and are the most potent source of antioxidants.

3. Peppers, including chili peppers and cayenne pepper, add great spiciness and flavor to many dishes. As such, they help to satisfy your appetite with smaller quantities of food. The hot flavor is from Capsicum baccatum, which contains antioxidant and anti-inflammatory compounds.

While we are on the subject of peppers, let me address the broader issue of "nightshades". Peppers, tomatoes and eggplant are all Unlimiteds that are part of the nightshade family. This group has gotten an undeserved bad reputation. There are many in our culture who caution against nightshades as pro-inflammatory. This is because they contain alkaloids, and alkaloids in high concentrations are toxic.

However, the amounts of alkaloids in these foods are very small, generally not enough to cause inflammation. In fact, the Arthritis Foundation lists them as among the "best vegetables for arthritis".[179] They do caution that a small minority of the population may be allergic to them, which could cause inflammation. Consuming any food you are allergic to will cause inflammation. Simply put, don't eat anything you are allergic to.

---

[179] "Best Vegetables for Arthritis." Arthritis Foundation, https://www.arthritis.org/health-wellness/healthy-living/nutrition/healthy-eating/best-vegetables-for-arthritis

However, popular nightshades also contain a number of strongly anti-inflammatory nutrients. In fact, anatabine, an alkaloid found in nightshades, has been found to be anti-inflammatory and is used as a supplement to fight inflammation.[180]

4. Cruciferous vegetables such as broccoli, kale, spinach, collard greens, cabbage, Brussels sprouts, cauliflower, turnip greens and many others are chock full of powerful phytonutrients and very few calories by volume. They fill you up and satisfy you. But they are especially known for their powerful cancer-fighting qualities.

Cruciferous vegetables have several carotenoids -- including beta-carotene, lutein, and zeaxanthin-- and vitamins C, E, and K, folate and minerals.[181] They also are a good fiber source. Of special interest is the high amount of glucosinolates, which are a big part of their flavor and which have been found to fight the development of bladder, breast, colon, liver, lung and stomach cancer in laboratory animals.

5. Citrus fruits are highly nutritious and have a moderate Glycemic Index value, meaning the carbohydrates in them turn to blood sugar relatively slowly. All citrus has vitamin C, which is a powerful antioxidant. By neutralizing many free radicals, vitamin C takes away some of the causes of inflammation. C also helps the body metabolize fat in weight loss, and it helps the immune system.

[180] "Effects of Dietary Supplementation with the *Solanaceae* Plant Alkaloid Anatabine on Joint Pain and Stiffness: Results from an Internet-Based Survey Study." Lanier et. al., October 21 2013, *The Journal Impact 2019-2020 of Clinical Medicine Insights: Arthritis and Musculoskeletal Disorders*, National Institutes of Health, https://www.ncbi.nlm.nih.gov/pmc/articles/PMC3825642/
[181] "Cruciferous Vegetables and Cancer Prevention." *National Institutes of Health National Cancer Institute*, https://www.cancer.gov/about-cancer/causes-prevention/risk/diet/cruciferous-vegetables-fact-sheet

Citrus, like nightshades, is a food that is extremely healthful for most people, but that may cause intestinal discomfort or other allergic reactions in others. Again, if you find that you are one of the small minority that is allergic to citrus, then don't eat it.

6. Turmeric is a commonly used spice that contains about 3% curcumin. This is a powerful antioxidant that has been associated with improved brain function, lower risks of heart disease, less depression, less cancer, and improvements to pain-free mobility with arthritis.

7. Tomatoes are flavorful, super low-caloric density, and high in Vitamins C and A. Vitamin A is both anti-inflammatory and pro-metabolic increase. Lycopene in tomatoes is anti-cancer.

8. Cocoa (unsweetened) contains procyanidin, a potent antioxidant thought to help in fighting heart disease, stroke, and cancer. It can be used in recipes, or it can flavor a beverage that already has some natural sweetness such as from darkly pigmented berries. If you need more sweetness, avoid refined sugars, but choose a zero-calorie sweetener such as stevia (also an Unlimited)

9. Beets are anti-inflammatory, and they are loaded with beneficial nutrients such as vitamins A, C, and B plus iron, calcium, magnesium, and potassium. They are fiber rich and very tasty. Beets can be cooked and eaten by themselves, and they are an excellent addition to soups and salads.

10. Green tea is flavorful and enjoyable to drink. It contains epigallocatechin-3-gallate, a polyphenol that has been found to inhibit inflammation. Drinking green tea hydrates and helps with weight loss.

11. Probiotics are foods such as fermented beets and sauerkraut that provide or encourage the growth of helpful bacteria in the digestive tract. This can reduce inflammation, especially in the gut such as irritable bowel syndrome. They also help resolve leaky gut syndrome, which is linked to leptin resistance, so they indirectly help to suppress appetite and boost the metabolism. These foods tend to be nutrient-rich and low-caloric density. The bacteria are living organisms, so it is best to consume them in whole foods as opposed to supplements.

12. Kelp contains fucoidan, an anti-inflammatory that helps with osteoporosis, arthritis and other bone problems. Its antioxidants fight free radicals. **It is high in iodine, magnesium, calcium, potassium, iron and fiber, and it has a small amount of omega-3 fats.** Fucoidan helps prevent internal blood clots, so it offers some protection from strokes and heart attacks. Kelp goes well in soups, salads and with mixed vegetables.

13. Mushrooms are extremely varied, but many are known to have tremendous anti-inflammatory benefits. Anti-inflammatory compounds in mushrooms include polysaccharides, terpenoids, phenolic compounds, and many others.[182] Mushrooms are a great addition to salads, are super low calorie, and add bulk and texture to many delicious dishes.

14. Ginger root is well known as an anti-inflammatory reliever of stomach upset. It has a pleasing flavor and offers a cleansing transition from one flavor to another in traditional Japanese meals. Ginger has gingerols, which are very strong anti-inflammatory compounds. Regular ginger root consumption helps reduce arthritis pain and improve mobility in arthritis sufferers.

---

[182] "Mushrooms: A Potential Natural Source of Anti-Inflammatory Compounds for Medical Applications." Elsayed et al., November 23 2014, *Mediators of Inflammation*, National Institutes of Health, https://www.ncbi.nlm.nih.gov/pmc/articles/PMC4258329/

Countables

1. Avocado has great mouthfeel in a salad, in guacamole or by itself. No diet would be complete without it, because it is so healthful. Although it is high in fat, the fats are almost all monounsaturated, which are the healthy kind. In fact, most of the fat is oleic acid, which is anti-inflammatory. It is low in carbohydrates and loaded with vitamins and minerals, especially vitamins K, C and B6, folate and pantothenic acid.

2. Nuts are a staple in the Mediterranean Diet because they are packed with antioxidants, but they vary in their nutrient contents. Almonds are especially rich in magnesium, manganese, and vitamin E. Walnuts are high in alpha-linolenic acid, which is an omega-3 fat. However, nuts have extreme caloric density, so eat them sparingly.

3. Grass fed beef has a higher ratio of omega-3 to omega-6 fatty acids, and it has significantly more of a variety of other healthier fatty acids than grain-fed beef. Unless it is labeled as grass fed, you can be pretty sure that the beef you buy at the grocery store came from grain feeder lots.

Omega-6 in small portions is good for the body's ability to fight rheumatoid arthritis, diabetic neuropathy and allergies, but most Americans get way too much of it, and in larger amounts it is inflammatory. Meats from grain fed animals have much higher omega-6 content.

Omega-3 helps to reduce inflammation, which is helpful in preventing osteoporosis, heart disease, some forms of cancer, and asthma. It is extremely beneficial to brain and eye health. EPA (EicosaPentaenoic Acid) and DHA (DocosaHexaenoic Acid) are long-chain fatty acids that are a part of omega-3. DHA especially is an important part of the process of growing and maintaining cells for the brain and retina.

Grass-fed beef also has precursors for vitamin A and E and other cancer fighting antioxidants. It is lower in overall fat content than grain-fed beef.[183]

4. Fatty fish, especially salmon, are well known for their EPA and DHA content, so they are associated with good health, brain food, and healthy fats. Chilean sea bass has the highest content of EPA and DHA.[184]

At the grocery store, you will have to pay more for wild caught than farm raised. As you decide which to buy, realize that farm raised have higher overall fat content but also have more EPA and DHA, according to the Harvard Health blog.[185]

It is generally thought that the ratio of omega-3 fatty acids to omega-6 is higher in wild caught. If you are thinking about buying a supplement for good brain health along with anti-inflammatory qualities, fish oils with very high EPA and DHA content are a good option.

5. Choose **free-range eggs** over the standard commercial eggs, because they contain a significantly higher proportion of omega-3 fatty acids. Besides, they taste better, and some believe they come from happier chickens. So feed your brain and cut down on

---

[183] "A review of fatty acid profiles and antioxidant content in grass-fed and grain-fed beef." Daley et al., March 10 2010, *Nutrition Journal*, National Institutes of Health, https://www.ncbi.nlm.nih.gov/pmc/articles/PMC2846864/

[184] "Fatty acid profiles of commercially available finfish fillets in the United States." Cladis et al., October 2014, *Lipids*, National Institutes of Health pubmed, https://www.ncbi.nlm.nih.gov/pubmed/25108414

[185] "Finding omega-3 fats in fish: Farmed versus wild." Julie Corliss, December 23 2015, Harvard Medical School, *Harvard Health Blog*, https://www.health.harvard.edu/blog/finding-omega-3-fats-in-fish-farmed-versus-wild-201512238909

inflammatory omega-6 as you imagine the freedom of the chickens that laid them.

6. Soy products are anti-inflammatory (despite the common misconception to the contrary).

"Soy and its products are high in polyunsaturated fat, fiber, calcium, and vitamins, but low in saturated fat. In particular, soybeans and soy-based products are the richest dietary sources of isoflavones, the most common and extensively studied phytoestrogens in human diets. Consumption of soy foods has been shown to have beneficial effects on multiple aspects of human health, including reduced risk of inflammation-related diseases, such as cardiovascular disease, diabetes, and certain cancers. It has been hypothesized that the anti-inflammatory and antioxidative activity of soy constituents might explain some of its health benefits. Studies have shown that soy and its isoflavones can inhibit cell adhesion molecule expression in cultured endothelial cells, reduce production of proinflammatory cytokines, and decrease oxidative stress in animal models. Several recent clinical trials have found that a soy-rich diet substantially lowers levels of tumor necrosis factor-α (TNFα), interleukin (IL)-6, C-reactive protein (CRP), IL-18, and nitric oxide, although results are not entirely consistent."[186]

In plain English, soy helps your health.

7. Canola and other monounsaturated oils such as olive oil are featured in many studies showing great health benefits of cutting down substantially on saturated fat and replacing it with essential fatty acids found in monounsaturated fats and polyunsaturated fats.

---

[186] "Soy Food Intake and Circulating Levels of Inflammatory Markers in Chinese Women." Wu et al., July 2012, *Journal of the Academy of Nutrition and Dietetics*, National Institutes of Health, https://www.ncbi.nlm.nih.gov/pmc/articles/PMC3727642/

Canola oil is higher in omega-3 fatty acids than most vegetable oils.[187]

As a word of caution, generally avoid heating either olive oil or canola oil above 200 degrees Fahrenheit. Both are generally very healthy oils, but at high temperatures they give off toxic fumes. Canola oil performs worse than olive oil in this regard. [188] The test for how well cooking oils avoid such fumes is generally their smoke point, so oils such as grapeseed oil, avocado oil, peanut oil and sesame oil are good choices for higher heat cooking, because they contain monounsaturated fats and have higher smoke points. Olive oil and canola oil have strong health characteristics when kept at lower temperatures.

Avoid

1. Avoid heavily-processed foods with lots of chemical additives.

Chemical additives often promote inflammation. There is no limit to the different ways this can happen, because there are so many different food processes and additives, but many of them rob helpful enzymes, interfere with normal digestion, and introduce unnatural chemicals to the body that naturally induce a protective response by the body.

---

[187] "A healthy approach to dietary fats: understanding the science and taking action to reduce consumer confusion." Liu et al., August 30 2017, *Nutrition Journal*, National Institutes of Health, https://www.ncbi.nlm.nih.gov/pmc/articles/PMC5577766/

[188] "Comparison of volatile aldehydes present in the cooking fumes of extra virgin olive, olive, and canola oils." Fullana et. al., August 11 2004, *Journal of Agriculture and Food Chemistry*, National Institutes of Health pubmed, https://pubmed.ncbi.nlm.nih.gov/15291498/

Sadly, this is no small or theoretical issue. Processed foods overall make up 76.9% of calories in the American diet.[189]

Ultra-processed foods make up the majority:

"About 55 percent of Americans' daily calories come from eating ultra-processed foods, a new study found. And the more calories that came from ultra-processed foods, the worse heart health was, the findings suggested."[190]

The results of following that American diet are catastrophic:

"[A] 10% increase in the proportion of ultra-processed foods in the diet was associated with a significant increase of greater than 10% in risks of overall and breast cancer."[191]

Ultra-processed foods are items like potato chips, sodas, candy, meal replacement shakes and bars, ready-to-eat and ready-to-heat meals, and almost every kind of food you are likely to see in a vending machine or convenience store. In 2019, Hall et al. conducted a study of these foods:

"Ultra-processed foods have been described as 'formulations mostly of cheap industrial sources of dietary

---

[189] "Is the degree of food processing and convenience linked with the nutritional quality of foods purchased by US households?" Poti et al., June 1 2015, American Society for Nutrition, *The American Journal of Clinical Nutrition*, https://academic.oup.com/ajcn/article/101/6/1251/4626878

[190] "Ultra-processed foods linked with higher risk of heart disease." Serena Gordon, November 12 2019, *UPI Health News*, https://www.upi.com/Health_News/2019/11/12/Ultra-processed-foods-linked-with-higher-risk-of-heart-disease/2371573584241/

[191] "Consumption of ultra-processed foods and cancer risk: results from NutriNet-Santé prospective cohort." Fiolet et al., January 10 2018, *The BMJ*, https://www.bmj.com/content/360/bmj.k322

energy and nutrients plus additives, using a series of processes' and containing minimal whole foods..."[192]

Many heavily-marketed weight-loss programs rely on ultra-processed foods. However, such foods may use chemical additives that are pro-inflammatory.

Hall et al. found that "eliminating ultra-processed foods from the diet decreases energy intake and results in weight loss, whereas a diet with a large proportion of ultra-processed food increases energy intake and leads to weight gain." That is a huge reason to avoid these foods.

They also described the damning results reported in many other studies of ultra-processed foods:

"The rise in obesity and type 2 diabetes prevalence occurred in parallel with an increasingly industrialized food system characterized by large-scale production of high-yield, inexpensive, agricultural 'inputs' (primarily corn, soy, and wheat) that are refined and processed to generate an abundance of 'added value' foods. Ultra-processed foods... now constitute the majority of calories consumed in America and have been associated with a variety of poor health outcomes, including death.

"Ultra-processed foods may facilitate overeating and the development of obesity because they are typically high in calories, salt, sugar, and fat and have been suggested to be engineered to have supernormal appetitive properties that may result in pathological eating behavior. Furthermore,

---

[192] "Ultra-Processed Diets Cause Excess Calorie Intake and Weight Gain: An Inpatient Randomized Controlled Trial of *Ad Libitum* Food Intake." Hall et al., May 16 2019, *Cell Metabolism*, https://www.cell.com/cell-metabolism/fulltext/S1550-4131(19)30248-7

ultra-processed foods are theorized to disrupt gut-brain signaling and may influence food reinforcement and overall intake via mechanisms distinct from the palatability or energy density of the food."[192]

In other words, ultra-processed foods may make you yearn for them because of short-circuits they create in your body, not just because they taste good.

2. Avoid refined sugars. Processed sugars are highly inflammatory. In addition to causing fat gain and diabetes, regular sugar intake is linked to heart disease, depression, cancer, impaired cognitive function, and dementia. It is highly addictive. Despite being seen as an energy source, a spike in blood sugar leads to a drop in energy shortly afterwards. It can cause tiredness, drowsiness, anxiety, irritability, and mood swings.

3. Avoid drinking two or more alcoholic drinks a day. Recent studies have shown that up to one drink in any given day can be good for you, but any amount beyond that contributes to weight gain, subjects the body to elevated risk of many chronic health syndromes, and shortens your life expectancy.

4. Avoid food allergens. Ridding your diet of foods that cause inflammation because of your allergies is a very personal quest. Almost any type of food – even ones known to be very healthy for most people -- can cause severe allergic reactions in a minority of folks who ingest them. Common allergies include gluten, dairy, peanuts, shellfish and citrus. There are many others. The good news is that just because other people are allergic to something does not mean you are. If you suspect you are allergic to a specific type of food, then avoid it by all means, see if you feel better, and consult with your physician.

Be careful though, because indiscriminate elimination of certain foods, if it lasts long enough, can make you intolerant to that food even if you had no problem with it before. So only eliminate the foods you are confident your body does not tolerate.

5. Avoid too little or too much sleep. Being short on sleep, or sleeping too much, causes all manner of negative health syndromes and leaves you much more susceptible to disease and inflammation.

6. Avoid artificial fragrances. Artificial fragrances are marketed as pleasant smelling, but an increasing number of people are reporting serious negative reactions to them, and with good reason:

"A survey of [25 scented air fresheners, laundry detergents, fabric softeners, dryer sheets, disinfectants, dish detergents, all-purpose cleaners, soaps, hand sanitizers, lotions, deodorants, and shampoos many of which were top sellers in their category] showed the products emitted more than 100 volatile organic compounds (VOCs), including some that are classified as toxic or hazardous by federal laws. Even products advertised as 'green,' 'natural,' or 'organic' emitted as many hazardous chemicals as standard ones…

"[P]eople report a variety of respiratory, dermatological, and neurological problems they attribute to scented products: 'Children have seizures after exposure to dryer sheets, and adults pass out around air fresheners,' she says. [Anne] Steinemann [, a professor of civil and environmental engineering and public affairs at the University of Washington, Seattle] and colleague Stanley M. Caress have written elsewhere that 19% of respondents across two U.S. telephone surveys reported health problems they attributed to air fresheners, and nearly 11% reported irritation they attributed to scented laundry products vented outdoors."[193]

---

[193] "INDOOR AIR QUALITY: Scented Products Emit a Bouquet of VOCs." Carol Potera, January 2011, *Environmental Health Perspectives*, National Institutes of Health, https://www.ncbi.nlm.nih.gov/pmc/articles/PMC3018511/

Keep in mind that any artificial fragrances that you use or wear may be impacting not only you but also people you care about and other people you do not even know.

Takeaways for Chapter 20

- **Chronic inflammation can shorten your life and cause obesity.**

- **Eating anti-inflammatory foods and probiotics can prevent or fight a wide range of illnesses at the same time that it brings about weight loss.**

- **Poor quality or inadequate sleep, too much alcohol, refined sugar, and food allergens are all pro-inflammatory and lead to negative health syndromes.**

- **Chemicals from processed foods and fragranced products induce chronic inflammation.**

Chapter 21

Planning Meals

Meals Can Take Five Minutes or Less

Time is the biggest challenge many people face when deciding whether to be healthy. This chapter will guide you to efficient ways to plan, prepare and eat meals that will take you to your goals.

If you live a busy life, you may be in the habit of eating only two or three times a day. This increases your hunger and slows your metabolism. Conversely, eating five times a day is associated with steadier blood sugar, ongoing satiety, and maximization of your metabolic rate.

Anyone who can eat three meals and two snacks can manage five meals. Why? Meals don't have to take longer than five minutes.

Five-minute meals

There are many kinds of meals that you can prepare and eat quickly. Some require virtually no preparation. Some require refrigeration. Some do not.

Milk and fruit or yogurt and berries are two examples of meals that require virtually no prep and can be eaten very quickly. There are endless possibilities for meals that are easy and quick, because they involve no prep and the foods, even though they may be natural whole foods, are ready to eat. Generally, you can pick a small amount of a ready-to-eat protein-rich Countable, a small amount of a ready-to-eat carbohydrate-rich Countable, some Unlimiteds that are ready to eat, and water or some other Unlimited beverage.

Some natural whole foods come from the store ready-to-eat, such as grapes, berries, and apples. You can cook other simple ingredients once or twice a week and have them on hand to mix and match for meals throughout the week.

Here are a few more 5-minute meals that require almost no prep time:

- Healthy, super lowfat deli meat (such as chicken or turkey breast), coarse grain bread, and Unlimiteds*

- Fat-free nut butter on toast with berries

- Lox on rye with tomato and cucumber. Unlimited fruits on the side

- 98% fat free pastrami and sauerkraut on rye with mustard and Unlimited fruit to the side

- Shrimp with cocktail sauce, pear and Unlimited fruit

- Sardines on a whole wheat tortilla with lettuce and tomato. Unlimited fruit on the side

*Note: Avoid deli meats with chemical additives.

There are hundreds more five-minute meals at topfitpros.com on the Manage Meals tab of the Eat As Much As You Want app.

Other ways to get five-minute meals

Whenever you cook more elaborate dishes, if you prepare more than you need in that meal, then you will have foods prepared that are ready to use in other meals.

I have clients who lead very busy lives and simply prepare certain basic ingredients such as cooked quinoa, cooked broccoli, kale, and chicken breast or fish once a week. They store these ingredients in containers in the refrigerator. Just before they leave for work each day, they pull out the ingredients called for in their planned meals and mix them together in different ways to make their meals for the day. This takes just a few minutes in the morning. That way, each meal takes less than five minutes when the time comes to eat it.

To make that work for you, just plan your meals for the week (which can be automated), then identify foods that should be prepared in advance. Set aside an hour or two, maybe on a Saturday or Sunday, and do the advanced prep.

Efficiency

Some extremely busy people allow their health to slide because they place their priority all on their work. This can lead to a long-term poor outcome in life. Conversely, others take care of business every day, but also take care of their bodies. These wise and highly successful people are far more likely to enjoy healthy and vibrant retirement years when the time comes.

The key to all of this is to be time efficient in both business and personal care, including food preparation.

Recipes

Advanced preparation of complex dishes saves a huge amount of time on the days we eat them. Making multiple portions of a favorite recipe means we have the additional portions available pre-cooked for days when we do not have time for cooking.

Date, label and freeze portions for use in future weeks. Some can go into the refrigerator for use over the next few days. Eat one portion when you make it, then save the rest.

The benefits of this approach multiply over time. I always have a ready pre-made supply of multiple recipes that I love. It hardly takes any more time to make a recipe big enough for five to 10 meals than it does to make it for one meal. The only limit is the amount of freezer and refrigerator space.

Refrigerator space

Efficient use of refrigeration space also helps with time efficiency. In the past, I was often frustrated by wasting precious time rummaging around in the fridge looking for foods I was sure were there, but took me a long time to find. Has that ever happened to you?

Now, I try to only put food in the refrigerator that I'll be eating over the coming week. Sure, there are some longer shelf-life items that I may have in there for two weeks, but it is counter-productive to keep things so long that they spoil.

That may seem like common sense, but I grew up in a household where foods gradually got shoved around and moved to the back, where they would spoil unattended. Now, I keep a close eye on what is in there. I either put it into a meal plan, or I get rid of it if it is unlikely to get eaten. That way, the space is only taken by foods that remain fresh. This also cuts down dramatically on spoilage.

Use appropriately-sized containers. All too often, we may put small amounts in large containers, then our cooling space fills up too quickly.

Try not to mix staple ingredients too far in advance. For example, over the course of a week, I may use cooked quinoa with fish, beef, chicken, broccoli, cabbage and any number of other ingredients. By keeping these pre-cooked ingredients separate, I can be more space efficient, and the dishes will taste fresher on the days that I consume them.

Freezer space

Most of us have lived with freezers that are much smaller than we would like. They often get filled with foods that will not be eaten for many months. Items at the backs of freezers often become forgotten, and there is no room for new foods.

It is easy to forget what is in the freezer. I am not as vigilant as with the refrigerator, but I periodically check to see what is in there. I then put forgotten items from the freezer into my weekly meal plan, especially if they have been in there awhile. If I come across items that will never be eaten, I get rid of them.

To avoid spoilage, always prioritize eating older items in the fridge first, then bring older freezer items into the meal plans for variety. The freezer is a staging area for meals I intend to have over the next two to four weeks. Most meals are made of fresh ingredients or pre-cooked foods stored in the refrigerator. The longer items stay in the freezer, the less space there is. Fast turnover is key.

Meal Structure

Healthy, efficient weight loss without hunger requires appropriate structure to each meal. Follow the right formula for planning and assembling a balanced meal that satisfies without causing you to consume too many calories.

Putting together a meal

Satiety and caloric restriction are critical elements of why the Eat As Much As You Want system works so well. The difference with this system is that you don't feel as if you have controlled calories, because you eat as much as you want and stay satiated. You just have to eat the correct kinds of foods in the right proportions.

To assemble a meal for weight loss, here are some basic requirements that will ensure satiety with appropriate fullness, macronutrient balance, plenty of phytonutrients, few calories, and lasting energy:

1. Countables ranges are met (Chapter 24). This means a small amount of protein-rich food, a small amount of calorically-dense carbs, and a modest amount of fat.
2. Have at least one serving of Must Haves. This way, you will have at least one phytonutrient-rich, low-Caloric Density, low-Glycemic Index fruit or vegetable.

3. The meal should have at least approximately two cups of food. The volume is important for satiety due to a resulting feeling of fullness and the amount of chewing required for a larger volume.

4. If part of the Countables is liquid (such as a Countable beverage or soup), then only count about half the volume toward your two cups of food minimum.

5. The meal should have at least about two cups of water or a beverage. Water content in any meal is important both for hydration and satiation. This is in addition to the two cups in item 3 above.

6. Additional Unlimited foods can be added for satiation without regard to calories after the first five requirements have been met.

Day planning principles

In a day's plan, strive for appropriate variety, nutrient balance, frequency and hydration to optimize health and keep your metabolism as high as possible.

Each day, have a serving or more of cruciferous vegetables (see "Appetite Suppressors" in the Unlimiteds lists in Chapter 9). These help satiate, and they also help fight various types of cancer and other diseases. Have at least one serving in each of at least three meals from any of the following lists: Appetite Suppressors, Sweet Super Foods and Anti-Agers. That ensures that you will take in a broad variety of health enhancing, anti-inflammatory phytonutrients.

For satiety[29,66] and a fast burning metabolism[65], women should have at least 96 fl. oz. of water each day, and men should have at least 120 fl. oz. This includes water in food, so it is actually a lot easier to achieve than most people believe. Note that it is possible to drink too much water, but that is rare, and it would mean having hundreds of fluid ounces of water a day.

Jump Starter Meals

If you have type 2 diabetes or are insulin resistant or pre-diabetic, then do not consume any Jump Starters or Rechargers. Avoid high-Glycemic Index foods.

For the rest of us, it is healthy to have small amounts of hi-GI foods at certain times of the day. By this, I *do not* mean refined sugar or white bread. I am talking about certain nutrient-rich whole foods such as mango, pineapple and watermelon.

When we have more than 4 ½ hours since our last meal, such as at breakfast, getting a little boost of blood sugar helps to even out our energy levels. Remember that the average person's bloodstream will only hold 80 to 100 calories of sugar at a time, so we do not need a lot. As a group, these meals that contain some hi-GI foods are called Jump Starter meals.

Workout Recovery

Eating a quick Jump Starter meal after a workout will accelerate workout recovery. As a personal trainer who leads small group workouts several times a day, this has been a very helpful fact to know. When I complete an intense workout and I must lead another group right away, sometimes I feel a little depleted. When that happens, I eat a handful of grapes, some fresh pineapple spears, or some other food from either the Jump Starter or the Recharger list, and I drink some milk. I bounce right back. The effect is immediate, and I am ready for the next fitness class. ("Jump Starters" and "Rechargers" are lists of good carbs that are hi-GI. See Chapter 12.)

There is a lot of science behind that little post-workout meal. Let me explain:

During a hard workout, our bodies release hormones such as adrenaline and cortisol that break tissues down for energy to feed our muscles. These are in the category of "catabolic" hormones. They are good, because they block inflammation and pain during the workout while breaking down muscle fibers.

Once we have finished our workout, we want recovery to start as quickly as possible. Recovery that starts more quickly is also likely to help us in other ways, such as making us want to stay more active for the balance of the day, and enabling us to do better in our next workout. Recovery is accelerated if we can mostly turn off the catabolic hormones and turn on the muscle repair and growth (anabolic) hormones. Insulin is an anabolic hormone, and insulin release is stimulated by an increase in blood sugar.

However, it is not helpful to have a massive spike in insulin. A little bump is effective, which you can get with a small amount of hi-GI carbohydrates along with some low-Glycemic Index carbs and some protein (like the handful of grapes and some milk that I mentioned before).

You can also boost insulin by consuming whey protein.[194]

Thus, a post-workout meal that combines a very small amount of whey protein (found in milk) and whole hi-GI fruits delivers valuable phytonutrients and a nice bump in insulin along with an excellent carb-to-protein balance. That makes milk, a Recharger and a Must Have a great combination for a post-workout meal (for example, milk, grapes and strawberries). If you are lactose intolerant, there are lots of other choices that do not include dairy, such as egg whites and rye bread with fermented beets or chicken breast and pasta sauce on lettuce with pineapple.

A 2003 study found *"...there is a period of rapid synthesis of muscle glycogen that does not require the presence of insulin and lasts about 30-60 minutes..."* after a workout. [195] This means that a small quick blood sugar boost after a workout accelerates the formation of stored muscle energy (glycogen) to speed recovery.

A 2018 study provided even more proof of enhanced recovery due to the kind of post-workout meal we are talking about:

> *"[A] high glycemic index meal, following a single... interval training session, can improve both sleep duration and sleep efficiency, while reducing in parallel sleep onset latency... [V]isual reaction time performance increased proportionally*

---

[194] "The insulinogenic effect of whey protein is partially mediated by a direct effect of amino acids and GIP on β-cells." Salehi et al., May 30 2012, *Nutrition & Metabolism*, National Institutes of Health pubmed, https://www.ncbi.nlm.nih.gov/pubmed/22647249

[195] "Determinants of post-exercise glycogen synthesis during short-term recovery." Jentjens and Jeukendrup, 2003, *Sports Medicine*, National Institutes of Health pubmed, https://www.ncbi.nlm.nih.gov/pubmed/12617691

to sleep improvements…. In particular, time to reaction was reduced by 8.9%…"[196]

Takeaways for Chapter 21

- **Meals can be prepared and eaten in five minutes or less.**

- **Once-a-week meal prep can leverage your time by giving you many more possible five-minute meals during the week.**

- **Efficient use of refrigerator and freezer space makes freshness and nutritional variety easy.**

- **Simple meal-planning principles provide a framework for satiety, a fast metabolism, good health and time efficiency.**

- **A Jump Starter meal right after a workout accelerates recovery in people who are not insulin resistant.**

---

[196] "Effects of High vs. Low Glycemic Index of Post-Exercise Meals on Sleep and Exercise Performance: A Randomized, Double-Blind, Counterbalanced Polysomnographic Study." Vlahoyiannis et al., November 2018, *Nutrients*, National Institutes of Health, https://www.ncbi.nlm.nih.gov/pmc/articles/PMC6267571/

Chapter 22

Creating Recipes

Popular Recipes Lead to Obesity

Our culture leads us to become obese, and recipes are a prime example. As a people, we have fallen in love with fats, bleached flours, and sugar. We pat ourselves on the back for choosing extra-virgin olive oil instead of butter or vegetable oil. We pride ourselves on using honey instead of refined sugar.

Unfortunately, olive oil adds just as many calories as butter or vegetable oil, and honey turns to blood sugar just as fast as refined sugar. Making those substitutions will not help us to lose weight. And weight loss, for most of us, is the most important change we need to make for our health.

"Healthy" Fats

Ironically, we tend to use even more olive oil than we would butter. I recently watched a friend praise his young son for dipping his bread into olive oil instead of putting butter on his bread. The bread came up literally dripping with fat, and father and son both thought that was a healthy choice. Think again.

As a culture, we have come to a general consensus that there are good fats and bad fats. It is true that some fats are better than others for brain health and other purposes. However, we should not increase our fat intake while we are increasingly struggling with obesity.

Ahh, but that is exactly what is happening. In 2004, about 31% of American adults were obese, and alarms were sounding that this was an epidemic. By 2015-2016, that number had climbed to 39.8%[197] The numbers have only gotten worse since then. By 2017-2018, 42.4% of all adults were obese.

---

[197] "Adult Obesity Facts." Centers for Disease Control and Prevention, https://www.cdc.gov/obesity/data/adult.html

Similarly, from 1988 to 2016 the average caloric dietary intake from fat has been rising, especially among adults over age 45.[198] The increases for the older population were only about 1% to 3.5% of overall calories depending on age and gender, but the migration toward greater fat consumption implies an increase in caloric density and overall calories.

About 70% of the US population exceeds the government's Dietary Guidelines for high-caloric density items such as added sugars and saturated fats.[199] At the same time about 80% fall short on consumption of low-caloric density items such as vegetables, fruit and dairy. According to an analysis done by *Business Insider* of data from the Food and Agriculture Organization of the United Nations, the average calories consumed by Americans each day rose from 2880 in 1961 to 3682 by 2013.[200] That is nearly a 28% increase in calories consumed. At 802 additional calories per day, if there were no change in calories burned, that would translate to a weight gain of over 83 pounds a year.

Unfortunately, the overall increase in fat consumption does not mean Americans are getting too much healthy fat. In fact, as a people, we are consuming less oil than the Dietary Guidelines recommend.[200] So while some health-conscious people such as my

---

[198] "Table 24. Mean macronutrient intake among adults aged 20 and over, by sex and age: United States, selected years 1988-1994 through 2013-2016." Centers for Disease Control and Prevention, https://www.cdc.gov/nchs/data/hus/2018/024.pdf

[199] "Current Eating Patterns in the United States." 2020, *Office of Disease Prevention and Health Promotion*, https://health.gov/our-work/food-nutrition/2015-2020-dietary-guidelines/guidelines/chapter-2/current-eating-patterns-in-the-united-states/

[200] "6 charts that show how much more Americans eat than they used to." Skye Gould, May 12 2017, *Business Insider*, https://www.businessinsider.com/daily-calories-americans-eat-increase-2016-07

friend and his young son are probably overdoing "healthy fat", over 70% are consuming less than is recommended.[200]

The overall increase in fat consumption and calories plus anecdotal evidence from my own experiences tells me the large majority of people are failing to be moderate when they consume fats. Weight control and good health demand that we tightly control our consumption of saturated fats (such as butter and omega-6 fats in meats and eggs), that we supplement fats only in small amounts, using only healthy oils, and that we eat more low-caloric density foods such as fruits and vegetables.

Fats and the Mediterranean Diet

As we learned in earlier chapters, fat does not satiate, and satiety hormones are the main drivers of your metabolic rate. Thus, it is likely that an increase in fat intake will translate to a proportionate increase in calories consumed without any offsetting boost to metabolic rates.

One tablespoon of olive oil is 119 calories. If we were to change nothing else about our diets but add 1 tbsp of extra virgin olive oil per day, that would equate to a fat consumption increase of 43,435 calories per year, which means a 12 pound weight gain each year. In 10 years, that is more than 120 pounds. (Of course, that is better than the 830 pounds per year that the actual caloric increases since 1961 imply.)

With the tremendous popularity of the Mediterranean Diet ("MD"), there is a common misconception that an uncontrolled increase in consumption of extra virgin olive oil is good for you.

Yes, we need to shift our fat intake balance more toward healthier fats such as omega-3 fatty acids, fish oils and polyunsaturated fats and away from unhealthy fats such as omega-6, saturated fats and trans fats. But do not increase your overall fat intake as a result.

The Mediterranean Diet ("MD") is extremely popular but also badly misunderstood by most people. The foods most preferred in the MD are all favored in the Eat As Much As You Want system also. However, oils and fats such as extra-virgin olive oil and nuts must be consumed in very small amounts if your objective is good health and weight loss.

Americans tend to mistake the idea that because something is good for you in small quantities, it must be great for you in large quantities. That is incorrect thinking both for fats and for alcohol. Quantities matter a great deal, and these are only good for you in small quantities.

The Eat As Much As You Want system and the MD are highly compatible. The danger of following MD without guidance on what should be limited and what should be unlimited is that you may consume certain fats and alcohol in quantities that a healthy, slender person in Greece would never have.

To create healthy recipes, look for ones that use foods that are on Unlimiteds lists and the favored Countables lists, then proportion the ingredients in the recipes in accordance with the Eat As Much As You Want system rules (Chapters 21 and 24). If there are ingredients that are not on the favored lists, then find substitutes that are.

"Healthy" Sugars

The addictive qualities of sugar and the damage that is done to our bodies as we inexorably move toward insulin resistance are just as great with honey, maple syrup and brown sugar as with cane sugar and other refined sugars. We cannot allow ourselves to be duped into believing we can simply change the form of the high-GI sugar we are consuming and make our problems go away.

The incidence of diabetes is huge, but prediabetes is even bigger:

> "More than 100 million U.S. adults are now living with diabetes or prediabetes, according to a new report released today by the Centers for Disease Control and Prevention (CDC). The report finds that as of 2015, 30.3 million Americans – 9.4 percent of the U.S. population –have diabetes. Another 84.1 million have prediabetes, a condition that if not treated often leads to type 2 diabetes within five years... [T]he disease continues to represent a growing health problem: Diabetes was the seventh leading cause of death in the U.S. in 2015."[201]

Hey, I love sugar just as much as the next person. But I have worked hard especially in the past two years to drastically cut down on sugar. Watching my father's last few years of his life was, and continues to be, a major driver in this decision.

Earlier I spoke about how some of my close relatives died, but I did not mention my dad. He had quite the sweet tooth, so he kept lots of fruit juices and other sweets around. He was a brilliant man, but he did not understand the sinister way that sugar can lure the human body into desiring what is unhealthy.

"I believe that the human body craves what it needs," he once told me.

---

[201] "Americans have diabetes or prediabetes; Diabetes growth rate steady, adding to health care burden." July 18 2017, Press Release, Centers for Disease Control and Prevention, https://www.cdc.gov/media/releases/2017/p0718-diabetes-report.html

This was his justification for consuming so much sugar. Instead of water, he drank fruit juice and sugary carbonated beverages. He loved pastries or pancakes for breakfast, which he had frequently. He spent the last years of his life battling type 2 diabetes, skin cancer, and pre-cancerous polyps in his colon.

He ended up dying of lung cancer. He had chain smoked for many years, but had quit 34 years earlier and had never been diagnosed with lung cancer until eight months before he died. He got plenty of exercise and remained basically healthy until his last few years.

All those decades, his immune system had prevented lung cancer. I suspect it finally got him because of a cascading failure of immunity. His body was fighting too many battles at once at the same time that his endocrine system was badly inflamed. Sugar is known to feed cancer, and I think the polyps in his colon were directly related to his years of sugar consumption.

Once any major area of endocrine function is compromised, health problems can multiply. We all have cancer cells in our bodies. While we are healthy, our immune systems are successful at killing the cancer cells faster than they can multiply. When our immunities falter or are overwhelmed by too many battles in different parts of the body, the body becomes less capable of overwhelming other threats.

There is no question that Dad's sugar addiction took its toll on his immune function. I can't help but believe he would have lived much longer if he had avoided diabetes.

Eat As Much As You Want System Recipes

I have spent untold hours searching the internet for healthy recipes. There are many authors who claim their recipes are healthy or that they help with weight loss. Some recipes have great ingredients such as healthy vegetables and grass-fed beef, wild-caught fish or free-range chicken. The trend is to always say "sea salt" or "kosher salt", but almost never plain salt. Almost all of them name trendy oils such as extra-virgin olive oil.

The problem is that most of them are very high in fat, sugar and salt. We are allowing ourselves to be duped into thinking we are eating healthily when we are not. Using fancy and healthy sounding names for ingredients does not undo the fact that these recipes have too much fat, sugar, and bleached flour.

A recipe can definitely be both delicious and healthy, but all too often chefs rely on fat and sugar to make them taste good. A truly good recipe should be delicious without having to be propped up by fancy names and unhealthy ingredient quantities. What is needed for good health is simple, natural whole foods that have a healthy balance of Must Haves, good carbs, lean proteins and low to moderate fat content.

Create your recipes in accordance with the Eat As Much As You Want system guidelines, and you can build healthy dishes that are satisfying and delicious.

Portions

One of the challenges of published recipes on the internet is that they say "Serves 4" or "Serves 6", but they do not take into account that each of us burns a different amount of calories. What might be a weight-loss portion for one person may be a weight-gain portion for another.

This may seem like common sense, but divide your recipes into portions that are specifically the right size for you and for your goal, so you can have meals that are in your Countables Ranges and that have at least one serving of Must Haves per portion.

Suppose your per meal Countables Ranges are nine to 16 grams of Countable Carbs, nine to 14 grams of Countable Protein, and no more than five grams of Countable Fat. Your recipe should contain Countables that fall somewhere in a multiple of these ranges. For example, if the recipe has 50 grams of Countable Protein, 60 grams of Countable Carbs and 20 grams of Countable Fats, then you could divide it into five portions, and each portion would be in your Countables Ranges with 10 grams of Countable Protein, 12 grams of Countable Carbs and four grams of Countable Fats. It helps of course to have an app to guide the balancing of your recipe and to tell you how many portions it makes.

Recipes in Recipes

Sometimes you may want to prepare a recipe, then use that one in multiple other recipes. For example, you may want to create a salad dressing, then use that for various salads. Just calculate the Countables in each portion of the salad dressing, and add those to any Countables from other ingredients in each portion of your recipe. Or, you can use an online application to make the calculations for you.

Recipe guidelines

- Divide the recipe into portions that are within your Countables Ranges.

- Include at least one full serving of Must Haves per portion.

- Make sure to have at least two cups of food per portion.

Takeaways for Chapter 22

- **Weight control and good health demand that we tightly control our consumption of saturated fats (such as butter and omega-6 fats in meats and eggs), that we supplement fats only in small amounts using only healthy oils, and that we eat more low-caloric density foods such as fruits and vegetables.**

- **Some popular diets such as the Mediterranean Diet use healthy ingredients, but you should apply the Eat As Much As You Want system guidelines for proportions of ingredients to achieve satiety, good health and weight loss.**

- **Just because ingredients have names that sound upscale and are popular among trendy people does not mean unlimited consumption is healthy or will lead to weight loss.**

- **High-GI sugars such as honey, brown sugar, and pure maple syrup can lead to insulin resistance and excess weight even though they are thought of as wholesome and natural.**

- **Balance and portion sizes are key factors in developing recipes that satisfy and lead to weight control.**

- **Follow the Eat As Much As You Want recipe guidelines when creating recipes.**

Chapter 23

Booby Traps

Beware: They're Inside Us!

Old misinformation lurks in our brains and sets us up for failure. Unlearning is sometimes more difficult than learning. We can understand new truths and still be influenced by the beliefs we used to have. Break the old patterns that led to failure.

The worst booby traps are set by beliefs we now logically understand to be false. We may have habits that need changing or temptations we are not even aware are luring us toward disaster. Let's get them out in the open. Forewarned is forearmed, as the saying goes.

Ending the yo-yo requires dedication and commitment. It also requires a change in belief about what constitutes dedication and commitment. That is the toughest part. Keep your eyes wide open; you can avoid the booby traps!

Wrong Ideals Lead to Failure

We have been taught to believe that certain broad ideals are worthy of aspiration and praise. We congratulate people on fast weight loss, tremendous willpower, and reaching their weight-loss goals. However, we fail to look at the longer-term picture.

When was the last time you looked at someone and said "Wow! You haven't gained any weight in the past five years! That's amazing!." Probably never. Yet keeping the weight off for all those years is a far greater accomplishment than losing it in the first place.

On the other hand, many people have looked at friends and thought "Oooh, you lost so much weight so quickly, but you've put back on a lot of weight since the last time I saw you. What happened to your willpower?" If you were thinking this, you probably would not say it out loud, of course. But just thinking it is an indication you have been drawn into the same set of misbeliefs that led to your friend's breakdown and yo-yo.

For sustainable weight loss, it is high time we shifted to strategic aspirations that are more effective than the ones that have led us to yo-yo. Speed, willpower, and arrival at our goal weights have left us vulnerable to gaining all the weight back. Think beyond the moment of reaching your goal weight. Carefully consider what life will be like after you get there. Picture yourself slender, healthy, and comfortable with your habits for the long term. Do not follow any strategy likely to only temporarily get you to your goal. Plan right at the start of your journey how you will make the vision of *staying at your goal* come true.

Booby trap #1: Worshipping sudden weight loss. Our culture worships fast weight loss. The bait for this trap is personal pride and potential bragging rights. It's fun to tell people about big amounts of losses in a very short time period.

This fantasy outcome is made especially tempting by the fact that we already know how to accelerate weight loss for the first several weeks. All we have to do is to cheat a little and make ourselves hungry. We know we'll lose weight more quickly that way because we have done it before.

Don't do it! Remember that a true yo-yo weight loss is fast loss followed by fast gain. If you have learned only one thing in this book, it should be that hunger and a slowed metabolism go hand in hand.

You can lose weight fast by depriving yourself of enough food to avoid hunger, but the next stop is starvation mode. It's no fun to get stuck in a plateau where you are hungry all the time but not losing any more weight. The Eat As Much As You Want system is a more gradual approach that allows you to go steadily all the way to your goal and keep the weight off forever.

Booby trap #2: Reliance on willpower. The number one reason people cite for regaining the weight they lost is lack of willpower. Usually, this is because they are subjecting themselves to constant hunger. Maintaining willpower is far easier if you avoid hunger by eating foods you like that fill you up and satisfy you.

Sugar and fats are the biggest temptations. If sugar is a problem for you, see Chapter 11 and complete the steps there, because if you flirt with your sugar addiction, your willpower is likely to weaken. Go also to Chapter 16. This will guide you to establish high levels of motivation.

We always need willpower. We do not however need to constantly test it unnecessarily with hunger. Based on what you have learned in this book, you already know that hunger is counterproductive. Make a strategic plan to eat right and avoid hunger, then use your willpower to maintain the commitment and discipline needed to follow it. End the yo-yo!

Booby trap #3: Bad exit strategy. Every popular diet out there can help you with weight-loss. There are no exceptions. Sometimes, they only get you to a point where you cannot lose any more weight because of a plateau. Other times, they may take you all the way to your goal. Then what happens? Is there a clear plan for how you break the plateau or stay at your goal? In other words, is there a plan that you are prepared to follow for the rest of your life?

Almost all weight loss plans claim to be "sustainable", but the habits they are promoting are not ones that anyone can or should maintain for a lifetime. As we have seen, a Keto diet is very unhealthy for the long term, and it can shorten your life expectancy. Simple calorie counting often leads to starvation mode. Eating according to the principles I teach in this book will help you to establish realistically achievable habits to keep the weight off healthily.

It is useless to set a weight goal without a vision for how you will stay there once you reach it. That is a huge trap that has caught many millions of dieters.

Think about all of the lessons you have learned in this book. Once you get to your goal, these lessons will still be applicable to your life, but you will not need to be as strict with yourself. Understanding the principles of sustained weight loss puts you back in charge of your body.

No matter what approach you choose to follow to achieve weight-loss, be sure you have a viable exit strategy from weight loss to weight management. Failed exit strategies cause yo-yos. The Eat As Much As You Want system equips you to avoid the yo-yo.

Unrealistic Expectations

Too many people charge into weight loss without preparing themselves for the rigors ahead. They fully expect all to go according to plan, and they believe that if it doesn't, they will just use willpower to overcome. We have been taught to believe that if we really want to lose weight, we will, and if we fail it is because either our genetics have stopped us or we are too weak. Both of these ideas are wrongheaded and will lead to failure.

Instead, we should prepare ourselves for the obstacles that will inevitably loom in our journey, and we should set expectations that are realistic. It should never be considered a personal failure when we do not get to our goal in a straight line. At the same time, we should make the journey as stress-free as possible. I have already spoken at length about the importance of avoiding hunger. Here are some additional pitfalls to avoid:

Booby Trap #4: Failure to establish coping tools. Habits are not formed overnight. Research suggests it can take nine or 10 weeks or more to form a new habit. Plan ahead about how you will handle setbacks. Ensure those setbacks do not define you. People who are successful at sustaining their weight loss are the ones who get back up after they have fallen down.

Having a strategy for coping with setbacks is important, so think through a variety of possible scenarios and how you will deal with them. In all cases, the key is to forgive yourself and those around you first, then to get back on track as quickly as you can.

The possible scenarios for setbacks are limitless, but allow me to give a few examples. Here's a recent one. You have been going to the gym, but an executive order from your state governor closes all gyms due to a pandemic. Do you give up on exercise? No! You find a way to workout at home, or you take up running or both.

Here's another. You travel for work, and you often find yourself with no other option than to eat at a fast food restaurant due to time constraints and availability. Do you simply resign yourself to always eating fast food and struggling with obesity? No!

When I travel, my first stop upon arrival is the grocery store. I carry Unlimiteds and Countables that will not quickly lose freshness, such as oranges, tomatoes, powdered nonfat milk, powdered nut butter, coarse grain bread, and tuna or sardines. There are many other examples. If you have a car with a cooler, then the list of possibilities grows even larger. Following this approach, you can never be stuck without options due to lack of time and lack of appropriate restaurants.

Think of every obstacle you face in your quest. Think through a solution. If you run into one you had not thought of, and you cannot immediately think of a solution, then sleep on it, and come up with a good solution for the next time. Over time, you will overcome many obstacles and may need to rise up from many failures, but that will make your coping tool kit more complete. This will ultimately make your journey to success easier the farther along you get.

Booby trap #5: Keeping temptations handy. I have had many clients tell me their houses are full of temptations. Some have the temptations because they cook for other people in their households who eat fattening foods. Others love to provide for church functions and for people in the community, so they prepare sweet baked goods.

I had one client who lost a lot of weight and looked great, but she decided not to tell her friends that she had sworn off of fudge. They knew she loved fudge, and they had a tradition of giving it to her for Christmas. Not surprisingly, she received a lot of fudge that Christmas, then insisted that it would be insulting to her friends if she did not eat it. She gained back all the weight she had lost.

If she had told her friends in advance what she was trying to do, she could easily have avoided the fudge temptation without hurting anyone's feelings. Without that temptation, she need not have regained all that weight.

If you can keep bad food choices out of your house, do so. The less convenient temptations are, the more likely you will be to resist. If you cannot keep bad food choices out of your house, at least make sure they are located somewhere that requires you to work to get to them. Some possibilities include a shelf that is higher than you can reach or a locked cabinet. The more inconvenient the temptations are, then less likely you are to succumb to them.

If you only have the foods there because you like to do for other people, cook healthy foods for them instead of sweets. Remember, sweets are just as bad for them as they are for you.

Booby trap #6: Unforgiveness. It is counterproductive to kick yourself over and over when you mess up. Time after time, forgive yourself. Everyone messes up.

Set your goals at reasonable levels. Your goals should be behavioral, such as the formation of good habits. Do not expect yourself to be perfect. No one is perfect. What is important is to keep getting back up and doing your best to stay on track to your target.

You own behaviors are what you can control. You cannot control the scale, but adherence to good habits is the most reliable way to get the scale to move. First, select a reliable strategy such as the Eat As Much As You Want system for how to get to your goal and stay there. Make sure your strategy is consistent with what scientific research says will work long-term and be healthy for you.

Next, plan your meals, then log your meals, activities, workouts, and sleep. Log your weight and measurements too, but really look at the other stuff to make sure you are doing what you need to.

Use the tools you developed in Chapter 8 to prepare for this moment: Look at the before pictures to see how you have changed. Look at the scale. Even if your weight is higher than last week, put it into the perspective of how far you have come since you started.

If you just started out, and you feel like you already did something wrong, refrain from self-criticism. Instead, focus on the baby steps of change. Have you been eating more of the Unlimiteds? Have you been getting more exercise? These new habits will start you on your journey, and you can build on that.

Losing Sight of the Long View

I have spoken at length about establishing habits that you can comfortably sustain. Remember that the first step is to think of how your weight loss will become permanent. It does no good to lose weight that you are going to gain right back. So whatever you do, it should be something you will feel good about doing for the rest of your life.

You can lose weight and keep it off. But first you must accept that the way you have lost weight in the past was incorrect because the weight did not stay off. So your approach must change. Accept that you did not know the right approach when you tried before. This book is teaching you the comfortable, sustainable way to lose weight.

People often lose sight of the long view before they even get started. Here are a couple of key examples:

Booby trap #7: Eating foods you hate. Make sure you pick foods from the Unlimiteds that you actually like. Do not eat any that you dislike. It's not sustainable to eat foods you don't enjoy.

Experiment with some recipes with fruits and vegetables until you find some you like. Then, only eat the foods you like, and eat enough to be satisfied. Never allow yourself to be hungry.

The sugar and processed foods exception: Do not decide what you like and dislike until you have kicked sugar and processed snack foods. Many people believe they hate all fruits and vegetables because their taste buds have been dulled by the constant onslaught of refined sugars, salt and chemical flavor enhancers in processed snack foods and other food products. These unhealthy addictions make it impossible to appreciate the natural sweetness and flavors of fresh whole foods.

The good news is you really can learn to enjoy fruits and veggies and to appreciate their wonderful flavors if sugar and junk food are not distorting your palette. Think back for a moment to Chapter 11, when I told you about the sugar rushes I would get from cakes and glazed cinnamon rolls. It got easier and easier for me to stay off of sugar once I kicked the habit, and my appreciation for the health benefits of whole foods has grown even greater.

End the Yo-Yo

Social pressures will often lead us to partake of unhealthy foods when we would not choose to do so on our own, so we also need to learn to navigate that. For example, two clients who are a married couple kicked the sugar habit due to underlying health issues. Their health improved, and they have been extremely happy with how good they feel now.

One of them recently told me she and her husband go periodically to dinner gatherings with friends who automatically serve prepared individual desserts to their guests once the dinner plates are cleared. With the desserts sitting in front of them, it is very hard to leave them uneaten for fear of offending the hosts. So they eat their desserts.

After they had been off of sugar for over a year, this same thing happened at a dinner party. They each had a small dessert, and they both felt the sugar rush. Afterward, they felt sick, didn't sleep well, and were reminded of all the reasons they quit sugar. Their now much-healthier bodies had become far more sensitive to the ill effects of sugar, and that gave them a greater appreciation for why they should continue to avoid it. They've decided from now on they will politely express their need to pass on dessert.

I have experienced the same thing myself whenever I have had a lapse and consumed a quantity of high-GI foods. (No, I am not perfect either.) I have had an uncomfortable sugar rush with a tingling pressure in my brain that reminds me of the terrible side effects of sugar consumption. I have used this as a reminder to make better food choices the next time. As a result, my lapses have become increasingly infrequent.

As discussed earlier, social support starts with communication. Your friends don't know how to support your efforts if you don't tell them. The couple I mentioned now plans to call the host ahead of the next party to say what sugar does to them, so the host will not serve the desserts to them at the party. Our society has evolved, and most people are happy to accommodate special dietary needs.

It is sad to think that sugar addiction is so rampant in our culture that going without is special, but it is also good that we can now express our needs without upsetting our friends.

So kick the sugar addiction, cut back on or eliminate ultra-processed foods, and find some fruits and vegetables you love.

Booby trap #8: Resignation. This is the worst booby trap of all, and it is extremely common. Resignation is giving up without even trying. At the outset of our coaching relationships, countless people have told me "I know what I need to do. I just don't do it."

If you have read this far, there is still hope for you. There is no good reason to accept failure. So let's talk about a couple of things all those folks who said that had in common.

First, they really did not know what they needed to do. They just thought they did. Most believed they needed to starve themselves and stop eating or drinking anything they like.

You already know that's untrue. Yes, you must give up refined sugars, high-fat foods and highly processed foods, then cut back on alcohol. But for everything we need to start saying no to, there are plenty of even more important things we can start saying yes to, because we will be healthier and stronger and more active. We can do more with our friends, children or grandchildren. We can do more things ourselves when we would otherwise have had to ask for help. Staircases will stop being daunting. We will become less vulnerable to sickness.

The possible satisfaction from having sugar and alcohol in your life is tiny when compared to the benefits of vitality, vigor, independence, self-confidence, improved attractiveness, and enhanced capabilities. And you definitely should never starve yourself. Eat as much as you want of the right foods and satisfy your hunger without gaining weight.

Second, they did not believe they could do it. They associated weight loss with feelings of great hunger, and they did not want to go through that. They did not believe they would have the willpower to sustain chronic hunger. Thus, their lack of belief in their own abilities to reach their goals was due to a lack of understanding that hunger is not the right path.

What sets you apart is that you have taken the time and the energy to learn the right way to lose weight. Knowing what you know now, this is a good time to decide whether you think you have the personal motivation to reach your goals. Does your weight-loss goal line up with your life's purpose? If it does, create your strategic plan, and get started.

Life offers too much potential joy for you to give up without trying. Neither hunger nor misery is necessary. Choose quality instead. Embrace a quality existence with purpose, meaning, good health, and no hunger.

Takeaways for Chapter 23

- **Resist the temptation to lose weight too fast.**

- **Before you start to lose weight, establish a strategy for keeping it off that includes habits you will establish now and maintain for the rest of your life.**

- **Anytime you fail to meet your own expectations, forgive yourself, get back up again, and return to the good habits you have been striving to establish.**

- **Eat only foods you like with one caveat: If your primary love is sweets and processed foods, that is unhealthy addiction talking. Kick those addictions first, then decide what you like.**

- Willpower is only as good as the strategy you are following. Using willpower to maintain a high level of hunger is counterproductive.

- Failures lie in the path of every great success. Your ability to keep getting back up again after failure is the true test of your ability to be successful. Establish tools for coping with potential setbacks. The more setbacks you overcome, the bigger your tool kit becomes, and the more successful you will be.

- Avoid temptations if at all possible. If not, then put the temptations as much out of reach as you can.

- Do not accept that the road to success will be too difficult for you. Educate yourself about how to reach your goals without hunger and with sustainable habits. Experience a high-quality life by making good choices.

Chapter 24

Your Sustainable Path

A Step-by-Step Guide

You want good health, a slender body, and a long, high quality life. And you want it to fit into the realities of your life. All of that is within your reach.

Having read this far, you now know a tremendous amount about what works for good health and sustainable, hunger-free weight loss. In this chapter, we will put it all together and give you a clear roadmap to success.

This book has shown you how to eat right and get the right kind of exercise for optimal health and longevity. You understand the long-term health consequences of making bad choices such as following the Keto diet or consuming lots of sugar, highly processed foods, or alcohol.

Listen to your heart. You are ready to make a change in your life. Look at your life's purpose. How does eating right, being healthy, and reaching your weight loss goal fit with your purpose?

Now is your time. Do not wait. This is a key turning point in your life.

Find your motivation

Before you start, write your life mission statement. Identify exactly how weight loss and a healthy lifestyle support your life's purpose.

Establish a social support network

Sign up for an online support group. Talk to family and friends about what you are doing. Enroll their support. Do not try to go this alone. Make sure your support group will be there long after you have reached your goal.

Begin to establish a habit of exercise

This is a long process. You cannot do it all at once. Just get started and ease into it.

Begin working on your sleep habits

Chronic hunger, low energy, and many other sleep-related problems can undermine your new eating habits once you start them. So look at what sleep strategies you are ready to adopt and begin to adopt them before you try to change your eating habits.

Even out your alcohol consumption

If you have been drinking more than one drink on any given day, cut back to one. Resist peer pressure or personal temptation to drink more. Ideally, you should make this change before you start changing a lot about how you are eating.

Each of these changes you are making will help you to have a better life and to either stop gaining weight or begin to have a slight weight loss. Remember that this is not a race. Make the changes incrementally at a pace you feel comfortable with.

Examine your lifestyle habits

Review Chapter 14 to see what habits you feel comfortable changing. Make modest changes to incorporate some of the things that the majority of successful weight-loss sustainers are doing in their lives. You do not need to make all of the changes at once or even before you start eating right. Just make a start, and become aware of what you would like to change in the future.

This should be evolution, not revolution. Have a plan for where you are headed, and take a couple of steps in the right direction.

A man came to me for fitness training. He was obese, but he said he knew how to lose weight, so he would do that on his own. He knew that I had coached a lot of people through sustained weight loss, and that I was a major proponent of healthy eating. He was convinced he had a better answer.

"I know what works for me," he declared.

"Okay, what is that?" I asked.

"Intermittent fasting," he replied with a knowing grin. "I only eat in the mornings. It works every time."

"How many times have you done it?" I asked.

"Plenty," he said. "Every time I want to lose weight."

"How does your current weight compare to other times when you've started losing it?"

"I'm the heaviest I've ever been," he said. "But the weight will come right off. You watch."

"I don't doubt you can lose it," I replied. "But how are you going to keep it off?"

He threw his hand toward me dismissively.

"I've read all kinds of books and studies," he said emphatically. "Intermittent fasting works."

He was a very smart guy who was financially quite successful. It amazed me that he could see no problem with the fact he had gained all of his weight back every time he lost it. His entire focus was he could lose weight at will.

He regaled me repeatedly about his ease of weight loss over the next couple of months. He bragged when he hit 15 pounds down, then 20, then 30, then 40 pounds.

"It's really easy for me," he said one day with a mischievous grin. "And I eat whatever I want! Someone brought in chocolate chip cookies in the morning the other day, and I chowed down on them. Yet I lost five more pounds since then."

"You don't see a problem with the fact that you have done nothing to change your eating habits?" I asked.

"Why should I? I lose weight anytime I want to. Easy peasy."

Soon after that, he started missing exercise sessions.

"Where were you?" I asked.

"I've been seeing different doctors."

"Why? What's wrong"

"Cancer. And profound fatigue," he answered. "They can't figure out the fatigue."

"Have you told any of them about your high sugar intake?"

"This has nothing to do with that," he said with great assurance.

"So you still see nothing wrong with the way you're eating?"

"No. Like I said, I'm losing weight."

I bit my tongue. There was no point in repeating my observation that he always gained the weight back. Or that poor eating leads to poor health. Or that sugar highs lead to profound fatigue, especially if you fast afterwards. He had already heard me say all of these things repeatedly.

He did not change his habits at all. He never did. But his health problems caught up to him, and he stopped exercising. He regained all of the lost weight, but the cancer and fatigue remained.

Don't repeat this client's mistakes. Step back and really examine your personal lifestyle habits in light of what you have learned in this book. Are you doing the things which will lead to good health, high energy and sustained weight loss? Repeating the same failing behaviors over and over again and getting the same results isn't smart.

Kick the sugar habit

Are you addicted to sugar? You cannot reliably plan meals and change your eating habits as long as your sugar addiction controls you. Do not try to start losing weight or go on a new diet and simultaneously attempt to stop eating sugar.

Kicking the habit requires focus and attention specifically on the sugar problem without taking on other dietary challenges at the same time. Follow the strategy laid out in Chapter 11 until the sugar habit is vanquished. Some of the rules of the Eat As Much As You Want system will apply to help you get over sugar, such as eating Unlimiteds. And, when sugar is no longer a problem, then you will be ready to adopt the rest of the rules.

Identify and eliminate other sources of inflammation

Our modern culture exposes us to many sources of inflammation in addition to sugar: chemical food additives, chemical fragrances, and food allergens. Seriously consider whether you are experiencing inflammation from any of these sources. Our genetics direct our bodies to be on guard against foreign substances entering the body, and our natural immune response is to attack them. A big part of the immune response is inflammation.

Food allergies or intolerances may cause our bodies to see otherwise healthy foods as foreign. The catch 22 is that if we cut out certain foods long enough, then our bodies will start to see those as foreign even though our bodies were handling them just fine before making the cut.

Common examples of this pattern are gluten and dairy. Most people handle them just fine, but many are intolerant or allergic. If you experiment with cutting these or other foods out of your intake, then you should do it very temporarily, just long enough to see if it makes a difference in how you feel. If it does, then consult a medical professional for guidance.

Choose appropriate alternatives for food allergens

Our popular culture often leads us to seek out direct equivalents for foods we cannot eat. This is not always the best solution. For example, when we are lactose intolerant, we should cut out all dairy that contains lactose. However, that does not mean we must seek out foods that are non-dairy that are called by dairy names such as "milk" or "cheese".

One of my nieces was lactose intolerant as a child. Thus, her parents kept soymilk and almond milk on hand for her to drink instead of milk. This way, she could easily fit in with the rest of the family and with her friends. When everyone else drank milk, she could drink "milk" too. From a social and child psychology standpoint, this made total sense.

However, as adults, we should be aware that neither almond milk nor soymilk is actually milk. If you choose such substitutes, fit them into your meal plans based on their Countable Carbs, Countable Protein, and Countable Fat contents and based on which Countables lists they are on. Nutrition should be your guide. Don't go by the names marketers assign to their products.

Let's examine some nutrition facts that bear on how items called "milk" may or may not fit into your eating plans. A protein is complete if it has all of the amino acids we need in the right proportions for our bodies to use to build and repair lean tissues. The completeness of the protein directly relates to whether the body uses it for protein synthesis, or breaks it down to glucose to be burned as calories and uric acid to be eliminated as urinated. Protein from cow's milk is complete. Protein from soymilk is nearly complete. Protein from almonds is incomplete.

Nonfat cow's milk has a balance of complete protein and slow digesting carbs with almost no fat. Light soymilk has a good balance of protein and carbs with a low amount of fat, but it is a little faster to digest than real milk, so it will tend to elevate blood sugar more than real milk. "Lowfat" unsweetened almond milk may have three times as much fat as either protein or carbs, and it has very little protein or carbohydrate. Oatmilk has over five times as much carbohydrate as protein. In short, neither almond milk nor oatmilk has even close to the same nutritional characteristics as milk. Nutritionally speaking, soymilk may be a reasonable substitute for real milk.

When you can, plan meals that don't require anything like the food that inflames you. Always plan your meals based on the rules below. If you want something similar to the old familiar food that you know causes inflammation, then choose it based on its Eat As Much As You Want system list and based on the balance of Countable Carbs, Countable Proteins and Countable Fats.

The app has a substitution function that will provide a list of healthy substitutes for almost any food you can think of, or you can simply pick meals you like that do not include the offending ingredients. Whether or not you use the app, stick to the following guidelines:

Eat As Much As You Want System Guidelines

Here are some rules to go by:

1. Plan your meals. Too much can and will go wrong if you do not plan ahead.

2. Eat five meals a day spaced about three to four hours apart. As many of these as you need to be can be five-minute meals.

3. Eat at least one serving of a Must Have with every meal, and include at least one serving from the Appetite Suppressors list per day.

4. Have at least two cups of liquid with every meal (soup, water, or other unlimited beverages). If part of the Countables is liquid (such as a Countable beverage or soup), then only count about half the liquid volume toward your two cups of food minimum.

5. In every meal, **consume Countables within your Countables Ranges** (discussed later in this chapter).

6. Consume *at least* your minimum calories each meal and each day. (See Caloric Minimums Appendix.)

7. Include probiotics such as fermented foods in one or more meals during the week.

8. Once you have satisfied rules 1 through 7, you may **eat and drink as much as you want from the Unlimiteds lists**.

9. Have at least a total of 96 oz of water per day if you are female **or 120 oz** if you are male. All water contained in your food and beverages counts.

10. Log your meals, TV watching, sleep, workouts and weight.

Optional:

1. You may also have up to one 12-oz 5% beer, one 5-oz glass of table wine, or one shot of 80 proof liquor per day.

2. If you are not insulin resistant, you may have one serving from the Jump Starter list (Countable) or the Recharger list (not Countable, but limited to one serving) at breakfast or with any meal immediately following a workout.

Countables Ranges

The Countables Ranges enforce a healthy balance of macronutrients – carbohydrates, proteins and fats – while still putting you in full control of your weight.

Countables are the foods that are not unlimited; these are foods that are typically more calorically dense than Unlimiteds, so they have grams of carbohydrates, protein and/or fat that must be counted. You should not try to live on Unlimiteds alone. Countables are vital to ensure that you reach satiety and macronutrient balance in accordance with the scientific research I have shared with you throughout this book.

I have coached weight-loss clients for many years. In the early years, after a client completed a questionnaire, I used the data from that to calculate Countables Ranges including ranges for grams of Carbs, Proteins and Fats for each meal. In each and every meal, your intake of Countables should be within your ranges for each of those three major macronutrients.

All of this is done automatically by the Eat As Much As You Want app now, so if you would like to have your Countables ranges calculated, then sign up for a free account at topfitpros.com, and answer the same questions my clients have answered. This will cost you nothing, but it will give you valuable information to be able to launch your sustained weight-loss journey. It will provide you with your Countables ranges, and it will calculate the Countables contained in any food you want to check.

Self-Assessments

If you prefer to go it alone without using the application for precise measurements of your specific Countables ranges, then you can use some general rules of thumb for Countables Ranges, and estimate your Countables Ranges based on the examples of a few of my clients who lost weight following the Eat As Much As You Want system.

The "Countables Ranges Examples" tables later in this chapter show the starting calculations for seven males and seven females, including their self assessed starting condition and exercise levels. The top nine lines in each table include information that contributes to the calculations. The bottom five lines show the actual Countables Ranges for each of the people featured.

Genetic Metabolism

Assess yourself based on your own perception of your genetic metabolism. Is it very slow, slow, average or fast? Here are the categories in greater detail:

Naturally fast. Select this if you have gained weight due to chronic overeating, but in the past when you have cut back on intake you have found it easy to lose weight. During your youth, you were quite slender without trying to be, but in your late twenties or later you began to put on some extra pounds.

Athletic or average metabolism. Select this if you have been generally muscular or if you have found it easy to put on muscle, but when you eat too much for too long a time you also put on some fat. It has generally not been terribly difficult to lose weight, but you have had to be disciplined if you wanted any sustained success in keeping the weight off.

Chronically slow metabolism. Select this if you have dieted off and on all your life, struggling with excess fat even as a young child. Trying to lose weight has always been a challenge. If you have had enough willpower, and you were extremely careful about what you ate, you could lose two or three pounds in a week. However, whether it was after two weeks or six months, your willpower always eventually broke down, and you regained the pounds that you had lost before.

Chronically very slow metabolism. Select this if 1) you have been diagnosed with a hypothyroid condition, or 2) you have struggled and dieted all your life, but even losing a pound a week has been a monumental achievement. You have cut your intake drastically and tried to eat healthily, and you have exercised, but the weight has refused to come off any faster than at a snail's pace. Whenever you take a two- or three-month break from the struggles, and you stop saying "no" to the foods your crave, you typically balloon up to a new personal record of excess weight.

Fitness level

Sedentary. Select this if you spend your days almost entirely sitting, and you have not worked out on a regular basis in the past year.

Deconditioned. Select this if you have been trying to find time for exercise, but have been hit-and-miss in the past year. You walk regularly, but if you try to run you are quickly out of breath. When you have worked out, catching your breath has been difficult, so you must keep yourself to a slow pace to make it through the workout.

Active. Select this if you exercise regularly at a moderate pace, and your life is full of activities that keep you on your feet.

Fit. Select this if you exercise regularly, often at intense levels of exertion. You have good stamina and endurance, you have strong muscles, and you still feel good the rest of the day after putting in a one-hour workout that would leave the typical adult exhausted.

Extremely Fit. Select this if you are able to sustain extraordinary levels of intensity for 50 minutes to an hour. You are slender, strong, fast, and agile.

Exercise

The next three self-ratings you see in the tables are for exercise quantity and intensity. The number for each of these is the number of minutes the client was doing in the average week at the time the client filled out the questionnaire. Here are the definitions for each one:

Moderate exercise should raise your heart rate and cause you to breathe harder.

Challenging exercise should feel difficult to maintain for a full 50 minutes.

Intense exercise should be so difficult that it causes you to breathe very hard. It requires strong willpower to workout for 50 minutes at this intensity before stopping to stretch.

Standing and ideal weight

The next row on the table is the average number of hours per day spent standing. For the purposes of these tables, "ideal weight" is your most slender weight when you were in high school or your twenties, less the amount you were overweight at that time. If you were underweight at the time, meaning you were at a weight that would be unhealthy for you to return to, then do not treat such a weight as your true ideal. Shoot for a healthy weight as your goal.

KEY

Metabolism: "NF" = "Naturally fast", "AA" = "Athletic or average", "CS" = "Chronically slow", and "VS" = "Chronically very slow".

Fitness: "S" = "Sedentary", "D" = "Deconditioned", "A" = Active, and "F" = Fit.

Countables Ranges Examples: Females1

Client	1	2	3	4	5	6	7
Metabolism	VS	CS	CS	NF	AA	AA	AA
Fitness	D	D	D	D	A	A	F
Age	58	39	46	53	44	69	47
Moderate	300	120	270	100	50	420	120
Challenging	0	180	0	150	30	120	120
Intense	0	0	0	0	20	0	120
Standing	4	5	5	4	6	12	10
Starting Weight	170	163	184	200	144	146	130
Ideal Weight	140	105	125	150	124	118	120
Countables:							
Protein min	8	9	9	10	10	12	13
Protein max	12	14	14	15	15	18	20
Carbs min	8	9	9	10	10	12	13
Carbs max	14	16	16	17	17	21	22
Fat max	4	5	5	6	6	7	7

Countables Ranges Examples: Males

Client	8	9	10	11	12	13	14
Metabolism	VS	VS	CS	AA	AA	VS	AA
Fitness	F	D	S	S	A	F	F
Age	51	64	56	60	59	44	17
Moderate	200	120	30	0	240	600	0
Challenging	200	200	150	120	60	240	60
Intense	0	150	0	180	60	0	160
Standing	8	4	12	6	8	9	2
Starting Weight	283	243	289	211	222	209	230
Ideal Weight	178	185	185	160	165	205	180
Countables							
Protein min	9	11	11	12	13	14	16
Protein max	14	16	16	17	19	21	23
Carbs min	9	11	11	12	13	14	16
Carbs max	16	18	18	20	21	24	26
Fat max	5	6	6	6	7	8	8

Extrapolate your Ranges

As you look at the ranges for each of the 14 clients in the tables, you should note a few patterns. Males burn more calories than females, so their ranges are higher on average. However, the ranges for some females are higher than for some males depending on the other factors. The slower your genetic metabolism, the lower your ranges are. Youth is associated with higher ranges. The more fit you are the higher the ranges. The more exercise you get, and the higher the intensity of your exercise, the higher the ranges. The higher your ideal weight, the higher your ranges, because more lean tissue means more calories burned each day.

It would be too complex to write about the precise formulae that I have created to calculate Countables Ranges, but you do not necessarily need that. You can self-assess and compare your self-assessment answers to those of the clients in the tables. That should give you a very good idea of what your ranges should be.

Generally speaking, weight loss is most successful and sustainable when you are getting at least 150 minutes a week of challenging or intense exercise per week plus another 270 minutes a week of moderate. It's not a problem if you start far below these levels of exercise.

Start where you are and work to first establish a habit of exercise. That is key. If the amount of exercise you are currently getting is a lot less than the amounts of any of these successful weight-loss clients, do not fret. If you are female, just start with ranges of 8 to 12 grams per meal of Countable Protein and 8 to 14 grams per meal of Countable Carbs and a maximum of 4 grams per meal of Countable Fat. If you are male, start with 9 to 14, 9 to 15, and 5 respectively. Those are minimum levels for maintaining your metabolic rate, and you should not go below them.

Calorie Counting

If you want to count calories, you may, but I do not recommend it. The Eat As Much As You Want system works extremely well if you just eat according to the rules and allow your body to tell you when you have had enough to eat.

The risk in counting calories is that you may be tempted to allow yourself to become hungry just to stay within budget. Do not do that.

Instead, allow your body to tell you when you have had enough to eat. You do not need to know what your caloric budget is because if you follow the rules, your body will tell you when you have had enough to eat before you have eaten too much.

However, if you want to fine-tune your choices of Unlimiteds to find ones that satisfy your appetite best and keep you satiated the longest with the fewest calories, it can be useful to track how many calories you have consumed each day compared to your caloric budget.

For example, suppose you add an apple to a meal, and that causes you to go over your caloric budget. If that happens, either add the apples anyway or choose a different Unlimited instead such as baby carrots or a salad with zero-calorie dressing.

If you find that you are still hungry after the salad, but you are not hungry when you eat an apple, then have the apple. In other words, do not eliminate the Unlimiteds that work best to satiate you. No substitute is a good substitute if the result is that your hunger is not satisfied.

Hunger slows your metabolism and sets you on a course to a potential weight loss plateau. Satiety, on the other hand, speeds your metabolism, and may cause you to burn more than the extra amount of calories that you consumed when you are eating the right way.

What Constitutes Sustainability?

Judge sustainability by how your habits impact your quality of life, both now and in the future. This is not just about weight loss. A high quality of life includes good health and avoidance of chronic hunger. It also includes a good sleep strategy, a strong social safety net, appropriate decisions about sugar and alcohol consumption, and personal goals that are in line with a clearly-defined life purpose.

Exercise is crucial because it keeps your body capable, and it makes health, vitality and the realization of many goals realistically achievable.

A high quality of life does not come from weight loss alone. If you are constantly hungry and suffering from cravings, that is not a high quality of life no matter how much weight you lost. And if you gain all the weight back in a yo-yo, how have you improved your life? Ending the yo-yo means keeping your own hormones from defeating you.

Early in the book, I quoted someone who said "Keep your eyes on the prize" in social media. This quote is troubling because so many people have their eyes on the wrong prize.

The real reward for weight loss is that it supports your life's purpose, and it helps you to attain a high quality of life. However, you can only realize that prize if you keep the weight off without hunger, and if you fully integrate healthy habits in your life so that they become comfortable.

The kind of life I want includes positive feelings such as ongoing satiety, a sense that my life has meaning, high energy throughout each day, and the sure knowledge that I can stay at my ideal weight without a struggle. To build such a life, I follow strategies for healthy sleep, very moderate alcohol consumption, a strong fit body, social support, and excellent nutrition. The Eat As Much As You Want system is more than a diet plan. It is a roadmap for a better life.

Takeaways for Chapter 24

- There is a clearly discernable path to your goals, and you have the map.

- If what you have done in the past has only worked temporarily, then it really has not worked at all for you. Choose a permanent solution.

- What works consistently is a comprehensive strategy that incorporates life purpose, eating habits, sleep strategy, regular exercise, moderate alcohol consumption, and avoidance of refined sugar, food allergens, and other sources of inflammation.

- The Eat As Much As You Want system guides you to the right eating habits.

- You can self-assess and extrapolate your Countables Ranges, or you can use an app.

- Calorie counting can be used as a tool for refinement of what you are doing, but it should never govern you. Listen to your body and eat if it says you are hungry.

- True sustainability can only be achieved with a system that promotes health without hunger.

Appendix:

Caloric Minimums

Calories to Maintain Metabolic Rate

My extensive coaching experience helping a lot of people lose weight and keep it off tells me that when people consume too few calories, their weight loss stops. This table is my effort to quantify what is the least amount of calories someone needs to maintain an optimal metabolism and avoid starvation mode. It is based in part on National Weight Control Registry studies and in part, on my own experience with my clients.

Note that males of a given metabolic speed tend to need more calories than females. Note also that the more overweight you have been, the lower your caloric minimums. And finally, remember these minimums only work to keep your metabolism up if you are faithfully following all of the other rules of the Eat As Much As You Want system.

My recommended caloric minimums are structured to encourage you to keep your intake relatively consistent throughout each day. Of course, you will not consume exactly the same number of calories in every meal, so each day's minimum is more than five times the per-meal minimum.

People with genetically faster metabolisms need to consume more calories than those with genetically very slow metabolisms. The recommended minimums reflect this reality.

It is also well established that people whose peak body weights have been substantially higher than their goals require lower minimums than people who have never been more than a few pounds overweight.

To be clear, caloric minimums are not caloric budgets. They are not the amounts that we recommend that people consume. They are merely minimums put in place to help people avoid metabolic crashes that disrupt their weight-loss and weight-maintenance efforts.

Each table represents the caloric minimums for a given goal, whether it is weight loss, weight maintenance, or weight gain. The left-hand column of the table ("Peak – Goal") indicates the difference between the highest amount that a person has weighed and the amount they would weigh if they were not overweight:

Weight Loss

Peak - Goal	Metabolism	Min cal/meal (Women)	Min cal/day (Women)	Min cal/meal (Men)	Min cal/day (Men)
≥30	Fast	130	775	161	930
25 to <30	Fast	135	800	167	960
20 to <25	Fast	145	850	179	1020
15 to <20	Fast	155	900	191	1080
10 to <15	Fast	170	975	209	1170
5 to <10	Fast	195	1100	239	1320
<5	Fast	215	1200	263	1440
Peak - Goal	**Metabolism**	**Min cal/meal (Women)**	**Min cal/day (Women)**	**Min cal/meal (Men)**	**Min cal/day (Men)**
≥30	Athletic	120	725	149	870
25 to <30	Athletic	125	750	155	900
20 to <25	Athletic	135	800	167	960
15 to <20	Athletic	145	850	179	1020
10 to <15	Athletic	160	925	197	1110
5 to <10	Athletic	185	1050	227	1260
<5	Athletic	195	1100	239	1320
Peak - Goal	**Metabolism**	**Min cal/meal (Women)**	**Min cal/day (Women)**	**Min cal/meal (Men)**	**Min cal/day (Men)**
≥30	Slow	100	625	125	750
25 to <30	Slow	115	700	143	840
20 to <25	Slow	115	700	143	840

End the Yo-Yo

Peak - Goal	Metabolism	Min cal/meal (Women)	Min cal/day (Women)	Min cal/meal (Men)	Min cal/day (Men)
15 to <20	Slow	125	750	155	900
10 to <15	Slow	140	825	173	990
5 to <10	Slow	165	950	203	1140
<5	Slow	175	1000	215	1200

Peak - Goal	Metabolism	Min cal/meal (Women)	Min cal/day (Women)	Min cal/meal (Men)	Min cal/day (Men)
≥30	Very slow	86	555	108	666
25 to <30	Very slow	105	650	131	780
20 to <25	Very slow	110	675	137	810
15 to <20	Very slow	100	625	125	750
10 to <15	Very slow	115	700	143	840
5 to <10	Very slow	140	825	173	990
<5	Very slow	150	875	185	1050

Weight Maintenance

Peak - Goal	Metabolism	Min cal/meal (Women)	Min cal/day (Women)	Min cal/meal (Men)	Min cal/day (Men)
≥30	Fast	205	1075	248	1290
25 to <30	Fast	210	1100	254	1320
20 to <25	Fast	220	1150	266	1380
15 to <20	Fast	230	1200	278	1440
10 to <15	Fast	245	1275	296	1530
5 to <10	Fast	270	1400	326	1680
<5	Fast	290	1500	350	1800

Peak - Goal	Metabolism	Min cal/meal (Women)	Min cal/day (Women)	Min cal/meal (Men)	Min cal/day (Men)
≥30	Athletic	195	1025	236	1230
25 to <30	Athletic	205	1075	248	1290
20 to <25	Athletic	210	1100	254	1320
15 to <20	Athletic	220	1150	266	1380
10 to <15	Athletic	235	1225	284	1470
5 to <10	Athletic	260	1350	314	1620
<5	Athletic	270	1400	326	1680

Peak - Goal	Metabolism	Min cal/meal (Women)	Min cal/day (Women)	Min cal/meal (Men)	Min cal/day (Men)
≥30	Slow	175	925	212	1110
25 to <30	Slow	190	1000	230	1200
20 to <25	Slow	190	1000	230	1200
15 to <20	Slow	200	1050	242	1260

End the Yo-Yo

Peak - Goal	Metabolism	Min cal/meal (Women)	Min cal/day (Women)	Min cal/meal (Men)	Min cal/day (Men)
10 to <15	Slow	215	1125	260	1350
5 to <10	Slow	240	1250	290	1500
<5	Slow	250	1300	302	1560

Peak - Goal	Metabolism	Min cal/meal (Women)	Min cal/day (Women)	Min cal/meal (Men)	Min cal/day (Men)
≥30	Very slow	161	855	195	1026
25 to <30	Very slow	180	950	218	1140
20 to <25	Very slow	185	975	224	1170
15 to <20	Very slow	175	925	212	1110
10 to <15	Very slow	190	1000	230	1200
5 to <10	Very slow	215	1125	260	1350
<5	Very slow	225	1175	272	1410

Weight Gain

Peak - Goal	Metabolism	Min cal/meal (Women)	Min cal/day (Women)	Min cal/meal (Men)	Min cal/day (Men)
≥30	Fast	365	1825	438	2190
25 to <30	Fast	370	1850	444	2220
20 to <25	Fast	380	1900	456	2280
15 to <20	Fast	390	1950	468	2340
10 to <15	Fast	405	2025	486	2430
5 to <10	Fast	430	2150	516	2580
<5	Fast	550	2750	660	3300

Peak - Goal	Metabolism	Min cal/meal (Women)	Min cal/day (Women)	Min cal/meal (Men)	Min cal/day (Men)
≥30	Athletic	355	1775	426	2130
25 to <30	Athletic	365	1825	438	2190
20 to <25	Athletic	370	1850	444	2220
15 to <20	Athletic	380	1900	456	2280
10 to <15	Athletic	395	1975	474	2370
5 to <10	Athletic	420	2100	504	2520
<5	Athletic	530	2650	636	3180

Peak - Goal	Metabolism	Min cal/meal (Women)	Min cal/day (Women)	Min cal/meal (Men)	Min cal/day (Men)
≥30	Slow	335	1675	402	2010
25 to <30	Slow	350	1750	420	2100
20 to <25	Slow	350	1750	420	2100
15 to <20	Slow	360	1800	432	2160

End the Yo-Yo

Peak - Goal	Metabolism	Min cal/meal (Women)	Min cal/day (Women)	Min cal/meal (Men)	Min cal/day (Men)
10 to <15	Slow	375	1875	450	2250
5 to <10	Slow	400	2000	480	2400
<5	Slow	480	2400	576	2880

Peak - Goal	Metabolism	Min cal/meal (Women)	Min cal/day (Women)	Min cal/meal (Men)	Min cal/day (Men)
≥30	Very slow	321	1605	385	1926
25 to <30	Very slow	340	1700	408	2040
20 to <25	Very slow	345	1725	414	2070
15 to <20	Very slow	335	1675	402	2010
10 to <15	Very slow	350	1750	420	2100
5 to <10	Very slow	375	1875	450	2250
<5	Very slow	435	2175	522	2610

Jim Frith

Takeaways for Minimum Calories Appendix

- Eating too few calories leads to Starvation Mode

- Meeting your minimum calories requirement is only one factor in keeping your body out of Starvation Mode so you can steadily march toward your goal weight.

- Your specific minimums are different from other people's.

- Factors that help guide you to your minimum include a) how heavy you have been less your reasonable weight goal, b) your genetic metabolism, and c) whether you are male or female.

- If you do not meet your caloric minimums each day and each meal, your metabolic rate is likely to crash.

Appendix:

Exercise

Why Multiplanar Exercise?

Exercises that are in all planes of motion are referred to as "multiplanar". To keep from losing muscle tissue during weight loss, it is extremely important to work out in all planes of motion. There are about 700 different muscles in the human body, and every one of them should be worked if you want to keep them all intact and strong. And all of the fibers in those muscles need to be challenged.

Running and bicycling will not to do that. Not even close. Those are aerobic exercises that are straight ahead and primarily use the legs. Treadmills and stationary bikes are the same way. Elliptical machines at least use the upper and lower body, but they leave out a lot of smaller stabilizer muscles because there is little rotation and no lateral movement, and they generally do not fire Type IIX fibers. (Remember that Type IIX fibers are the strongest, least used and least vascular muscle fibers, and they are the most vulnerable to sarcopenia if not used.)

Many of your muscles are very small, and they only get worked when you are twisting, turning, or moving sideways. In life and in athletics, injuries most commonly occur when you are changing direction, so strengthening the muscles involved in direction changes helps to prevent injuries.

One of the goals of multiplanar training is to involve as much lean tissue as possible in each exercise. Incorporate balance and stability challenges to work the smaller stabilizer muscles and to train your central nervous system to coordinate your body in complex movements.

Planes of motion

The primary planes of motion are sagittal, frontal and transverse. The sagittal plane is straight ahead, frontal is side-to-side, and transverse is rotational. Frontal and transverse plane exercises are most important in injury prevention because these are the planes of motion where most non-contact injuries occur in life and in athletics.

Sagittal plane exercises are more traditional straight ahead exercises such as push ups, sit ups, sprints, squats, lunges, and burpees. Most traditional free weight exercises are also in the sagittal plane such as deadlifts, bench presses, power cleans and upright rows.

People love to hate burpees, shown here, but if you want to get your heartrate up, this one is highly effective for that. Start standing, then squat low with your hands on the floor, throw your feet back

438

into a pushup position, some up as explosively as you can muster, then just in the air. This is for very athletic, fit people. Don't do it if you are beginning to get back into exercise after having been sedentary for a good while. This is not for the faint of heart!

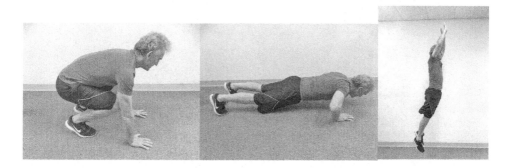

Fortunately, this, like just about any other exercise, can be modified to suit your current fitness level. Instead of going all the way down to the floor, try squatting down and reaching as low as you can, then coming up and reaching overhead. As time goes by, you can get lower and incorporate a jump. Eventually, you may go all the way down for a pushup. As you build a workout for yourself, always modify your exercises to be within your safe execution range considering your current level of fitness. Don't risk getting hurt!

When I lead workouts, whether online or in person, I do not generally incorporate burpees. I prefer exercises that are easily and quickly adaptable so they are the appropriate challenge for each participant.

Frontal plane exercises are side to side. One example is a side lunge. Hold a dumbbell in each hand, step to your left and squat down reaching your dumbbells to either side of your left knee. Return to upright, and lift your left foot, then curl and press the weights overhead while you stand on one foot.

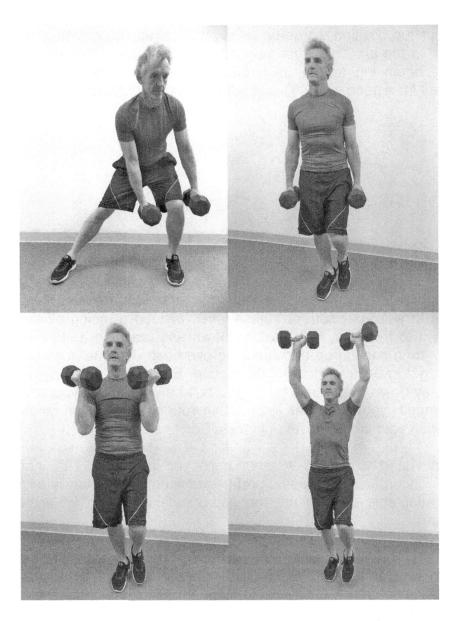

Other examples of frontal plane exercises are 1) side crunches, which you can do on a stability ball, a Bosu®, or the floor; 2) side walking with exercise tubing under your feet; or 3) side C's with a TRX®; or 4) "up and overs" (which are side steps up and side steps down changing feet at the top) with dumbbells and an aerobic step.

Here are side crunches on a stability ball:

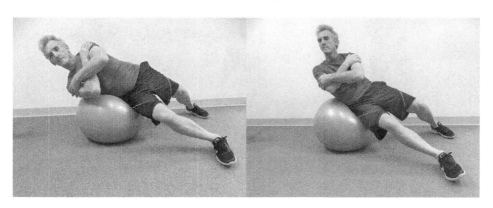

Side walking is an exercise just about everyone who has reasonably good balance can do. Just curl up your arms with your elbows in front of your ribs, then try to keep your hips and shoulders level as you lift your lead leg and step out to the side:

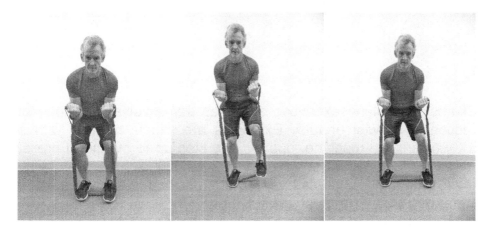

Each exercise can be done at an easier or a more intense and challenging level. Here are some pictures showing how to do an explosive, intense version of up and overs:

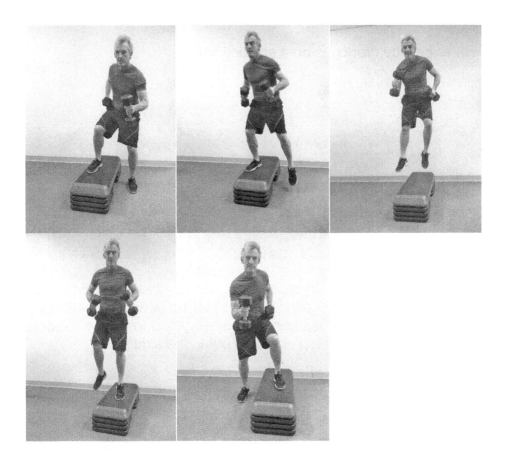

Transverse plane exercises are ones that involve a change of direction or a twist or turn. Examples are simple rotation with a TRX® or a cable machine, quarter turn step-up to overhead press, quarter turn box jumps (see Plyometrics below), or "press-bys" with exercise tubing. With press-bys, you start facing the anchor, make a quarter turn step, then push the tubing handles past you to one side as you rotate your torso.

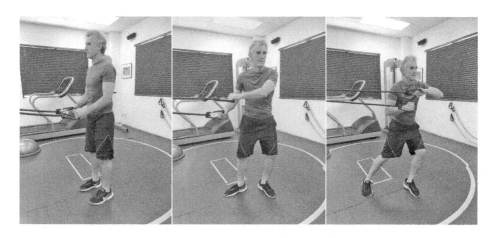

Here is what simple rotation looks like when performed on a cable machine. Just keep your hands straight out about a foot in front of your sternum and turn your body. You can do these with elastic exercise bands/tubing also:

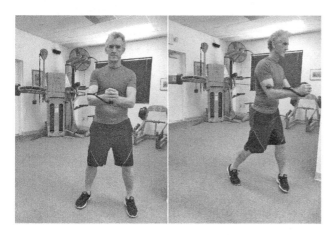

A quarter turn step up to overhead press has you stand beside a step. It could be an aerobic step like the one pictured, or a sturdy footstool, or the bottom step of a staircase. Hold weights in your hands. Take a quarter turn toward the step, bring your lead knee forward so your bodyweight is centered over the foot on the step, draw in your stomach, and stand up on one leg. Curl and press, then unwind the whole thing in reverse and start over again.

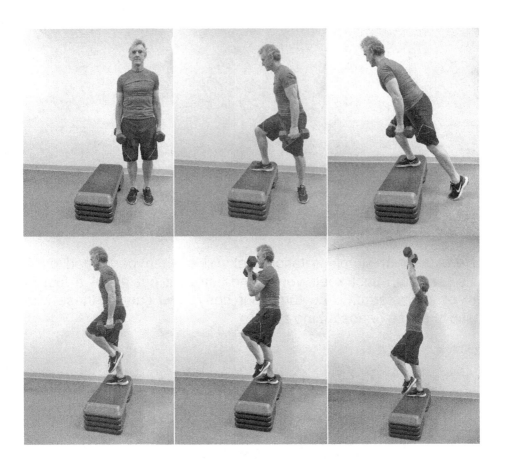

Another kind of multiplanar exercise is a "dynamic stabilization" exercise. With these, you hold rotational muscles still (such as those in the spine) as you create a dynamic force against them. Examples are "infinities" (or sideways figure-8s) on the battle ropes, side walking with a cable machine, and single arm dumbbell rows with one knee on a Bosu®.

Here is a single arm dumbbell row in the "pointer position" on a Bosu®. Draw in your abdominal muscles (i.e. suck in your gut) to support your back and solidify your core and balance while you do this:

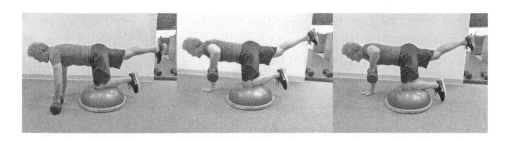

There are also combination exercises that use multiple planes of motion in a single exercise. Wood chops with a cable machine and "chop and stop" with a medicine ball are examples of this.

If you take fitness classes, I recommend one-hour classes using a wide variety of multiplanar exercises throughout each workout. By the time each workout is finished, you will ideally have done 20 to 25 different exercises, and virtually every muscle in the body will have been challenged. Broad utilization of lean tissue in a single workout naturally boosts testosterone and growth hormone release, and it provides a rigorous overall challenge to the participants. In addition to training stamina, endurance, strength, balance and stability, your trainer can help you to challenge Type IIX muscle fibers by interspersed use of plyometrics and heavier resistance.

Plyometrics

Recruitment of Type IIX muscle fibers requires either heavy lifting or explosive movement. Plyometrics are sudden movements such as jumps, throws, sudden stops, throwing slam balls down, boxing, creating waves in ropes, or sprint and agility drills. While being sensible about injury avoidance, incorporating plyometric exercises into a workout is important for young and old, newbie or competitive athlete. They cause retention of Type IIX fibers while enhancing speed, improving motor nerve synapse firing, and increasing metabolic rates for 24 to 48 hours after the workout.

Below, I am shown doing a quarter turn box jump. Of course, you can choose to jump a shorter height or no height at all, or maybe you can jump higher. Whatever the height, it is the explosiveness of the movement that helps you recruit and keep your Type IIX muscle fibers, the strongest ones you have.

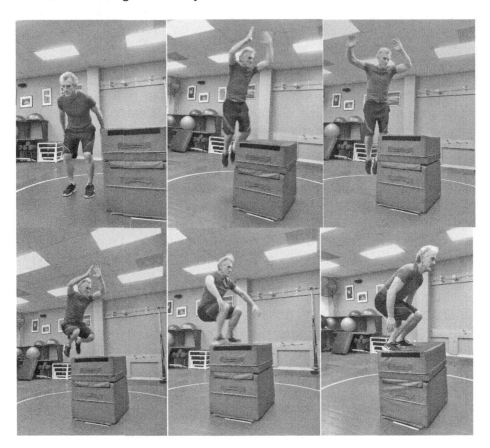

Why High Intensity Interval Training?

As your fitness levels improve, I highly recommend that you eventually try high intensity interval training (HIIT). Here are eight important reasons why HIIT has become extremely popular:

1. HIIT is more time efficient. In fact, you can burn the same number of calories with HIIT in about half the time as moderate intensity continuous training (MICT). MICT is something like riding on a stationary bike or running on a treadmill at the same moderate pace for a long period of time. Given identical energy expenditure, the fat losses and cardiorespiratory benefits are about the same between MICT and HIIT, but MICT requires a workout that is almost twice as long.[202]

2. HIIT causes much higher metabolic rates at rest. EPOC (excess post-exercise oxygen consumption) is much higher after HIIT than after MICT. Your EPOC is a measure of how much higher your resting metabolic rate is for 24 to 48 hours after your workout. If you have a higher EPOC, you are burning more calories at rest. Two minutes of sprint interval training produces about as much EPOC over the following 24 hours as 30 minutes of continuous endurance training.[203]

3. The right kinds of HIIT are more enjoyable than moderate exercise. If you ask a person who does not regularly workout whether it would be more enjoyable to workout at high intensity or moderate intensity, most people would say moderate. However,

---

[202] "Comparable Effects of High-Intensity Interval Training and Prolonged Continuous Exercise Training on Abdominal Visceral Fat Reduction in Obese Young Women." Zhang et al., January 1 2017, *Journal of Diabetes Research*, National Institutes of Health, https://www.ncbi.nlm.nih.gov/pmc/articles/PMC5237463/

[203] "Two minutes of sprint-interval exercise elicits 24-hr oxygen consumption similar to that of 30 min of continuous endurance exercise." Hazell et al., August 2012, *International Journal of Sport Nutrition and Exercise Metabolism*, National Institutes of Health pubmed, https://www.ncbi.nlm.nih.gov/pubmed/22710610

studies have shown that when people actually do the workouts, HIIT is usually perceived as more enjoyable.[204]

I must caution that not all HIIT is equally enjoyable. Very high intensity interval training ("Tabata"), while time efficient, is too challenging for most people to enjoy as a regular form of exercise. Tabata was designed to push people so hard that they could not continue for more than about four minutes. One popular interval for Tabata is 20 seconds of intense exercise followed by 10 seconds rest. Tabata was originally created for high-level performance athletes, and it is most appropriate for that group.[205]

Similarly, HIIT is less enjoyable with longer intervals. Clients enjoy intervals of 30 to 60 seconds, but they do not like 120 second intervals.[206]

I find this to be true in my own practice, so I try to stay with around 45 seconds of exercise per interval followed by 15 seconds

---

[204] "High-intensity interval running is perceived to be more enjoyable than moderate-intensity continuous exercise: Implications for exercise adherence." Bartlett et al., February 24 2011, Society of Health and Physical Educators (SHAPE America), *Journal of Sport Sciences*, https://shapeamerica.tandfonline.com/doi/abs/10.1080/02640414.2010.545427#.Xe0mmut7mu5

[205] "The Effects of High Intensity Interval Training vs Steady State Training on Aerobic and Anaerobic Capacity." Foster et al., December 2015, *Journal of Sports Science & Medicine*, https://www.ncbi.nlm.nih.gov/pmc/articles/PMC4657417/

[206] "Affective and Enjoyment Responses to High-Intensity Interval Training in Overweight-to-Obese and Insufficiently Active Adults." Martinez et al., January 2015, *Journal of Sport and Exercise Psychology*, https://journals.humankinetics.com/view/journals/jsep/37/2/article-p138.xml

of transition/rest for most of the workout. I find that I can keep my clients enjoyably engaged at this pace for longer durations.

4. Adherence is better with HIIT. Exercise is only good for you if you do it. It must be a lifetime habit, or the benefits rapidly fade. So the most important question in any type of exercise is "Will people keep doing it?" The answer with HIIT is yes much more often than with MICT. One study, for example, found that HIIT "participants spent significantly less time exercising per week, yet were able to maintain exercise enjoyment and were more likely to intend to continue."[207]

5. Enjoyment of HIIT increases over time. In many forms of exercise, people like the exercises less as time goes by. I find that by keeping the workouts fresh with a lot of variety, my clients like HIIT workouts more and more the longer they continue the habit of doing them. I balance the goals of variety and freshness against the clients' needs to feel competent, so I provide some repetition of specific exercises across the week and from one week to the next, but I give tremendous variety within each workout and from one workout to the next.

My experiences with my clients match the results of a 2016 study [208] that found that "enjoyment for high-intensity interval

---

[207] "High-intensity compared to moderate-intensity training for exercise initiation, enjoyment, adherence, and intentions: an intervention study." Heinrich et al., August 3 2014, *BMC Public Health*, https://bmcpublichealth.biomedcentral.com/articles/10.1186/1471-2458-14-789
[208] "Enjoyment for High-Intensity Interval Exercise Increases during the First Six Weeks of Training: Implications for Promoting Exercise Adherence in Sedentary Adults." Heisz et al., December 14 2016, *PLOS/One*, https://journals.plos.org/plosone/article?id=10.1371/journal.pone.0168534

exercise increases with chronic training". In contrast, the study found that enjoyment of MICT typically "remained constant and lower". Over time, clients develop a knowledge base and capabilities to properly execute HIIT exercises, and this gives them greater confidence. Positive feedback bolsters this confidence, and they develop favorable feelings toward the workouts.

6. HIIT lowers blood sugar. Countless times, following a few months of HIIT with me, clients have come in glowing about how great their doctors' visits have been. They have told me of dramatic reductions in cholesterol, blood pressure, and body fat. One of my favorite things to hear -- and I have heard it a lot -- is that their blood sugar levels have markedly improved. Some have even told me that they have "cured" their type 2 diabetes.

A 2015 study substantiates that my clients' experiences typical of HIIT participants. The study found *"There was a reduction in insulin resistance following HIIT compared with both"* a group of participants doing continuous training and a control group. *"HIIT appears effective at improving metabolic health, particularly in those at risk of or with type 2 diabetes."*[209]

7. HIIT improves immunity. Strenuous exercise enhances immune function in the body.[210] During intense exercise, there is as much as a tenfold increase in the number of immune cells in the body. Immediately following the workout, the extra immune cells are deployed out of the bloodstream to the places in the body such as

---

[209] "The effects of high-intensity interval training on glucose regulation and insulin resistance: a meta-analysis." Jelleyman et al., November 2015, World Obesity, *Obesity Reviews*, National Institutes of Health pubmed, https://www.ncbi.nlm.nih.gov/pubmed/26481101

[210] "Research debunks 'myth' that strenuous exercise suppresses the immune system." Andy Dunn, April 20 2018, *MedicalXPress,* https://medicalxpress.com/news/2018-04-debunks-myth-strenuous-suppresses-immune.html

the lungs where the likelihood of infection is greatest; thus they proactively go to work to protect you. A few hours later, if the extra cells are not needed where they were deployed, they return to the bloodstream to be used elsewhere.

8. HIIT is the best exercise to improve heart health. HIIT training does more than any other type of exercise to improve aerobic capacity, which is the best "predictor" of whether your future will be healthy and long-lived with a strong heart.[211]

Weightlifting

While multiplanar exercise is by far the most effective at preparing your body for daily life and athletics, traditional weightlifting is also healthy and useful, especially when it is a supplement to HIIT multiplanar exercises done every week. I personally like to vary my workouts with several multiplanar workouts a week, then trail running and traditional weightlifting each done once a week. That provides for outstanding overall general fitness.

However, how weightlifting does or does not fit into your life depends on your specific goals. If you think it may, then by all means read this subchapter.

---

[211] "High-intensity interval training for health benefits and care of cardiac diseases - The key to an efficient exercise protocol." Shigenori Ito, July 26 2019, *World Journal of Cardiology*, https://www.ncbi.nlm.nih.gov/pmc/articles/PMC6763680/

Weightlifting and goals

Depending on your goals, you can lift weights in the context of multiplanar HIIT workouts, or you can do it as a standalone separate workout.

Whatever types of exercises you are doing when lifting weights, rest time plays a big role. If your objective is maximum strength or muscle size, you may want to lift very heavy and take enough time between sets or exercises for your body to recover and your heart rate to come down. However, for the best aerobic results as well as improvements in stamina and endurance, it is best to minimize the time between sets or exercises and to only lift amounts you can manage with 15 or more repetitions per set.

For long-term health and fitness, we should all plan to keep our Type IIX muscle fibers. For general fitness, I recommend exercises that increase stability, stamina and endurance. These also develop better nerve synapses, increase the tensile strength of ligaments and tendons, improve vascularity to the muscle tissues, and prevent the burning of Type IIX fibers for energy.

There are lots of online resources to teach you about traditional weightlifting. If you want to pursue that, I recommend you look for training videos. For general fitness, I recommend you do high repetitions (15 or 20 per set) and take no more than about 30 to 60 seconds rest between sets. There is no way I can teach you proper lifting in this one chapter, so I recommend that you find someone who can.

To build muscle endurance, do repetitive exercise such as distance running, swimming, or bicycling. Upper body muscle endurance can be enhanced with low weight, high repetition exercises, typically with 25 repetitions or more per set. Be sure you do exercises in all planes of motion to work all the smaller core muscles in your spine, shoulders and elsewhere. That means doing twisting, turning and lateral movements, not just straight ahead.

For stamina, especially in athletics, make sure you do a lot of whatever it is that you want stamina for. If you like tennis or basketball, play a lot of tennis or basketball. To use weightlifting to develop stamina, lift weights that you are able to lift in good form about 20 repetitions per set.

Weightlifting and adaptation

One of the themes I have taught you about in this book is the SAID principle ("specific adaptation to imposed demands"). Whenever you lift, your approach should be designed to elicit specific adaptation. To get adaptation with weightlifting, it is generally accepted that the best approach is to lift in good form as many times in a set as you can complete the movements without allowing your form to break down. In other words, pick a weight and do all the repetitions you can until you are just one short of failing to maintain good form. Refer to the previous section and adjust your weight to allow yourself to be one short of failure with the number of repetitions you are targeting for your specific goal.

In the past, we called that working to muscle failure. When we realized that failure would be going one too far, and the results of doing the exercise right are super positive, we started calling it working to success. So work to success!

For general fitness, your heavy weightlifting workouts should ideally be about an hour long. If you are doing only one heavy lifting workout a week, try to include a variety of sets that address muscles all over your body including legs, arms, shoulders, chest and back.

If you are doing more than one such workout a week, split the workouts into multiple days specifically addressing different body parts. Those are called splits, and you can look online for lots of recommendations on 2-day, 3-day, 4-day and 5-day splits. Splits are most appropriate if you are focusing most of your training on traditional weightlifting with the goal of increasing absolute size or strength. However, if your goal is general fitness, I recommend you just do the traditional weightlifting one day a week and focus most of your workout time on multiplanar interval training.

Muscle size

If your goal is to increase muscle size, then you need to decide how much time you have to devote. People who are going for maximum size generally believe that too much cardio will hold them back from maximizing their muscle growth. This is not the healthiest approach to fitness development, which is why I personally opt for general fitness.

However, there are certainly a lot of positives to having big muscles. Muscular athletes dominate some sports. Many people believe that big muscles are physically attractive, so that may be another reason to pursue them.

People who are truly dedicated to developing size tend to stay in the gym for at least two hours for each workout, often four to five times a week. However, you can make good progress with as little as three one-hour workouts a week. Depending on how much time you have to devote to it, look for a 3-, 4-, or 5-day split online, and you will find lots of options for what your workouts will look like.

For hypertrophy (muscle growth), try to lift heavy enough that you cannot lift more than four to 12 reps in a set in good form. Stop the set just one rep short of losing good form. The last thing you want is to get hurt, and that last rep in bad form is what will do it to you. Take at least two minutes rest between sets to ensure that you can get just as many reps with each set. Those long rests between sets are why people trying to maximize muscle size tend to spend so much time in the gym.

Competitive athletes

If your goal is to be a competitive athlete in a non-lifting sport, then be careful that the weightlifting you are doing matches up with your sport. Every different sport has its unique needs, and you should have professional advice about what is the best overall training plan to maximize your performance. In many sports, too much bulk can undermine performance.

Keep in mind also that lifting weights is not just vertical lifts. As we have seen in the section on Multiplanar Exercises, you can use cable machines and exercise tubing to create horizontal resistance challenges as well as twisting, lateral and diagonal challenges so that your muscles are being worked in all planes of motion. This kind of training is especially important in strengthening that mimics the movements and stressors that you will encounter in your sport.

For muscle size and absolute strength use enough weight that you would not be able to lift more than somewhere between four and 12 repetitions in good form. When you are able to do more than 12 reps at a given weight, move up on your weight.

If you are also trying to improve explosive speed, be sure to incorporate plyometrics such as throws, jumps and punches. The same Type IIX muscle fibers your body recruits when you lift heavy weights are also recruited for explosive movements. Any athletes whose sports demand both strength and speed should do both of these two distinctly different types of exercise.

Cautions

Do not regularly lift any amount of weight that is too heavy for you to get four good reps. Super heavy weights – the ones you could not lift in good form at least four times in quick succession -- can tear your muscle fibers more than your body can recover from between workouts. Keep in mind that all of the improvements to your strength and other adaptations happen during recovery, so if you do not recover fully between workouts, you start moving backwards. This abuse of your muscles can cause serious injuries, especially if it is done repeatedly.

In my years as a trainer, I have come into contact with a wide variety of people with different backgrounds and experience. Two different clients have come to me to strengthen, years after tearing a bicep (upper arm muscle) completely off the bone. Another came to me years after tearing one pectoralis major (chest muscle) off the bone. Weightlifting that tears your muscle off the bone is completely counterproductive to any goal you may have, so use good judgment about how much to lift.

If an accident has destroyed muscle tissue, all is not lost. I have seen tremendous recoveries that doctors have predicted could not happen. One client's leg was crushed when he was leaning into the trunk of his car and a truck struck him from behind. Another client broke 17 bones in her foot during a fall. Both were told they would never walk again, and both were eventually able to lift very heavy weights, run, and do high box jumps while training with me. This was the result of shear grit and determination from each of them. They would not quit trying just because their doctors told them they would never be able to do it.

However, pushing yourself to the point of self-destruction as my clients did by lifting too heavy (before meeting me) is a bad idea. Weightlifting should not be about ego; it should be about health, vitality and strength. Do it intelligently.

Note that some bodybuilders intentionally tear more muscle fiber than can recover by the next workout because scar tissue creates bulk. Such scarring makes the muscles look bigger, but it also weakens them. I strongly discourage that approach. Having huge muscles that are weak is unhealthy, and it will be unhealthy in the long run.

I much prefer to be as strong as possible rather than to have the biggest muscles possible, so I stick with being able to always get at least four good reps, and I do most of my exercises in the 15 to 20 rep range.

Exercise is Worth It

Most people think of exercise as a burden until it becomes a habit. Then they realize how great it is. I have had many, many clients tell me stories of the fantastic differences exercise has made in their lives. These stories typically include elements such as going up steps without huffing and puffing, having great medical reports, experiencing situations where they are certain they would have been seriously injured were it not for their training, and generally having much higher quality lives.

"You changed my life for the better!" is a refrain I have heard many times.

My life would not be nearly as great now if I did not exercise regularly. Considering my previously high blood pressure, I imagine my health would be very poor right now. Instead, I can do things many people in their twenties cannot do. I love what exercise does for me.

Years ago, I received a call from a client's doctor. The doctor thanked me for training his elderly patient.

"If it were not for your training," the doctor said, "he wouldn't still be alive."

It felt awesome to receive that call.

The doctor who called me has long since retired. His former patient, however, is still going strong at age 85. In fact, he just left a vigorous training session with me a few minutes ago.

Takeaways for Exercise Appendix

- **Exercises that have you twist, turn and move sideways are extremely important in preserving muscle tissue that gives you stability and protects you against injuries.**

- **A well-designed workout challenges your muscles to play all of their vital roles including balancing, stabilizing certain parts of your body while other parts of your body move, moving you repetitively at a low level of intensity, moving explosively, and moving heavy objects.**

- **If your body is able to tolerate it, higher intensity workouts confer tremendous health benefits.**

- **Studies have shown that a higher percentage of participants enjoy High Intensity Interval Training and stay with it than moderate intensity exercise.**

- **Heavy lifting and explosive movements are necessary to preserve certain muscle fibers, strength, and a variety of abilities.**

- **Exercise is extremely rewarding, and it is a vital part of any quest for a higher quality life.**

Epilogue

My Dream

I deeply appreciate you for spending this time with me. I have shared not only the science of weight loss and sustainability but also of myself. I have intentionally made myself vulnerable in the hopes that I could reach a few people such as you to make your lives better.

Weight loss and weight management can be a pleasant journey or a tumultuous odyssey. Now you are able to choose which it will be for you. The yo-yo brings an unnecessary and bitter ending to what may have been a great struggle. I don't want anyone to have to struggle. My dream is that it will become common knowledge that hunger and a battle against food cravings are part of a false path that leads away from both sustained weight loss and greater quality of life.

What I want for you is the easier path that promotes satiety with fewer calories and engineers a metabolism so healthy and fast you naturally lose weight and keep it off. I want you to have a longer, better life. How you can achieve all of this is truly what this book is about.

I have spoken from my heart in order to fulfill my life's purpose. What is your purpose, and how can you best fulfill it? We may or may not ever meet, but I feel deep satisfaction knowing that I have opened a path for you to experience a substantially positive change in your relationship with your body and in the quality and meaningfulness of your life. Thank you for affording me that opportunity. May you successfully navigate the path that takes you where you want to be and allows you to stay there.

ABOUT THE AUTHOR

Jim Frith

Jim invented the Eat As Much As You Want system (EAMAYW®) first for himself. In 2008, he lost 40 pounds and has kept it off ever since. Since then he has helped countless clients to achieve sustainable weight loss.

Jim owns two fitness businesses, Ascending Fitness and TopFitPros.com, home of the EAMAYW® app. Long ago, he earned the Master Trainer designation by the National Federation of Professional Trainers. He believes that successful weight loss must be part of a much bigger picture if it is to last. He spends his days helping others to reach their health and fitness goals. He integrates multiple sciences to provide a holistic approach to fitness, including exercise science, nutrition, and healthy lifestyle choices.

His fitness and weight-loss recommendations are based on many years of research and experience with clients. In this book, he shares the science that will end the yo-yo of dieting forever.

Jim's Credentials:

National Federation of Professional Trainers

- Master Trainer
- Certified Personal Trainer
- Advanced Sports Nutrition Specialist
- Advanced Endurance Training Specialist
- Advanced Weight Training Specialist

National Academy of Sports Medicine

- Certified Personal Trainer
- Corrective Exercise Specialist
- Performance Enhancement Specialist

Center for Massage and Natural Health

- Certified Massage Therapist
- NC LMBT #14700

Body Therapy Institute

- Certified Medical Massage Therapist

Harvard University

- Bachelor of Arts, Economics

Made in the USA
Monee, IL
21 April 2021